LESSER WRITINGS

WITH

THERAPEUTIC HINTS

BY

E. A. FARRINGTON, M.D.,

Author of 'Clinical Materia Medica', Professor of Materia Medica at the Hahnemann Medical College of Philadelphia, Editor of the Hahnemannian Monthly, Chairman of the Bureau of Materia Medica and Member of the Editorial Consulting Committee of the 'Cyclopaedia of Drug Pathogenesy',
U. S. A.

B. Jain Publishers (P) Ltd.
USA—EUROPE—INDIA

LESSER WRITINGS WITH THERAPEUTIC HINTS

18th Impression: 2018

NOTE FROM THE PUBLISHERS
Any information given in this book is not intended to be taken as a replacement for medical advice. Any person with a condition requiring medical attention should consult a qualified practitioner or therapist.

All rights reserved. No part of this book may be reproduced, stored in a retrieval system or transmitted, in any form or by any means, mechanical, photocopying, recording or otherwise, without any prior written permission of the publisher.

© with the publisher

Published by Kuldeep Jain for
B. JAIN PUBLISHERS (P) LTD.
B. Jain House, D-157, Sector-63,
NOIDA-201307, U.P. (INDIA)
Tel.: +91-120-4933333 • *Email:* info@bjain.com
Website: www.bjain.com

Printed in India by
B.B. PRESS NOIDA

ISBN: 978-81-319-0729-0

IN MEMORIUM

JANUARY 1, 1847, was the birth date of the great physician Dr. Ernest A. Farrington and he was born in that part of the city of Brooklyn, N.Y., then called Willimsburg, with which city he was, for the rest of his life, closely identified. From early childhood he manifested a fondness for study, and his education was carefully and judiciously directed. Nature seems to have endowed him with a ready perception and a retentive memory, and it is no wonder that he was always among the foremost of his schoolmates, with whom, indeed, his genial manners and readiness to help, made him a general favorite. His classical education was obtained in the Philadelphia High School, from which he graduated at nineteen years of age with the highest marks of approbation in every department, higher, in fact, than had ever previously been attained in that institution.

After a short interval, he began the study of medicine under the instruction of his brother, H. W. Farrington, M.D., and in the fall of 1866, matriculated from the Homœopathic Medical College of Pennsylvania. The following year he entered the newly established Hahnemann Medical College, from which he graduated in the spring of 1868. Throughout the whole course of his professional training, as in his earlier educational discipline, he maintained the same persistent application, the same earnest determination to excel, the same untiring enthusiasm. Having deliberately chosen medicine for his profession, he consecrated himself to a conscientious preparation for its responsible duties, as to a sacred calling.

The pre-eminence which had marked his standing among his classmates indicated his future functions as a teacher. Within a year after leaving college he was engaged as lecturer on forensic medicine in the same institution, and still later transferred to the chair of pathology and diagnosis.

On the 13th of September, 1871, he was married to Miss Elizabeth Aitkin, of Philadelphia, an event which brought more than usual joy, as in his wife he found a most congenial and helpful spirit, both as to his professional and religious life. This union was blessed with four children, three boys and one girl.

The dignified positions already secured by Dr. Farrington were but stepping stones to that most important and difficult department of homœopathic medicine, the chair of materia medica, to which he was elected in 1874, upon the resignation of Prof. Guernsey.

But it was not alone in his admirable qualities as a public teacher that Dr. Farrington contributed to the promotion of our art. He was an active worker in various societies for the cultivation of medical science, and the author of many valuable papers in the journals of our school. His contributions to our literature are of great practical merit, and combine completeness of statement, cogency of reasoning and conciseness of expression, in a remarkable degree.

He was a member of the State Society and joined the American Institute of Homœopathy in 1872. In 1884 the Institute appointed him a member of its Editorial Consulting Committee on the new "Cyclopædia of Drug Pathogenesy". In all these relations he was an assiduous and conscientious worker. In debate he was a ready speaker, logical in argument, choice in expression. No labor seemed too great, no effort too severe, so long as it ended to promote the advance toward that standard to which he felt the profession should aspire.

Naturally he possessed a strong and vigorous constitution; but, in December 1884, a neglected cold and subsequent unavoidable exposure, resulted in an attack of acute laryngitis. He continued his class lectures even with many warnings and thus a severe bronchitis developed. He then sailed for Europe in the hope that change of air and scene would cure him; but alas the disease steadily progressed, when he returned to Philadelphia and quietly passed into eternal rest on the 17th of December, 1885.

Conscientious, zealous and learned, he seemed destined to be a leader among men. He was early called to his work on earth— that work he faithfully performed. Early the call came to his work on high—confidently he entered thereon.

FOREWORD

The great philosopher of the Homœopathic Healing Art, Dr. Ernest A. Farrington, was destined to be a leader among his fellow-brethren. Within the short span of 39 years of life, which he was allowed by Providence to enjoy, he established a fame and reputation which would baffle time's tyrannic claim and will be sacredly commemorated in the heart of homœopaths all over the world, until eternity.

Possessed of superior analytical powers and the divine gift of a master-spirit, this able physician used to contribute various articles in different British and American journals on different intricate matters of our system of treatment and the present work is an exhaustive collection of these invaluable articles, collected and arranged with the most painstaking care. Many of the articles incorporated herein, it may be safely asserted, will not only be widely read with profit but will also give the readers a correct estimation of the great erudition of its eminent author.

In conclusion, we shall thankfully acknowledge the help we have readily received towards the compilation of this work from the different homœopathic concerns of the United States of America.

Our special thanks are due to Dr. Harvey Farrington, M.D., the prominent physician of Chicago (U.S.A.) and the illustrious son of the immortal author, for his kindly helping us with valuable suggestions throughout the time of its early preparation. Our sincere thanks are also due to Dr. T. S. Iyer of Basavangudi, South India, who apart from helping us through press matters, had personal interviews with Dr. Harvey Farrington concerning this publication while Dr. Iyer was on his tour to America.

The publishers will deem their labour well-paid if the book is as warmly received by the profession as it deserves.

SALZER & CO.

CONTENTS

	PAGE.
Homœopathy as a Science	9
The Elasticity of the Law of Homœopathy	15
Value of Hahnemann's "Totality"	20
Do medicines make functional changes?	21
A Syllabus of Materia Medica (Questions and Answers)	31
Modalities as arranged by Bonninghausen	59
Use of universal symptoms	64
Remarks on some of the acids	67
On several remedies more or less anæsthetic	74
Remarks on several summer remedies infrequently used	82
A brief repertory of medicines affecting the posterior nares, with comments and suggestions	84
Drugs affecting the occipital region	94
Remedies in neurasthenia affecting the lumbo-sacral region	166
Antipsorics in the atrophy of infants	178
Prognosis of pancreatic diseases	229
Manganese for women	234
Spasmus Glottidis	237
The mouth symptoms of the mineral acids	247
Notes on the treatment of Peritonitis	250
Indications for some of the metals in Neuralgia	256
Gout	258
Cuprum in defective reaction	265
Malarial Cachexia; Remote effects of Malaria; Treatment	267
Laceration of the Cervix Uteri (Preventive Treatment)	273
Discussion on the treatment of Intermittent Fever	280
Discussion on Dr. William Sharp's paper on "The foundations and boundaries of Modern Therapeutics"	296
Discussion on Dr. Richard Hughes' paper on "The value of Hydrocyanic Acid" in Epilepsy	299
Hahnemann and Misapplied Homœopathy	300
Correspondence	303
Confirmation of Symptoms	304
Dynamization of Drugs (Dr. Dudley's platform)	308

CONTENTS

	PAGE.
Is it justifiable?	314
Detection of Insanity	316
Suggestion for "A Model Materia Medica"	318
A Proving of Natrum Phosphoricum	338
Salicylic Acid: Additional Proving	355
Lac Caninum: Additional Proving	360
Provings of Linaria Vulgaris	361
Supposed Poisoning by Toad Stools (Agaricus Muscarius)	362
Is Laughing Gas injurious (Nitrous Oxide)	363
Rhus Poisoning	364
Merc. Iod. and Merc. Biniod (when Doctor's disagree who shall decide?)	365
A Synopsis of Quillaya Saponaria	367
Notes on Tarantula	370
Clinical Cases, etc.—	
A case of Puerperal Convulsions	373
A case with comments	376
A point in the etiology of Ophthalmia Neonatorum	378
An interesting post-mortem	380
Albuminuria	381
Atony of the Uterus	382
Bad Cold	383
Cases from Practice	384
Cholera Infantum	386
Cramps	387
Cure of a Hypopyon	387
Dizziness	388
Dropsy	388
Drowsiness	389
Dyspepsia	389
Epilepsy	390
Fever	391
Gelseminum in Albuminuria	392
Mental Derangements	393
Ovarian Tumour	394
Paralysis from Spasms	395
Pericarditis	397
Sanguineous Tumor	400
Scarlatina	401

CONTENTS

Clinical Cases, etc.—*contd*.
    St. Vitus' Dance 401
    Supposed Phthisis 402
    Syphilis 402
    Ulcer on Chin 402
    Varicella 403
    Vermicular Trouble 404
    Whooping-cough 405

HOMŒOPATHY AS A SCIENCE.

THE art of medicine claims great antiquity, but the science of medicine yet awaits a discoverer.

More than a century ago, Hahnemann's labors initiated the genuine art of medicine. But not one of his *theories* has ever stood the test of experience. What he stated as *facts* stand as firmly now as when they were promulgated. But science, defined as knowledge "methodically digested and arranged", was never aided by his theories. Where has he consistently explained the law of cure? Was his *psoric theory* scientific? True, the facts announced in his Organon as to the way to treat the sick, how to select and change the remedy, to make provings, etc., are undoubtedly correct. Equally true is it that remedies acting from within out, from more to less vital parts, will be most likely indicated in chronic diseases. But his *itch hypothesis* is readily disproved.

The same applies to all subsequent attempts at establishing Homœopathy as a science.

What is this? Is it because Homœopathy is not a science? No. It is because genuine science does not appear at the present day. It is because investigators are plunging more and more deeply into materialism.

Darwin's inexcusable offence does not consist in his promulgation of the absurd theory of the origin of man, but rather in the anti-spiritual direction of his whole line of study. With an utter contempt of revelation, he manufactures the moral sense of men out of the necessities of their living together peacefully. And yet we know that true morality springs not from man but from heaven.

But Darwin is not an isolated example of falsity in science. Huxley and Tyndall, Proctor, and indeed the entire corps of investigators from A to Z, turn their conceited minds earthward only, and so learn nothing of higher import than what appertains to the plan of their senses.

Now the same pall overhangs Homœopathy. Hahnemann did not belong to the materialistic school. To him the plant or root from which he made his tincture was not inert matter alone, but contained a living principle which was not nature but life. He knew that he was dealing with forces which transcended his natural senses, except in so far as their activities were displayed in their workings through matter. Hence his studies led him to the process of potentization of drugs. These are not claimed as spirit. We cannot escape from matter while we are in this world. So his method did nothing but rid spiritual forces of weighty matter, allowing them to act in the finest particles of matter only. Thus disinthralled, his remedies were free to act above the crude laws of physics, independent of gravity and of chemistry, but still within the bounds of matter.

We are gifted with remedies then which obey laws new to the physician. Their subtle movements are marvellous to him who has been accustomed to the more superficial phenomena of philosophy, chemistry, etc. He was wont to investigate drug action from his standpoint. He saw in a very general way, that certain medicines influenced certain functions or organs, and so constructed a chemico-physiological materia medica; one full of fallacies, because even what of truth it contained was perverted by misapplication.

The danger which threatens our system of medicine lies in the fact that we are being dragged into materialism. We are so wedded to Allopathy that we cling with obstinacy to her false and crude notions. We seem to think that Homœopathy rests on Allopathy as does a house on its foundation; and when we feel insecure in the superstructure, we descend to the cellar for aid. There is not one single truth in Allopathy *per se*. If there is, then just to that degree is our school false; for the two are diametrically opposite.

But, it may be asked, is there no truth in pathology and diagnosis, in the physiological investigation of drug effects, etc.? Emphatically no, as sciences.

To clearly apprehend the truth of this statement, we must acquaint ourselves with the genuine doctrine of order in nature.

Generals are formed of particulars, the latter being incomparably the most important.

Take, by way of illustration, the human body. In a very general analysis, it is composed of organs. Each organ is made up of tissues. Each tissue is divisible into molecules. Beginning with a single organ, as, for instance, a muscle, we find it composed of fibres, these of fibrillæ, and each fibrilla of smaller parts. As we pursue our analysis, we still find each miscroscopic portion a minute effigy of the whole. But just as in the potentized medicine so here the properties of the muscle are discovered much more clearly, and are seen to be numerous and quite different from what the undivided muscle would exhibit. We are accumulating particulars, and find them more and more complex as we advance.

The same applies to the practice of medicine. It is not alone sufficient to learn the general range of action of a drug or an outline of a disease, but also and pre-eminently the peculiarities of each. These when discovered so far outweigh the rest, that they must be used in every accurate prescription.

Pathology, as dogmatically taught, is not true. Arbitrary boundaries are given to diseases, and this artificial production is definitely named. Such a process of thought is too general to be practical and too superficial to escape the fallacies of appearances. A synthesis is correct only when its component elements are. *Baptisia* develops a picture of typhus; *Arsenic* of cholera Asiatica, *Bryonia* produces pseudo-membranes, etc.; but unless analysis reveals the individual symptoms in these cases respectively, the conclusion is vague and uncertain.

Objection, it will be seen, is not raised against pathological facts, many of which are true, but to the manner of their construction into a science.

Such facts enable us to interpret symptoms, and place some estimate on their relative value. They aid in the forming of the "totality". They assist in forming a prognosis. That they only assist, however, is because the course of a disease, subsequent to a Homœopathic prescription, is not the unqualified course it would pursue unmodified. A typhoid patient, for example, might exhibit an unmitigated fever, with evening exacerbation, bloody stools and tympany. But if, after the similimum, the mental symptoms lessen, or the latest become less intense, our prognosis is qualified thereby, despite the gravity of the remaining symptoms.

Schussler's offence does not consist in understanding physiology and pathology, but in dragging them into therapeutics and in recklessly misapplying them. Had he, at the suggestion of physiology, proved his twelve remedies, he would have acted rationally and effectively.

All medical questions find confirmation or refutation before the test of the laws of the Organon, not before Allopathic hypotheses or Homœopathic adoptions from the old school. Indeed we may go farther and assert that physiology itself must be tried before the same tribunal; for is not living power superior to the lifeless disclosures of the dissecting-knife or the torture-born phenomena of vivisection?

That pathology as at present taught is arbitrary is quite evident. A child suffering from membranous croup received, by the advice of the consulting physician, *Belladonna*. To the astonishment of the attending doctor the laryngeal spasms ceased, and the child rapidly recovered.

Now, in the language of pathology, croup is an inflammatory affection attended with the formation of a pseudo-membrane. Transferring this definition to therapeutics we must prescribe a drug which causes a false membrane. Teste says give *Bryonia;* Bæhr and Kafka, *Iodine,* because of their pathological relation. But such teachers are just the drags who would tie us to Allopathy. The attending physician in the case quoted agreed with them, and but for the genuine prescription of counsel the little sufferer would have fallen a victim to their eclecticism.

It is true that there was a pathological condition in which the *Belladonna* state closed, namely, the spasm of the glottis; but this state was not determinable from the arbitrary study of croup but from the analytical study of the individual case. Thus was formed a correct synthesis.

It is not so that our first duty is to our patient. Our first duty is to the truth, which, when loyally served, best enables us to do the greatest good to the sick.

We must learn the undiscovered rules that regulate the profound workings of our potentized drugs. We must extend our knowledge of the relations of remedies. We must study physiology from our new standpoint.

To aid us in our labors, to at least start us in the right direction, we must rationally comprehend and apply the rules which Hahnemann has left us.

This unwholesome fidelity to the researches of the old school is the legitimate result of materialism, which believes only in the tangible. It obscures thought and throws doubt over all interior mental operations.

So long as we keep our minds bound to the vague generalizations of the allopaths, we will never advance one step forward, and will sooner or later, utterly discard what has already been taught in the Organon.

The only hope for genuine medicine is in the unprejudiced investigation of high potencies. It is in their study that we shall find the complex phenomena of diseased processes—phenomena which will show pathology as now taught to be a tissue of fallacies, however true are its disjointed facts.

Until our united efforts tend in this direction, we need not hope for the establishment of Homœopathy as a perfect art, much less as an exact science.

THE ELASTICITY OF THE LAW OF HOMŒOPATHY.

TRUTH is not narrow and restricted; it is broad and, in its own sphere, universal. It manifests itself in degrees, from a most superficial presentation to the most profound comprehension. One thing, however, is requisite; its essential qualities must obtain, or it is proportionately defective or even destroyed.

So with the law of Homœopathy. In its sphere it is universal; in its acceptance it appears in all shades, from the crudest practice to the most skilful efforts of a Hahnemann. Still, there is a *sina qua non,* which is that there shall, somewhere, be a similarity between disease and drug.

Gradations in this law are not only such as may be expressed by the relative degree of fulness of acceptance—gradations comparable with the continuous fading of light from the brilliant centre to the boundary between light and darkness. Gradations in the law are also such as are expressed discretely, like the rounds of a ladder that represent distinct, progressive steps.

Two or three of these latter degrees are so clearly defined that I purpose considering them for a few moments in their bearing upon my theme.

Physicians, who depend solely or chiefly upon so-called pathological indications in selecting a drug, are certainly within the province of Homœopathy, because they are, in a way, applying its law. They are seeking for fixed and definite similarities between drug and disease. They are mounted on one round of the ladder of true medicine.

Physicians who depend solely or chiefly upon so-called nutritive remedies are, doubtless, within the pale of Homœopathy, for they are after a fashion applying its law. They seek the similar from among drugs that in normal quantities act physiologically, and in abnormal amount cause disease similar, in some features, to their known pathogenetic effects. They, too, are mounted on a round of the same ladder.

Physicians who depend solely or chiefly upon the Organon in prescribing are unquestionably within the domain of Homœopathy, for their aim is to discover what may be aptly termed the *similimum*. They are making the nicest possible application of the law of similars. They, necessarily, are mounted on a round of the ladder of the genuine medicine.

But what are the essential difference in these three gradations that mark them as discrete? And which of them is the highest round, nearest to the fountain of truth? Let us see. All three classes claim that they take the "totality of the symptoms" from which the desired remedy is to be deduced. But they differ severally in the method of deduction. One picks out as characteristic the pathological changes; another, nutritive changes; the third, "the more prominent, uncommon and peculiar features of the case." The first two rely mainly upon objective changes; the third upon subjective as well as objective. These essential distinctions characterize the three classes respectively when they, for one reason or another, step from their own round up or down on to another. If the pathologist gives any weight to a mental symptom, or to a drug effect he calls 'contingent', it is always held in subordination to the pathological lesions, it is always with the reservation that the latter must be subservient to what he terms characteristics. And this brings me to my second question: which of these is on the highest round?

Electively I decide for the Hahnemannian, and designate the round upon which he stands as that which gives the broadest and loftiest view of medicine ever yet obtained by mortal discoverer. His position is the only logical one, for he holds in his mental grasp all that is below him, and, moreover, knows just how to value every step below him, and so to determine their relation with the higher and the highest. He heralds with delight the discovery that *Arsenic* can cause endocarditis; *Bryonia,* pleurisy; *Mercurius Corrosivus,* Bright's disease; and *Kalmia,* almuminuria. If he cannot possibly do any better, he is at liberty to descend from his height and employ one or the other of these drugs accordingly. But usually his command *of other and more interior effects of drugs* leads him to proceed more intelligently and to act more comprehensively. "I see," he says, "certain subjective and less ultimated objective symptoms that call more emphatically for another drug—for *Pulsatilla.*" "But," comes up the objection from the round below, "*Pulsatilla* has not the pathological symptoms." "True, but it has the important symptoms, of the case, which I recognize as not mere reflex effects of the localized disease, but which rather bear a causative relation; and, besides, they are manifest in planes of molecular action, which necessarily hold to the coarser parts the relation of cause to effect, and any drug applied to the local symptoms only will have but a partial and palliative effect."

Continuing the conversational style I have almost unconsciously drifted into, let me presume the pathologist asks: "How can your method ever result in a tangible, fixed therapeutics? Are you not doomed always to remain in the speculative?" "No," the Hahnemannian answers, "we rest on *terra firma* as well as you, even if we are not so anxious to measure out precisely where shall be our footing. Our method develops an objective therapeutics." "How?" "To illustrate, the world-renowned *Aconite* owes its febrile usefulness to the method of Hahnemann. When Hahnemann first prescribed it, he knew little or nothing of its power to cause and cure synochal fever. He selected it from concomitant symptoms, guided by the rule of characteristics, and lo, soon it becomes an invincible fever-remedy. It does not clearly appear from the provings of *Hepar* that the drug can hasten the formation of pus; boils were developed, unhealthy sores suppurated, but the power of the drug over pus was deduced from such symptoms as intolerance of pain, parts feel sore as a boil, etc." "But", it is rejoined, "now that these objective and pathological facts are determined, are they not of paramount importance, and is it not Homœopathy to use them?" "It certainly is Homœopathy, but whether or not it is always pure Homœopathy is another question. The same process of deduction that gave these facts existence still rules. *Aconite* is doubtless similar to synochal fever; indeed, experiments since Hahnemann's time have proved that it can cause chill, fever, and sweat; but to be the *similimum* in a given case *Aconite* requires also the peculiar mental anguish and restlessness so distinctive of it, and not the quiet and torpor of some other inflammatory drugs." "Are not such subjective symptoms as you refer to incomplete, and when fully developed into their pathological ultimates do not the latter become all sufficient as indications?" "They certainly are incomplete in the sense that they are not ultimated; but since they originate the ultimates they do not cease their activity when the latter appear; they still hold the superior position of cause to effects; and, besides, they represent disease changes of a more interior character than do their ultimates—disease changes which, be it ever remembered, *may ultimate in more than one way;* hence, they are of a more universal value."

In this connection I cannot do better than quote the words of an allopath, Dr. Andrew Clark, who, while learning a wholesome lesson for himself is unwittingly re-teaching many a delinquent homœopathist what has long since been practically forgotten. I quote from the *Hahnemannian Monthly* of October, 1884:

"We are so much concerned with anatomical changes; we have given so much time to their evolutions, differentiations, and relations; we are so much dominated by the idea that, in dealing with them, we are dealing with disease itself, that we have overlooked the fundamental truth that these anatomical changes are but secondary, and sometimes the least important, expressions or manifestations of states which underlie them. It is to these dynamic states that our thoughts and inquiries should be turned: they precede, underlie, and originate structural changes; they determine their character, course, and issues; in them is the secret of disease; and, if our control of it is ever to become greater and better, it is upon them that our experiment must be made."

While, then, I admit that the law of Homœopathy is elastic enough to give me quite a range of treatment, it is clear to me that my duty demands my earnest endeavour to employ, whenever I can, the purest and highest method of applying that great boon to humanity —the law of similars.

VALUE OF HAHNEMANN'S "TOTALITY."

IF the students or the physicians comprehend the general qualities of a drug, they are prepared to apply its particulars. Given, for instance, a special symptom: sleepy, but cannot sleep—*Bellad., Apis,* if the general properties of these two remedies are known, the choice is easy.

Still, it must be remembered that it is only by the multiplication of particulars that the general character can be distinctively drawn, just as *a strange object becomes more and more familiar and separable from its similars as we recognize more the relation of its parts to the whole.*

Recognizing that the totality is to be employed rather than single symptoms, some teachers have neglected the latter, and have published descriptions of drugs, hewn out after the fashion of their own synthetic thought. This error arises from a misunderstanding of the procedures of the so-called symptomists. Few, if any, prescribe for one symptom; for, although such a single indication may lead them to a drug, their knowledge of the drug as a whole immediately comes into consciousness, and they intuitively fit the fact into its proper place. Now, because this understanding of the whole was acquired by a long and patient attention to details,—to characteristics,—they really have a more accurate mental picture than most of their accusers. A correct generalization of a drug, then, can only be made after a full and complete analysis of its particulars. The mental impress formed by a reconstruction of these particulars is the true general. Always afterwards in prescribing, when a single characteristic presents itself, it is to be measured by its relation to the whole. This is the true value of Hahnemann's "totality".

DO MEDICINES MAKE FUNCTIONAL CHANGES?

AT a regular monthly meeting of the Society held on May 11th, 1876, A. R. Thomas, M.D., President, being in the Chair, the following interesting papers were read by E. A. Farrington, M.D.: "Do medicines make functional changes?" being a reply to an article of Dr. Lippe in the May number of the *Medical Advance,* entitled, "The Last Departure of Homœopathy in the Physiological Livery," and by Pemberton Dudley, M.D., "On the Cimex Question."

In the May number of the *Medical Advance,* Dr. Lippe contributed an article entitled, "The Last Departure of Homœopathy in the Physiological Livery."

So far as the charges preferred in this article apply to me personally, they demand no reply. But so far as they compromise the integrity of the College in which I hold my professorship, I am bound to enter the contest in her defence.

In the early part of the winter I issued a syllabus containing some questions, arranged in sections. These questions comprised a goodly portion of the Materia Medica, certainly such portions as the beginning practitioner ought to thoroughly understand before he commences the practice of medicine.

To this syllabus Dr. Lippe raises several objections, *viz.*:—

> first, he considers that it reaches Schusslerism;
> secondly, that it is contrary to the teachings of Hahnemann;
> thirdly, that it is false because the answers to many of the proposed questions are impossible—cannot be true.

The words which seem especially obnoxious to him are these: "The intelligent application of Materia Medica requires a knowledge of the changes medicines make in functions and nutrition." For example, I asked, "What changes does *Lachesis* make in the blood?" This Dr. Lippe terms Schusslerism. He asserts, and misapplies Hahnemann to confirm his argument, that it is impossible to know what changes medicines make in function and nutrition.

The reply to his argument comprises three questions:
> first, what is Schusslerism?
> secondly, can we learn what changes medicines make in function and nutrition?
> thirdly, if he can, of what use is such information in the application of drugs?

First, if Schusslerism means the law which Dr. Hering discovered some thirty years ago, then I plead guilty to the charge. If it means floundering about with untried remedies, basing their symptomatology on their supposed physiological action, making a cure all of twelve substances—then I most emphatically deny the charge. Every question propounded in the syllabus is answered either from provings or from clinical experience. If Schusslerism means that medical substances act on tissues producing changes in function and nutrition, then again must I plead guilty.

And this brings us to the second question, upon the solution of which depends the maintenance of my position. A function is, literally, an act, a performance, and applied to physiology, "is the action of an organ or set of organs" (Dunglison). If I take a drug and symptoms result, are not these the expression of altered functions—altered in degree or quality? If, for instance, *Lachesis* causes hemorrhages with a settling like charred straw (Guernsey), or if it causes profuse bleeding, the blood will not coagulate (Lippe): is this not a nutritive change? And will this altered blood perform its normal functions? Let the answer be found in the gangrene, the erysipelas, or the impending typhoid state.

Were Dr. Lippe to ask how are the changes made, I would be compelled to answer, I know not. The secret workings of vital force are under infinite surveillance. Just how it works, mortal man may never know. We live in a world of effects, and it is only of these we can become cognizant.

The blood propelled by the heart, sweeps over the aortic arch and down the aorta, never dispensing its gifts until it reaches its ultimata in the capillaries. Nerves run to and from centres, giving no impressions until their termini are reached. The ulna, irritated at the elbow, tingles at its termination in little and and outer side of ring-fingers. So with every vital effort, it is in its fulness only when terminated in its appointed organ or organs.

Organs are made of tissues, tissues of molecules, and herein are consummated the complex vital phenomena which make up life. As Hahnemann says, the internal changes we cannot determine. But their effects, which appear normally in conscious sensation and motion, and abnormally in symptoms, are determinable. Whether these symptoms are subjective or objective, they express a change in function or nutrition, and bespeak the tissue or tissues involved.

If a function is truly defined above, will not the symptoms show a changed "action of an organ or set of organs?"

If I take a remedy, say *Rhus*, and it produces a vesicular eruption, will it be denied that a change in nutrition has taken place? And cannot we perceive what change has taken place? Or, still more to the point, if for a non-uniting fracture we prescribe *Calcarea Phos.,* and the callus quickly forms—a callus containing a hundred-fold more lime than we give—can we deny a tissue and a nutritive action?

We know that tearing, boring pains indicate an affection of bones or periosteum; that sharp, shooting pains indicate an affection of serous membranes. We know that *Aconite* acts on serous sacs, increasing their suction; while *Sepia, Iodine,* etc., relax serous and synovial sacs.

Equally sure are we that *Hypericum* acts on nerve tissue, *Arnica* on the capillaries, *Mercury* in the production and *Silicia* in the prevention of pus formation, *Conium* on adenoid tissue, *Graphites* in the dissolution of cicatricial tissue, *Creosote* on the mucous lining of the stomach, *Silicia, Chamomilla, Bryonia,* on connective tissue, *Ferrum* on the hæmatin, *Phosphorus* on the blood cells, and so on through the Materia Medica.

But thirdly, Are such facts of use in the application of materia medica? True, a physician may cure the *Lachesis* hæmorrhage without any other information than the mere words of the symptoms. But so long as man finds delight in the exercise of his God-given reason, he will demand the *why*—the why which anticipates every new truth—the why which led to Hahnemann's quinine experiments, and to every succeeding step in his discovery of Homœopathy.

No physician can intelligently apply medicines with simply a memorized materia medica. He is then like the industrious student who, in his attempt to learn French, memorized the dictionary but learned nothing of grammatical construction. Neither can the physician always succeed in obtaining the necessary totality of symptoms without an intimate knowledge of functional perversions. He must know from physiology what are the normal relations of organ with organ;

from pathology what changes diseases cause; from the history of diseases what are their probable course, duration and result. For example, delirium, photomania, singing, praying, making verses, will yield to *Stramonium;* but the same symptoms with retained placenta, demand *Secale.* Neuralgia in and over the left eye may yield to *Spigelia,* but if a tilted uterus exist, even though there are no subjective pelvic symptoms, the remedy will be *Actaea Rac.*

Gross in his "Comparative Materia Medica," gives as a symptom of *Apis,* "suppurations do not occur." Why? Virchow tells us that the production of pus demands an inflammation of the parenchyma. *Apis* only attacks surfaces, hence it seldom forms pus. The utility of this characteristic is evident in contrasting the remedy with *Belladonna,* which does attach the parenchyma; *Apis,* tonsils bright red, erysipelatous; *Bellodonna,* tonsils bright red, swollen threatening suppuration.

If a patient passes urine depositing a reddish sand, are we damaging Homœopathy if we search for the cause of this defective oxygenation of nitrogenous matter? On the contrary, will not the revealed symptoms help to complete the totality, and so help us to diagnose between *Lycopod., Natrum Mur., Ant. Crud.,* etc., all of which have such a urinary deposit?

If a newly proved drug causes white, flocculent urine, are we violating the precepts of the Master if we analyze this excretion and, finding phosphates in excess trace thence the relation of other symptoms produced? Let it be remembered, however, that symptoms have a relative value; and although we may make use of every known means in analyzing a case and collecting the totality of its symptoms, we must arrange our picture according to the well tried rules of the Organon.

The true physician, while he holds fast to the precepts of Hahnemann, neglects no fact which a progressive science might utilize, no discovery which bears the stamp of truth. If the new discovery contradicts his well confirmed laws—his creed it may be called—it must be false, for truth cannot invalidate truth.

DISCUSSION.

Dr. Jeanes agreed with Dr. Farrington, that in order to understand that which is abnormal, it is necessary to be acquainted with what is normal; and with Dr. Dudley, that disgusting remedies should not be introduced into our materia medica. The individual physician may experiment with them if he wishes, but they need not be put into our works. He had no doubt that many uncertain symptoms had crept into our materia medica, but he thought these could generally be traced to the recording of clinical symptoms with the results of provings; especially in the case of alterations in nutrition. *Graphites,* for example, was said to exert an influence on cicatricial tissue, but it had never produced it. As to the twelve tissue remedies, he was opposed to them as being against the principles of Homœopathy.

Dr. Korndoerfer would not like to go without the (potentized) bed-bug in his pocket-case. He had once succeeded in removing the symptom, "violent shooting pain along from vagina up towards left ovary, which had lasted six months," within one hour by one dose of *Cimex* 30. Ought we to be willing to sacrifice a remedy that can produce such a result? We already use the *Spanish fly* and *Musk,* which are hardly less disgusting than the *Cimex.* He did not approve of searching for new remedies of this kind, but we ought not to give up a good thing because it seems dirty. We should not be hypersensitive; if such things are real curative agents, that fact, and that only, should govern our action towards them.

Dr. Farrington said, in answer to Dr. Jeanes' remark in reference to *Graphites*, that of course it could never have caused cicatricial tissue, but it had caused induration of cellular tissue, which so nearly resembles it that it gave the basis of comparison.

He was sorry to have to disagree entirely with Dr. Dudley. He would not be willing to throw *Psorinum* to the dogs, his own experience with it had been too valuable; nor yet *Variolinum,* however disgusting their origin may appear. Nor would he wish to abandon the *Cimex*. In his opinion, the laity had nothing at all to do with the names of our remedies, nor with the substances used; and when potentized these all taste alike.

As to the unreliability of reported verifications of acute symptoms, spoken of by Dr. Dudley in his paper, we have no means of testing whether a group of symptoms has disappeared of itself, or has been removed by our remedy. If left to nature, the symptoms run a certain known course, and disappear in a certain order; whereas, the proper Homœopathic remedy will prevent this course, and cause the symptoms to disappear in a contrary order. For example, in a case of poisoning by *Rhus.,* the vesicular eruption will spread in a certain direction. If, after the use of *Croton Tig.,* we find that the course is stopped, and the advanced stages begin to fade first; not those that first appeared, as would be the case if left to nature we may be sure that our remedy has done the work and not nature.

Dr. Dudley used to think himself a sort of pariah, a medical outcast, who agreed with no one, and with whom no one agreed except in adopting the law of similars; but he was glad to find that at least in one other point he could agree with Drs. Farrington and Korndoerfer. Dr. Korndoerfer, in his paper last month, has said that the Homœopathic remedy is not that one whose symptoms can be patched together, so as to agree with the symptoms of a disease. He certainly is correct in that. This evening, Dr. Farrington had carried same idea a step further, and has maintained that an acquaintance with the functional changes produced by our remedies is not possible, but necessary to an intelligent use of them.

The use of *Spanish fly* and of *Musk* does not, in his opinion, justify the use of *Cimex,* and the other disgusting remedies to which he referred in his paper. His argument against them is based upon the popular disgust; whereas, in the case of the other substances mentioned by Dr. Korndoerfer, there is no popular disgust; fashion has sanctioned their use. What can we think of that physician who goes to the lowest cesspools in search of his remedies? He, for his part, would not judge such a man worthy of credence. If driven by necessity, and there was nothing else left, he supposed he would use such remedies too, but only as a last resort.

Dr. Korndoerfer did not wish to be understood as advocating these lowest remedies; and yet, why should they not be used? No doubt we, and many others, have made involuntary provings of *Cimex;* but Dr. Wahle of Rome felt warranted in making a voluntary proving of it, which has certainly been productive of some good. What can be nastier than *Psorinum;* and yet he would not wish to be without it. In the case of a little child with a dirty looking eruption of its scalp, and an indescribably disagreeable smell from the person in spite of the greatest care, *Psorinum* cured in a week; and the same remedy also removed ugly pustules from around the finger nails of the mother, within the same time. Such an experience certainly ought to induce us to hold fast to the remedy.

Dr. Farrington would like to ask two questions:

(1) What would Dr. Dudley do, if, driven by necessity, he really wanted such a remedy? Ought he not to be able to find it somewhere, for example, in just such a work as Allen's Encyclopædia?

(2) Does anybody know any remedy that had horribly offensive black watery stools at night? He had met stools of such a kind in many cases of cholera infantum, and the children had been cured by *Psorinum*. Should they have been sacrificed, because *Psorinum* is nasty?

Dr. Dudley answered the first question by saying, that if *Cimex* were not recorded, probably some better drug would be; and, that if a case occurred in which this other drug could not help, there would be many others where it would, and *Cimex* would not.

Dr. Korndoerfer reminded him by the proving of *Cimex,* one remedy was added, and it did not interfere with the introduction of another.

Dr. Jeanes: In olden times the Homœopathic physician was contended with about 80 remedies; and now, from 800 to 1,000 have been experimented with; and this is not the one-millionth part of the substances which can operate upon the human system to change its action.

Dr. Dudley said chemistry could furnish any number of drugs, and potent ones, if we were in need of new remedies.

Dr. Farrington: True; but we must not forget that there exist differences between substances of the animal, vegetable, and mineral kingdoms, which are not represented by a difference in their chemical formulæ.

Dr. Korndoerfer stated an incident that proved there was a difference between the action of the Phosphate of lime, derived from the mineral kingdom, and taken from the animal.

Dr. A. R. Thomas had seen in the Journal of the College of Pharmacy, some five years ago, a detailed method for the preparation and administration of the "measuring worm", and a method for extracting therefrom a crystalline substance. He did not think, then, that the old school could sneer at us on account of some substances found in our Materia Medica, as they are in the habit of doing.

The Society then adjourned.

(The following questions were formulated by the late Dr. E. A. Farrington and published by him without answers, in pamphlet form, in January, 1876.)

FOREWARD

The time is ripe and has long since been ripe for us as Homœopaths to take to ourselves somewhat of the enthusiasm of our foregoers in our materia medica. A world renowned surgeon has taken a strong step for the establishment of at least the plausibility of our method of therapy. Harvey Cushing, in the Cameron Prize Lectures, delivered in 1925 at Edinburgh, says:

"And now that the smoke of battle has cleared and we no longer hear the barrage of the shot gun prescriptions of our predecessors, we may even salute the infinitesimal Hahnemann and look upon Osler's contempt for most drugs as indirectly a great benefaction of practical therapeutics."

Let us avail ourselves of our heritage. That sincere but biased antagonist of Homœopathy, Oliver Wendell Holmes, in a lecture before the Harvard Medical School, once said:

"I firmly believe that if the whole materia medica could be sunk to the bottom of the sea, it would be all the better for mankind and all the worse for fishes."

We admire Holmes, both as a physician and a literateur. We disagree with him in the use of the word "whole" instead of the word "much". Had the latter word been used we would have been in hearty accord. We feel after a perusal of some Homœopathic literature that a certain stimulus may be given to the more enthusiastic study of our materia medica, if we publish a series of questions formulated by Farrington some fifty years ago and answer the questions from certain symptoms confirmed with accord by Hahnemann, Hering, Lippe, and the elder Raue and Korndoerfer.

AUG. KORNDOERFER, JR.
CLARENCE BARTLETT,

Section I.

1. *What changes are made in the blood by Lachesis?*

    High grade hemolysis and anticoagulant action.
    Indicative symptomatology: Hæmorrhagic diathesis.
    Blood dark, noncoagulable; small wounds bleed much.

2. *What changes are made in the blood by Apis?*

    Indicative symptomatology; Phlebitis, echymotic spots, varicose veins, dropsies.

3. *What changes are made in Serous Membrane by Bryonia?*

    Inflammations (dry).
    Indicative symptomatology: Tearing stitch-like pain in chest in region of diaphragm and various joints.

4. *What changes are made in the Skin by Rhus Tox?*

    Inflammation—Vesicular, macular, papular, pustular lesions.
    Indicative symptomatology: Intolerable itching, red measly rash all over body. Urticaria, ivy poisoning, pemphigus.

5. *What changes are made in Capillaries by Hamamelis?*

    Relaxation of capillary circulation (venous). Venous congestion. Passive hæmorrhage.
    Indicative symptomatology: Venous hæmorrhage from all orifices of the body.
    Varicose veins.

6. *What changes are made in Buccal Mucous Membrane by Arum Tri?*

   Inflammation.
   Indicative symptomatology: Excessive acrid saliva, buccal cavity raw, sore, bleeding.

7. *What changes are made in Mucous Membranes by Lycopodium?*

   Catarrhal inflammation.
   Indicative symptomatology: Oversensitiveness to hearing and smell. Mouth and tongue dry, without thirst.
   Bitter taste in morning.

8. *What changes are made in Mammary Glands by Conium?*

   Inflammation and tumefaction.
   Indicative symptomatology: Tumors of mammæ with piercing pain worse at night; gland abnormally tender.

9. *What changes are made in the Urine by Bryonia?*

   Renal inflammation (complicating acute infectious disease, scarlet fever).
   Indicative symptomatology: Urine loaded with albumin.
   Face bloated below the eyes, burning in the urethra when not urinating.

10. *What changes are made in the Glands by Mercury?*

    Inflammation, with or without suppuration.

11. *What changes are made in the Skin by Arsenic?*

    Anæmic appearance, pasty; later, yellow and scaly. Dryness, burning, itching, inflammation and ulcerated; associated with the appearance of petechiæ.

Indicative symptomatology: Herpetic eruption, itching and burning. Petechiæ. Blue spots. Urticaria.

12. *What changes are made in the Throat by Belladonna?*

Acute inflammation.

Indicative symptomatology: Dryness of the mucous membrane. Feeling as if throat were too narrow for deglution. Tearing pain, worse when swallowing liquids. Liquids may be regurgitated through the nose.

13. *What changes are made in the Nails by Graphites?*

Finger nails black, rough, matrix inflamed, with soreness, throbbing and numbness. Finger nails thick and deformed. Ingrowing toe-nails.

14. *What changes are made in the Intestines by Veratrum Album?*

Condition stimulating high grade acute inflammation.

Indicative symptomatology: Stools—watery, greenish, mixed with flakes. Gushing, profuse rice-water discharges. Colic; cutting as from knives. Cholera morbus, worse at night, cold sweat on the forehead. Vomiting and purging at the same time; after fruits.

15. *What changes are made in the Stomach by Kreosote?*

What symptomatology seems to indicate it might be called for in ulcers and malignant conditions.

Indicative symptomatology: Corrosive fetid ichorous discharges from mucous membrane, vitality greatly depressed. Rapid emaciation. Vomiting. Tension over stomach; tight clothes intolerable.

16. *What changes are made in the Lungs by Phosphorus?*

   Would seem to be associated with congestions and even specific inflammations. Hæmorrhagic diathesis. There appear no symptoms confirmed by Hering, Raue and Lippe, as a group, although the following have been confirmed individually by Korndoerfer, Sr., and the others.
   Indicative symptomatology: Worse lying on the left chest, better when lying on the right side. Heaviness of the chest, as if weight were lying upon it. Congestion of the chest; oppression; anxiety; worse from emotion. Pain between scapula.

17. *What changes are made in the Nerves by Hypericum?*

   Injury to parts rich in sensory nerves, especially fingers, toes and matrices. Lacerations, when intolerable pain shows nerves are severely involved.

18. *What changes are made in Cellular Tissue by Apocynum?*

   Œdema and dropsy.

19. *What changes are made in Peristaltic Action by Asafoetida?*

   Increased peristalsis. Flatus passing upwards, none down. Offensive eructations. Constipation.

20. *What changes are made in Structure of Tongue by Muriatic Acid?*

   Inflammation even to ulceration.
   Indicative symptomatology: Taste acrid, putrid, like rotten eggs, with ptyalism.
   Tongue sore, bluish; ulcers with black bases and blisters. Tongue dwindles, looks shrunken.

21. *What changes are made in Heart Muscle by Coffee?*

   No organic changes, but functional.
   Indicative symptomatology: Palpitation, violent, irregular with trembling of the limbs.

22. *What changes are made in Spine by Strychnine?*

   Strychnia has a stimulating effect on the central nervous system, but especially upon the motor tracts of the spinal cord. In overdoses it increases the nervous reflexes, and causes nervous irritability and sleeplessness. In toxic dose it causes tetanic spasms and opisthotonos.

23. *What changes are made in Heart by Digitalis?*

   Inhibition of heart action through irritation of pneumogastric nerve.
   Indicative symptomatology: Pulse small, irregular, slow. Feels that heart would stop beating if he moves.

24. *What changes are made in Mucous Secretion by Pulsatilla?*

   Catarrhal inflammation.
   Indicative symptomatology: Discharge bland, white, yellowish-green, thick.

25. *What changes are made in the Teeth by Fluoric Acid?*

   Rapid caries. Fistula dentalis.
   Indicative symptomatology: Teeth exquisitely sensitive to touch.

26. *What changes are made in the Bones by Silicea?*

   Inflammation, swelling, suppuration and necrosis.

27. *What changes are made in Cartilages by Silicea?*

   Inflammation, especially the knees.
   Indicative symptomatology: Fibrous parts of joints, especially of the knees, inflamed.

28. *What changes are made in the Blood by Arsenic?*

   Anæmia.
   Indicative symptomatology: The skin, nervous symptoms and general condition of the patient all suggest this. Skin pale, pasty-like. Anæmia.

29. *What changes are made in functions of Mucous Membrane by Allium Cepa?*

   Acute catarrhal inflammation with profuse secretion from eyes and upper respiratory tract.
   Indicative symptomatology: Profuse bland lachrymation. Constant sneezing, with profuse acrid coryza. Fluid coryza, headache, lachry-

mation, cough, thirst, loss of appetite, fever, worse in the evening. Profuse acrid watery discharge from nose with bland lachrynation.

30. *What changes are made in functions of Spine by Cocculus?*

   Paralytic weakness of motive nerves of the spine (and sensory).
   Indicative symptomatology: Paresthesia of the hands and arms. Lower limbs nearly paralyzed. Paralysis of the limbs. Symptoms are more suggestive of functional rather than organic changes.

31. *What changes are made in Nutrition by Iodine?*

   Improper assimilation of food.
   Indicative symptomatology: Emaciation with good appetite. Cachetic condition, profound debility and great emaciation. Eats freely, but loses weight all the time.

32. *What changes are made in Mucous Secretions by Natrum Muriaticum?*

   Hypersecretion; secretions are altered in quantity; character remains mostly moral; pus may be found.
   Indicative symptomatology: Catarrh, when secretion is clear. Loss of smell. Nose sore; interior of the alæ nasi swollen

33. *What changes are made in Portal Circulation by Sulphur?*

   Congestion of single parts or any organ, more especially at the climaxis. "Scroflous" diathesis; subject to venous congestion, especially of the genital system. Chronic alcoholism;

dropsy and ailments of drunkards. Frequent desire for stool (more marked than in Nux Vomica), constipation—or early morning diarrhœo-hæmorrhoids.

34. *What changes are made in Cerebrum by Opium?*

Congestion; inflammation; appolexy.
Indicative symptomatology: Delirious talking. Eyes wide open, face red, puffed up. Thinks she is not at home. Imagines parts of the body are large.

35. *What changes are made in functions of Nerves by Phosphorus?*

Nervous asthenia; lowered vitality; mental hyperactivity; hallucinations.
Indicative symptomatology: Oversensitiveness to external impressions; fears loss of reason; restless fidgety, moves continuously, cannot sit or stand still a moment. Excitable, easily angered and vehement, from which he suffers. Mind over-active.

36. *What changes are made in Nutrition by Ferrum?*

Mal-assimilation; wasting due to hæmorrhage, etc., chlorosis, anæmia.
Indicative symptomatology: Extreme paleness of the face, lips, tongue and mucous membrane of the mouth. Weakly persons with fiery red face. Least exertion or emotion causes flushing of the face.

37. *What changes are made in Skin by Graphites?*

Chronic inflammation; pruritis; fissure-vesicles; pustules; ulcerations.

Indicative symptamotology: Cracks and fissures at the end of fingers, nipples, labial commissure, anus and between toes. Unhealthy skin. Every injury suppurates. Old cictoes. Unhealthy skin. Eczema in the hollow of the knees; finger nails thick and chippled. Finger nails black, rough, matrix inflamed, sore, throbbing, numbness; no suppuration.

38. *What changes are made in Spinal Circulation by Belladonna?*

    Inflammation.
    Indicative symptomatology: Loss of co-ordination of muscles of both upper and lower extremities, very like the heaviness and helplessness of movement observed in the first stages of progressive paralysis of the insane.

39. *What changes are made in Color of Skin by Argentum Nitricum?*

    Indicative symptomatology: Skin blue, gray, violet, bronze color, to a real black. Skin brown, tense, hard.

40. *What changes are made in Urine by Lycopodium?*

    Hæmaturia, from gravel and chronic catarrh. Red, sandy sediment in the urine. Foamy urine.

41. *What changes are made in Connective Tissue by Silicea?*

    Stimulates fibrosis and cicatrization in chronic suppurative inflammations.

42. *What changes are made in the Solar Plexus by Carbo. Veg.?*

Farrington attributed the abdominal symptomatology of *Carbo. Veg.* to a hypothetic action on the solar plexus. His indicative symptomatology was as follows: Indigestion of low type, especially cases resulting from debauchery, indulgence in table luxuries and from bad effects of wines and liquors and all kinds of dissipation. In the bad effects of dissipation, it was held to be indicated by headache, especially in the morning when awakening from sleep; dull headache referred to the back part of the head with a great confusion of mind; humming or buzzing in the head; aggravation in the warm room, pain going from the occiput into the head and into the eyes, giving a dull, heavy aching in that locality. Nausea and weakness referred to the stomach, usually a burning sort of distress referred to the epigastrium; unable to take milk because it produces flatulence; stomach feels heavy; flatus; belching and borborygmi both offensive. Constipation with flatulence, which are aggravated after every spree. Morning diarrhœa with stool which is watery and thin; peevish, easily angry. Vertigo reflex from gastric disturbance; worse after a debauch.*

43. *What changes are made in Skin by Petroleum?*

Inflammation. Intertrigo, eczema.

Indicative symptomatology: Humid soreness behind the ears, eczema. Skin hard, rough, cracked, tips of the fingers rough. Deep

---

*Here we have quoted direct from Farrington's *Clinical Materia Medica.*

rhagades on hand; thick crusts worse during winter. Hot swelling of the soles of the feet. Feet tender, bathed in a foul smelling sweat. Ulcers, stinging pains. Ulcers heal slowly.

44. *What changes are made in Mucous Secretion by Kali Bich.?*

Inflammation of mucous membrane with plastic exudate; pseudomembrane; excessive activity of glands and profuse section of mucus. The excessive secretion rapidly is converted into a fibrous exudate—and formation of a so-called false membrane.

Indicative symptomatology: Tickling as from a hair high up in nose. Pressing pain at the root of the nose. Discharge of large quantities of mucus from nose when blown. Stiches in the right side, and a sensation as if two loose bones rubbed against each other. Scabs on septum—ulcerations of the septum.

45. *What changes are made in Cicatrices by Graphites?*

Graphites has an excellent effect in reducing or even removing cicatricial tissue. This therapeutic use of the remedy originated in an observation that workers in graphite experienced very ready healing of wounds on the hands, and cicatricial contraction of the eyelids following wounds and surgical operations. *Graphites* may also be used successfully for the absorption of indurated surfaces.

46. *What changes are made in the Urine by Benzoic Acid?*

Strong odor like horse urine (hippuric acid).
Indicative symptomatology: Urine when passing is hot and has strong, pungent, fetid odor.

Urine high coloured; increased specific gravity; hot, scalding. Ammoniacal and very offensive. Enuresis nocturna of children.

47. *What changes are made in the Larynx by Bromine?*

Inflammation, and formation of exudate.

Indicative symptomatology: Cold sensation in larynx; cold feeling when inspiring. Asthma worse during the night. Rattling of mucus long before it can be expectorated. Wheezing and panting with violent cough. Difficult expectoration of tough, stringy mucus. Membranous croup. Cough worse on dressing, better on getting warm in bed. The peculiarity of this discharge is its thick, stringy nature, and difficulty of detachment. It stretches out into long strings.

48. *What changes are made in the Blood by Cinchona?*

The specific action of cinchona (quinine) on the blood with the exception of its specific antiplasmodium malariæ destructive action is rather poorly developed.

Indicative symptomatology: Hæmorrhages from the mouth, nose, lungs, and bowels, with a longing for sour things. Metrorrhagic dark blood.

49. *What changes are made in Nutrition by Natrum Mur?*

Mal-nutrition. Emaciation.

Indicative symptomatology: Emaciation even when living well, great weakness, relaxation of all bodily and physical powers from least exertion.

50 *What changes are made in Bones by Aurum?*

Exostosis of bones in skull and other bones.
Indicative symptomatology: Boring pains in bones; especially after the administration of mercury. Pains driving to desperation. Pains wander from joint to joint. Tearing pains in the metatarsal joints. Laming twinges in toes of the right foot.

51. *What changes are made in the Blood by Pulsatilla?*

Hæmorrhages. Blood dark, easily coagulating. *Pulsatilla* is an invaluable remedy in amæmias, but is indicated more for the collateral symptoms than by reason of an anæmia producing action *per se*. Chlorosis is a particular sphere, the symptoms of which it presents to a characteristic degree; chlorotic or anæmic women, always complaining of sensations as of chills, and yet find relief for their ill-feelings in the open air and cannot tolerate a warm room. Pains are associated with chilliness. Chlorosis after failure of iron. Late and scanty menstruation. Fickle appetite, and especially for indigestible articles, as pickles.

52. *What changes are made in Functions of Nerves by Caulophyllum?*

Hysterical and epileptiform spasms at puberty; with menstrual irregularities, especially in hysterical females.

53. *What changes are made in Spinal Cord by Conium?*

In poisoning cases, conium produces a progressing paralysis starting from below and proceeding upwards without loss of consciousness. Associated symptoms are prickling sensations in the muscles, pain in the head, twitching and tremors together with stiffness and rigidity of some of the muscles. Movements weak and unsteady, gait staggering. Nausea and occasionally vomiting with profuse salivation. Deglutition difficult. Respiration at first accelerated, later becoming slow and labored, weak and irregular and finally ceasing.

NOTE: Seguin utilized the depresso-motor effect of *Conium* in the treatment of obstinate tics, but it seems to have produced little permanent good effects.

54. *What changes are made in Functions of Nerves by Gelsemium?*

Motor paralysis.
Indicative symptomatology: Complete relaxation and prostration of whole muscular system. Great weakness and trembling of the tongue, hands, legs and entire body.

55. *What changes are made in Nutrition by Calcarea?*

The apparent changes in calcium and general mineral metabolism.
Indicative symptomatology: Bones-swelling, softenings and curvature. Caries. Stinging pains.

56. *What changes are made in the Portal Circulation by Nux Vomica?*

Nux Vomica produces congestion of the portal circulation as indicated by its beneficial influence over hepatic and gastric disturbances arising from the excessive use of alcoholics, highly seasoned foods and the use of purgative medicines. The liver is often found to be swollen and hard and sensitive to the pressure of the clothing.

57 *What is the action of Calcarea Phosphorica in Fractures of Bones?*

It has been noted that where bones have a suture or joint, there *Calcarea Phosphorica* has an action. It causes pains along the sagittal suture, and again at the sacroiliac symphyses. In the case of fractures we may assume that there is an artificial joint for the time being. And so we reason that with delayed union *Calcarea Phosphorica* may be a remedy, and clinically we get results. It promotes union in delayed healing of fractures, especially in a person of the *Calcarea Phosphorica* constitution.

58. *What changes are produced in the Urine by Colchicum?*

The urine is made dark and turbid; in some cases it is almost black from admixture of altered blood. It is highly albuminous.

59. *What changes are made in the Larynx by Iodine?*

Iodine produces an inflammation of the larynx, either specific or non-specific; including diphtherial, syphilitic or tuberculous. The indications are hoarseness lasting all day; phlegm in small quantities and tough; constant hemming and hawking; dry morning cough from tickling of the larynx.

Section II.

1. *When is Cactus the Remedy in Heart Affections?*

    Cactus is indicated in the so-called cardiac neuroses (angina pectoris) and in cardiac hypertrophy. Its special characteristic symptom is a sensation of constriction about the heart.

2. *When is Ipecac the Remedy in Cough?*

    In the bronchial catarrhs of infants and chubby children; cough with inclination to vomit; constant coughing without expectoration though chest is apparently full of mucus; cough with strangling; with much accumulation of mucus in the chest; cough with gagging and vomiting.

3. *When is Cheldonium the Remedy in Cappillary Bronchitis?*

    Capillary bronchitis following measles or whooping cough; the characteristic hepatic symptoms are present. The face is of a deep red; great oppression of the chest; one foot hot, the other cold; cough usually loose and having a rattling sound; expectoration raised with difficulty; sharp stitching pain under the right scapula.

4. *When is Belladonna the Remedy in Cerebral Congestion?*

    In the milder cases, when there is sensation of heat about the head, the feet being cold. In the violent form; Face red and conjunctivæ injected; severe throbbing headache; patient may be drowsy or wakeful; or the drowsiness and wakefulness alternate; rouses from slumber as if startled; jerking of the limbs; twitching of individual muscles of jerking of entire limbs; violent throbbing of the carotid arteries; pupils dilated; scanty urine.

5. *When is Rhus Toxicodendron indicated in Rheumatism?*

   Rhus is the remedy more for the rheumatic diathesis than for typical rheumatic fever. In the rheumatic diathesis it is inicated by its characteristic modalities, *i.e.,* aggravation in damp weather, and relief from continued motion. Prominences of bones, as those on the cheeks are sore to the touch. *Rhus* affects especially the sheaths of muscles, and has a special affinity for the back. It is our best remedy for lumbago.

6. *When is Cantharis the Remedy in Dysuria?*

   The symptoms of *Cantharis* may relate to the entire urinary tract. There are: Burning pains extending from the kidneys down either ureter to the bladder; persistent violent urging to urinate; violent cutting pains extending along the spermatic cords to the testicles; burning in the glans penis. Urine does not pass copiously but dribbles drop by drop; bloody urine; pain in the region of the kidneys; region of the kidneys sensitive to touch.

7. *When is Elaps the Remedy in Haemoptysis?*

   When there is a feeling of coldness in the chest after drinking; cough accompanied by intense pain in the chest, especially on the right side in the apex; sputum consists of dark blood;

right lung more involved than the left; morning pain sufficiently severe to prevent patient from getting up.

8. *When is Psorinum the Remedy in Cholera Infantum?*

Child wakes up from sleep as if frightened; cries out in sleep. Diarrhœa; stools profuse, watery and offensive and black; stools of green mucus, mixed with blood; aggravation at night; odor almost putrid. Nervousness and fretfulness precede the diarrhœa by two or three nights. Pale, sickly, delicate children; lack of reaction.

9. *When is Ustilago indicated at Climaxis?*

Vertigo. Hæmorrhages at climaxis; metrorrhagia; bright red blood, partly fluid and partly clotted; or, oozing of dark blood with small coagula.

10. *When is Sepia the Remedy in Over Exertion of the Mind?*

The indicative symptoms are mainly mental. They include indifference to one's family; anxiety with fear; great irritability alternating with indifference; flushes of heat over the face.

11. *When is Secale the Remedy in Cholera?*

Patient cold; almost pulseless; spasmodic twitching of the body here and there; cannot bear being covered. Collapse, face sunken, distorted, particularly the mouth; crawling sensation as from ants. Stools watery, slimy; stools greenish, discharged rapidly with great force or even involuntarily; stools painless without effort and with prostration.

12. *When is Apis Mellifica the Remedy in Dropsies?*

Dropsies of renal or cardiac origin. In renal cases, waxen hue to the surface of the skin; transparent whitish or slightly yellow tinge. Urine scanty. Thirstlessness. After scarlatina with nephritis; swelling of the eyelids. Urine scanty and albuminous; surface of the body feels sore and bruised. In cardiac cases, the dropsy is especially manifested in the feet.

13. *When is Psorinum the Remedy in Typhoid Types of Fever?*

When the general condition is such that the physician feels assured that so far as organic changes are concerned the patient is safe; and the patient is mentally depressed or low spirited, or hopeless of recovery. At the same time he is weak of body. Weakening night sweats; defective reaction to ordinary apparently well indicated remedies.

14. *When is Theridion the Remedy in Headache?*

For nervous headaches generally, and in hemicrania. Throbbing over the left eye and across the forehead; sick headache, with aggravation from persons walking across the floor or from slight noises. Nausea aggravated on rising from lying posture. Sensation of pain in the vertex, as if patient could lift off top of the head. Hemicrania; flickering before the eyes and then blurring of vision, nausea aggravated by closing the eyes, and by noise.

15. **When is Cantharis the Remedy in Erysipelas?**

    In erysipelas of the vesicular type. Characteristically the rash appears first on the nose with or without vesicles. From this point it spreads to one or the other cheek with formation of vesicles, which break and discharge an excoriating fluid.

16. **When is Sepia the Remedy in Prolapsus Uteri?**

    Prolapsus uteri with congestion; yellowish leucorrhea. Prolapsus with inclination to left side causing numbness in left half of the body with pain; pain in the pelvic region relieved by lying, tenderness of the os uteri; pressure as if everything would protrude through vulvæ.

17. **When is Sepia the Remedy for Ulcers?**

    Small ulcers appearing about the joints of the hands, and especially on the fingers. These ulcers are painless.

18. **When is Apis Mellifica the Remedy in Urticaria?**

    Useful especially in acute rather than in chronic cases. Sudden appearance of long white or pinkish white wheals, attended by itching, burning and stinging; intervening skin is of deep scarlet. Especially indicated in cases caused by eating shell fish.

19. **When is Cantharis the Remedy in Diphtheria?**

    Diphtheria attended by burning or raw feeling in the throat; great constriction of the throat and larynx, amounting almost to suffocation on any attempt at swallowing; debility pronounced; especially indicated in cases in which dysuria is present.

20. *When is Lachesis the Remedy in Tonsillitis?*

    In tonsillitis with suppuration when the pus is of a dark, thin and offensive character. The inflamation starts on the left side, and spreads to the right. The throat is of a bluish red hue; frequent sense of constriction; sensation as of a lump in the throat, which must be constantly swallowed; throat externally very sensitive to touch; excepting in cases with pronounced swelling patient finds relief from swallowing solids and aggravation from liquids, or empty swallowing.

21. *When is Sepia the Remedy in Ozena?*

    In cases in which large lumps of yellow greenish mucus or yellowish green crusts with blood are discharged from the nose; loss of sense of smell; fetid odor from the nose.

22. *When is Apis the Remedy in Diphtheria?*

    The case is generally one of insidious onset and insidious progress; prostration is profound with high fever and drowsiness; the pulse is rapid and not strong. The throat presents a varnished appearance; the membrane is thick and looks like wash leather; œdema of the uvula; rim of the glottis is swollen and œdematous causing breathing to be hard or labored; burning, stinging pains in the throat; blisters on the border of the tongue. Often associated with œdema in other portions of the body. Red rash over the body in some cases. The throat externally may be swollen and œdematous.

23. *When is Tarentula the Remedy in Hysteria?*

Patient jerks the limbs and body generally. She becomes quiet when attention is directed away from her. Lively music tends to promote activity of movements.

24. *When is Lachesis the Remedy in Typhoid Fever?*

In adynamic cases with low delirium of the low muttering type; increasing mental torpor with coolness of the extremities; tremor of the hands and feet; tongue protruded with difficulty and trembling, or it catches on the teeth; tongue coated brown, sometimes with small blisters on its tip; lips crack and ooze a dark blood; loquacity followed by depression. Diarrhœa usually present; stools characteristically of a highly offensive odor.

25. *When is Naja the Remedy in Heart Affections?*

When in infectious disease, as diphtheria, there is impending paralysis of the heart. The patient is blue; wakens from sleep gasping; pulse intermittent and thready.

26. *When is Apis the Remedy in Ovaritis?*

When the right ovary especially is involved. Extreme soreness of the right ovary with burning, stinging pains or sensations. Some tumefaction detected by examination per rectum or vagina. Sometimes associated with pain in the left pectoral region and cough. Sharp lancinating pains extending down the right thigh.

27. *When is Secale the Remedy in Cholera Infantum?*

Stools large and contain undigested food; stools watery and offensive; sudden spasmodic expulsion of watery stool followed by great prostration.

28. *When is Lachesis the Remedy in Constipation?*

In any diseased condition in which constipation may exist when the following symptoms are present: *Lachesis* may be indicated: Costive, ineffectual urging to stool; anus feels closed. Stools offensive even when formed. Sense of constriction of the sphincter. Throbbing at the anus. It also may be indicated in constipation with hæmorrhoids, especially in cases occurring at climaxis, in women with scanty menstruation or in **drunkards**.

29. *When is Sepia the Remedy in Amenorrhoea?*

Amenorrhœa at puberty or later; pains in the uterus, bearing down; crosses the limbs to prevent protrusion of the parts. Uterine induration.

30. *When is Coccus Cocti the Remedy in Cough?*

In whooping cough or pulmonary tuberculosis when the cough has a morning aggravation and is followed by the vomiting of long ropes of stringy mucus. In tuberculosis there are sharp, stitching pains beneath the clavicles.

A SYLLABUS OF MATERIA MEDICA

31. *When is Cantharis the Remedy in Dysentry?*

Stools are slimy and bloody, and contain flakes that look like scrapings of the intestines, but which really consist of fibrinous formations. Tenesmus is pronounced and may be attended by dysuria. Pains are of colicky character; cutting, burning, gripping pains of wandering character.

32. *When is Sepia the Remedy in Dyspepsia?*

Dyspepsia incident to uterine disease associated with an empty, gone feeling in the epigastrium or abdomen with sour or bitter risings or taste in the mouth; longing for pickles and acids, indulgence in which seems to relieve. Tongue coated white. Bowels constipated; stools hard, dry and insufficient. Abdomen swollen and distended with flatus. Soreness in the hepatic region from congestion of the liver.

33. *When is Apis Mellifica the Remedy in Tuberculous Meningitis?*

Early in the case when there is effusion. Patient cries out with a piercing shriek. Child is sleepy, and awakened from sleep with a shrill cry; it may be wholly or partly conscious; sleepy but cannot sleep; spasms of the flexors so that the big toes are turned upwards. Child bores its head into the pillow. Body convulsed and other side as if paralyzed. Strabismus. Pulse rapid and weak.

34. *When is Lachesis the Remedy in Heart Affections?*

In organic affections and in functional disturbances at climaxis. Palpitation with sense of constriction as if held by a cord. Oppression on awakening; inability to lie down. Hydrothorax; hydropericardium. Horrible sensation of smothering feeling about the heart on awaking from sleep, forcing patient to get out of bed.

35. *When is Ustilago the Remedy in Uterine Haemorrhage?*

Usually in cases characterized by passive uterine congestion. Bright, red blood, partly fluid and partly clotted. Uterus indurated; the examining finger causes bleeding. Hæmorrhages at climaxis or during labor.

36. *When is Variolinum the Remedy in Small-pox?*

Appears to be traditional or empiric; most standard text-books silent on subject.

37. *When is Psorinum the Remedy in Eruptions?*

In cases presenting a constitutional defect by reason of which the illness fails to respond to well selected remedies. Eruptions essentially of a herpetic character, and accompanied by great itching, which is aggravated as soon as the patient gets warm in bed. Later the skin has a dirty, dingy appearance, as though the patient had not been properly washed. Skin may present a coarse look as if it had been bathed in oil. Eruption moist. In children especially about the scalp, but characteristically from the scalp down either side of the face, involving the cheeks and ears, like tinea capitis. Eruption at times moist, and oozes an offensive secretion; at other times is dry, or furfuraceous. Ulcers on legs, usually about the tibia and around the ankles or other joints.

38. **When is Cantharis the Remedy in Gonorrhoea?**

    Chordee in the course of gonorrhœa; complicating cystitis with the usual *Cantharis* symptoms.

39. **When is Sepia the Remedy in Leucorrhoea?**

    Discharge of a yellowish green color and somewhat offensive, with bearing down pains in the abdomen and in the small of the back; feeling as if everything will be forced out through vulvæ; backache referable to the lumbar or sacral region, decidedly worse when patient is standing or walking. Burning pains in the uterus, and sometimes pains of a sharp character shooting upwards, or there may be a sensation as if the uterus was clutched by a hand. Menses usually late and scanty.

40. **When is Lachesis the Remedy in Ovaritis?**

    Ovaritis when the left ovary is affected; tenderness to pressure of clothing. Menses scanty, feeble; blood lumpy and black and very offensive; pains in the hips; bearing down in the left ovary. Uterus intolerant of the least pressure.

41. **When is Aranea Diadema the Remedy in Aggravation from State of Atmosphere?**

    All the symptoms of *Aranea Diadema* are characteristically worse in damp weather or from dwelling in damp localities.

42. *When is Secale the Remedy in Spinal Congestion?*

   Secale produces a passive congestion of the spinal cord, and hence prolonged use of it or chronic poisoning by ergot may be followed by a train of symptoms strongly simulating those of tabes.

43. *When is Apis Mellifica the Remedy in Heart Disease?*

   In cardiac affection and inflammation with dropsy or œdema; dyspnœa; sudden lancinating or stinging pains; restlessness, anxiety. The restlessnes is of a fidgety character.

44. *When is Lachesis the Remedy in Erysipelas?*

   When the rash is most pronounced on the left side. The face at first is bright red but soon assumes a bluish hue; considerable infiltration of the cellular tissue; pulse is accelerated and weak; feet are apt to be cool; patient drowsy; muttering delirium.

45. *When is Tarantula the Remedy in Spinal Irritation?*

   Excitability of the peripheral nerves; hands in constant motion; headache, relieved by burrowing the head into the pillow; enlargement of the uterus and ovaries.

46. *When is Psorinum the Remedy in Imperfect Reaction?*

   In Psoric constitution, and after acute exhausting illnesses; usual remedies though well indicated failing to act satisfactorily.

MODALITIES AS ARRANGED BY BONNINGHAUSEN.

ONE of the most useful chapters in Bonninghausen's "Therapeutic Pocket-Book" is that which comprises the modalities, the conditions of aggravation and amelioration.

But unfortunately they are not sufficiently individualized. They are rather treated as general characteristics, applicable to the entire range of action of the drugs.

When the book was being written, Dr. Hering urged its author to state just what symptoms or group of symptoms were affected by a given condition. For instance, instead of writing "worse from motion, *Bryonia*", Dr. Hering desired that it should be stated what symptoms were worse from motion.

But Bonninghausen refused to comply with this request as reasonable as it was; so his book was crippled, and we have lost, probably irreparably, the particulars of his vast clinical work.

This is greatly to be regretted for many reasons, one of which is the aid such work might give in the construction of a systematic Materia Medica.

Symptoms are, as it were, threads of one fabric, which fabric is the entire drug. Hence symptoms must possess certain common relations, to discover which, is to discover the woof of the whole cloth.

Now very few of the modalities have a universal application. They rather belong to definite groups of symptoms. To clearly discriminate in such cases, requires not only a general knowledge of drug effects but a particular knowledge; and just here, Bonninghausen's clinical studies would be of the greatest service.

But since we are not so favoured, it should be the agreeable duty of each practitioner to make observations for himself, and communicate the results to his colleagues. Let me illustrate what I mean.

An oft-confirmed condition of *Sepia* is amelioration from violent exertion of the body. The full symptom reads: "The complaints disappear during violent exercise such as walking in the open air, fencing, etc. (horseback riding excepted), and appear most frequently and severely when sitting quiet, forenoon and evening."

How far is this modality applicable, and what is its explanation?

We find as well confirmed, aggravation from walking quickly and less frequently, worse from exercise; worse from motion. Also, relieved in a recumbent posture; better lying down, etc.

Examining particularly into its symptoms, we observe that the headaches, sacro-lumbar pains, heaviness in the abdomen, and faint, weak state, are all emphatically aggravated from motion. Bearing down in the pelvic region induces a desire to remain sitting or lying, with the eyes closed. Prolapsus uteri, better sitting with the limbs crossed or lying on the right side.

One form of pelvic distress seems to necessitate motion. It is described as a distress in the hypogastrium as from a distended bladder, worse from continued sitting and lying, better on walking about. But this same patient was also relieved momentarily by lying on either side, with the thighs fixed on the abdomen.

Another prover complained of pain across the lower part of the bowels, relieved by passing urine; felt only on lying down.

On the other hand, we notice that palpitation of the heart is diminished by "walking a long distance and walking fast." And if the nervous weakness is not too great, if the patient is tired, languid, feels bruised, parts laid on go to sleep, she feels worse while sitting; and although stiff and sore on beginning to move, walking soon relieves.

It is well-known that *Sepia* affects the nervous system and causes, through vaso-motor relaxation, venous congestions. The connective tissue all over is likewise relaxed. From this arise: "Fulness, venous fulness, in various parts; empty, gone, sensations; feeling as if the joints were slipping out of place; prolapses of the viscera; and, through overfilled veins bruised sore feelings in the muscles, numbness, paralytic weakness, etc."

Now exercise, by favoring venous return and stimulating lax tissues, tends to relieve just the pathological state upon which many *Sepia* symptoms depend. But horseback riding since it jars the sensitive parts, and even tends, like the motion of a ship, to retard venous return, necessarily aggravates the *Sepia* patient.

This, I submit, is the explanation of the modality under consideration.

Confusion sometimes arises from modalities which are opposed to each other; as *Magnesia Muriatica* better from pressure, worse from pressure—*Calc. Carb.*, worse from washing; better by cold bathing—*Bryonia,* worse from motion; better from motion—*Sulphur,* worse or better on an empty stomach—*Petroleum,* better or worse when stretching out the diseased limb, or when drawing it up.

These aparent contradictions may spring from the two-fold action of the drugs. But they also may arise from the fact that nearly all modalities have but a limited range belonging to the same remedy.

How, then, can they be discriminated, if the plan of Bonninghausen is to be continued?

If we consult the provings of the above-cited remedies we find a solution to our difficulties. *Mag. Mur.* has relief of headache from pressure, but aggravation of hepatic symptoms. In general the *Calc. Carb.* patient is made worse by bathing, but in colic and peritonitis, cold-water applications give prompt relief, and so on.

Still another defect in Bonninghausen's method arising from generalization, is his imperfect presentation of a symptom.

Thus, under *Alumina* we read: "Inclination for open air." But the complete symptom requires the further statement that, nevertheless, neither cold nor warm can be borne well.

There is an underlying system, according to which modalities can be arranged, and we should find it. We know that complaints involving muscular tissue are increased by motion, while affections of fibrous structures are improved by continued motion. Many variations of symptoms accord with diurnal, weekly, and annual changes, barometrical vicissitudes, etc., all of which are acknowledged to be exhibitions of natural laws. For instance, *Natrum Mur.* has its acme at 11 A.M.—just the hour of daily maximum electric tension; *Lycopodium* has its acme from 4 to 8 P.M.—just the hours of minimum electric tension; *Nux Vom.* has arousing at 3 A.M.—an hour when *Bryonia, Arsenic, Sepia, Sulphur,* and other remedies, which act on the intestinal contents, also offer symptoms. *Rhododendron, Natrum Carb., Petroleum, Phosphorus,* etc., are worse before a thunderstorm, when the air is poor in ozone, and when constitutions needing an abundance of this form of oxygen, must necessarily suffer.

A west wind, in our latitude, is, in winter, frequently cold and dry; a south wind warm and relaxing; and an east or north-east wind cold, raw and damp.

Consistently herewith, we have one set of remedies, *Aconite, Hepar, Spongia, Causticum,* in exacerbations from one wind; *Ipecac, Bryonia, Carbo Veg.,* for the next; and *Sepia, Allium Cepa, Dulcamara,* etc., for the last.

Gelsemium, Bryonia, and *Quillaia,* picture a cold which is the effect of a relaxing atmosphere; *Nux, Aconite, Belladonna,* catarrh caused by cold, crisp weather. *Ipecac* portrays a wheezing, rattling bronchial catarrh, with loose but difficult expectoration, just such a cold as a debilitated lax-fibred patient might contract under the depressing influence of a southerly, warm, thawing wind. *Hepar,* on the contrary, displays the rough hacking cough or the croupy rattle which one might expect to follow exposure to piercing cold winds.

Many more instances might be cited, tending to prove the harmony of the effects of provings with the numerous accidents and contingencies of our checkered existence.

Try to investigate them thoroughly.

USE OF UNIVERSAL SYMPTOMS

IT is patent to all that the remedy for a given case is the one which covers the characteristic symptoms. Hence no rule of practice is a correct sequence from the law of cure that in any way whatsoever disputes the selection from the totality of the symptoms. But theory and practice do not always agree; that is, their agreement is not always evident; so Hahnemann and his followers have all along striven to discover sub-rules that shall aid in the difficult task of curing disease. For example, the Organon instructs us how to proceed when one drug will not cover the totality, when constitutional taint obscures, when epidemic influences are at work, etc. And, further, still more in accommodation to circumstances, Hahnemann suggests as often needed as usually required, etc., *Thuja* in sycosis, *Sulphur* in psora, etc. Now, of course, it is not to be inferred here that such drugs must be given for the respective "constitutions;" for the recommendation is ever subservient to the exacting law. Still, their suggestion is very helpful, because it represents a principle, and because it expresses the results of experience. It simply means, use such remedies as are best adapted to the removal of the underlying taint that is complicating and perpetuating the illness; generally, *Thuja* or *Sulphur* will do, because so often proved useful; but here, as always, characterizing symptoms must decide.

Agreeably to all this, physicians have, at times, when unable to fit "the totality", chosen a remedy that suits those characteristics upon which the entire disease seems to depend.

In this manner we have learned to employ *Collinsonia* for many diseases when a congestion of the lower bowels with piles obtains. Employing such characteristics as piles bleeding, feeling of sticks in the rectum, stool in light-colored lumps, uterine affections, varices, irritable heart, etc., have yielded readily to the drug, just as though they depended for their existence upon pelvic stasis.

Similarly we have seen palpitation, vertigo and dyspepsia vanish under the influence of *Pareira Brava* selected for its grand characteristic, "Must get down on all fours and strain to pass water; pains go down the thighs." So, too, *Berberis* relieves a host of ailments when selected for its radiating renal pains, "Pains into the hips; urine with yellow, loamy sediment." *Anisum Stellatum* has cured hæmoptysis when selected by its key-note, "Pain at the junction of the third right rib with its cartilage". *Myrtus Communis* has retarded phthisis when there was present sharp pain through the upper part of the left lung; *Ceanothus* has removed leucorrhœa when in addition there was sharp pain in the splenic region. And so on almost indefinitely.

Now in all such cases there is, of course, a connection between symptoms treated as central and the others that disappear along with them, though often we are not able to detect it.

In some instances, however, the symptom or group of symptoms employed plainly exhibit a universal quality of a drug; as when we select *Bryonia* in cases worse from motion; *Thuja* for nervous phenomena depending upon affections of skin and mucous membranes, or for warts; *Rhus* for complaints of fibrous tissues, better from continued motion; *Causticum* for paretic aphonia, even if of catarrhal origin and so on.

In such cases we are not prescribing for a single symptom, we are making use of a universal, characteristic property and wherever in the human body tissue like that under treatment exists, there the medicine can have an effect. And as metastases usually occur from similar part to similar part we prevent such a catastrophe by the universal scope of our drug. To explain further, suppose we examine into the application of the modality of *Bryonia,* worse from motion. It is universally present in all tissues that are generally affected by exercise; as in muscles, serous and synovial membranes, and inflamed joints. *Bryonia* depresses the sensorium, producing dulness and want of desire to use the brain; hence naturally the patient has aversion to motion. Now fibrous tissues are generally relieved by continued exercise, and, consistently, the "fibrous pains" of *Bryonia* are exceptions to the modality under consideration. Nervousness is a symptom that generally impels one to move; and accordingly, the *Bryonia* patient, when nervous, is compelled to move, though thereby he intensifies other sufferings. *Thuja,* as is well-known, affects epithelia everywhere, first making them grow excessively and later, causing their absorption; hence, if the wart is that characteristic of the arbor vitæ, *Thuja* does not suppress it, but cures it, acting consentaneously upon the whole "epithelial" man.

Rhus affects notably fibrous tissue; hence its modality, better from continued motion; but the purely muscular pains of the remedy, and the prostration, are worse from motion. If then, we prescribe for the modality better from motion, *Rhus,* we do not really depend upon one symptom if the case concerns chiefly joints, tendons, sheaths of muscles, and kindred structures.

When, therefore, we employ what we may term universals, we are not guilty of selecting a single symptom to the rejection of the rest. But when, as is, alas, too often done, we prescribe for an isolated symptom, simply because we recognize it as characteristic of a certain remedy, forgetting that what is charac-

teristic in one connection may not be in another, and
that a characteristic of a drug may not be an important
symptom in a given case, we do violence to the principles
of the Organon, and violate common sense. A case
is published in a journal. The reader sees clearly
enough what remedy should be given, and so is
astonished to find that drug is claimed to have cured
which has only one symptom of the case, and that a mere
modality; for instance, worse after sleep, *Lachesis.*
When we use proper discrimination, then will we have
creditable clinical reports.

REMARKS ON SOME OF THE ACIDS.

YESTERDAY in finishing my remarks on the acids
in general, you will remember that I divided them
into two classes, the vegetable and mineral. Then I
referred to the debility characteristic of acids *in toto,*
and observed that in vegetable acids debility is marked
by a soft, feeble pulse, whereas that of the mineral
acids is marked by irritability, the pulse being rather
wiry. I next drew your attention to the dietetic value
of acids and also to their general medicinal properties.
I referred to their power of increasing the alkaline
secretions and of diminishing the acid. Therefore they
increase the flow of saliva and lessen the secretion of
the gastric juice. I referred to the use of acid drinks
during the course of fevers for the purpose of pro-
moting the flow of saliva, and spoke of the pseudo-
membranes which many of these acids, notably *Lactic*
and *Acetic Acids,* can produce. I referred to the power
of *Lactic Acid* to dissolve even the enamel of the teeth.
Speaking of the vegetable acids, I gave you a few hints
regarding the use of *Citric Acid* in hæmorrhages. This

acid is often employed as a Homœopathic remedy for a peculiar state of mind in which careful house-keepers suddenly become indifferent to all that formerly interested them. This symptom does not come from simple stubbornness, but is the result of a debilitated condition. You will here recall a similarity to *Sepia,* which has indifference, not only to household matters, but also to persons, formerly loved. I incidentally referred to symptoms of a rheumatic character produced by *Lactic Acid,* namely, inflammation, redness and swelling of the joints, especially of the smaller joints, with profuse sweating; also to hawking of mucus and to swelling of the tonsils, with pain and sense of constriction which are worse from swallowing. There is a pseudo-membrane in the throat.

I also referred to the grape-cure; stating that grapes were useful for the purpose of diminishing obesity, and also in dropsy when it came from sluggishness of the circulation rather than from organic disease. At the same time I remarked that the abuse of these vegetable acids may develop their characteristic debility; the patient will then have diarrhœa, the mouth will become sore and filled with aphthous ulcers, the saliva run from the mouth, and symptoms of scorbutus appear.

To-day I invite your attention to two of the mineral acids, *Phosphoric* and *Sulphuric Acids. Phosphoric Acid* causes and therefore cures, a peculiar debility, a debility which is not a simple weakness, such as occurs when one is worn out by work, but which comes from alteration of the fluids of the body (particularly of the blood), as after long-lasting weakness of digestion, malnutrition, etc. *Phosphoric Acid* differs materially from *Phosphorus.* I cannot, therefore, agree with those who assert that the latter becomes oxidized in the system, and that when we are taking what is called *Phosphorus* we are in reality taking *Phosphoric Acid*. This is asserted by Heinigke in his "Outlines of Materia Medica," and by Hempel. While we cannot deny that *Phosphorus* quickly appropriates oxygen, it is certain that its effects potentized are different from those of the acid. No one is willing to admit that *Phosphoric Acid* can be replaced in typhoid fever by *Phosphorus*.

Phosphoric Acid at first causes an increase of vitality. True to its *Phosphorus*, it is at first slightly stimulating. This, however, is soon followed by the opposite condition, in which the sensorium seems to be very much depressed, so that we have developed a condition of complete apathy. Not only is there dulness of thought, but also want of feeling apathy. This sensorial apathy is usually accompanied by more or less drowsiness and indifference to one's condition. When not extreme, you will notice that the predominant mental state is one of melancholy or sadness. These symptoms have led to the use of the drug for the effects of disappointed love and for jealousy, and also for the protracted effects of grief. You will recall *Ignatia* as a remedy for the acute effects of grief, and *Opium* for the immediate effects of fright. The *Ignatia* woman is introspective. She sits brooding over her trouble, and suffers from nervous complaints as a result. In *Phosphoric Acid* mental and bodily depression result from the grief. There are frequent sighing, heat, and a crushing weight on the top of the head, perspiration in sleep, or from every little exertion or mental excitement, palpitation of the heart, etc. The body seems to emaciate steadily. The nearest ally here is *Natrum Mur.*, which also in the protracted effects of grief has its same sort of headache.

You may use *Phosphoric Acid* in a peculiar kind of headache which occurs in school children. The pain is constant and is of a dull depressing character, with blurring of vision. These symptoms always disappear during the holidays, but return again as soon as studies are resumed.

Phosphoric Acid has a marked effect upon the stomach and abdomen. You may give it with confidence in diarrhœa when the movements are watery, whitish or grayish-white, often containing undigested food and accompanied by constant rumbling and gurgling in the bowels. It seems as if the patient's abdomen had become converted into a yeast-pot. Now you will read in the books that the great key-note of this diarrhœa, in addition to this rumbling and distension of the abdomen, is that despite the long continuance of the disease there is but little prostration. I do not deny this. It is a legitimate inference from one of the symptoms which reads something like this: "The prover is astonished that his symptoms last so long, and yet he does not feel weak." This has been crystallized into a characteristic of the drug. But you will go astray if you depend too much upon it. *Phosphoric Acid* can cause a distressingly debilitating diarrhœa, and I do not hesitate a moment to prescribe it when the patient is greatly prostrated, if he has bloated abdomen and undigested stools, particularly if the latter are watery and whitish. Accompanying this diarrhœa, especially in children, you will notice the mouth becoming sore, and the tongue is pale and clammy rather than bright red or dry. The face is pinched, there are dark rings around the eyes and other evidences of exhaustion.

Phosphoric Acid is used for the complaints of women when menstrual irregularities are associated with dull pressure in the right hypochondrium,—probably from passive congestion of the liver.

Phosphoric Acid, like *Phosphorus,* sometimes acts on the lungs. It is very useful in some of the stages of phthisis. There is a tickling cough, which seems to come from the pit of the stomach, accompanied with burning in the chest, passive congestion. The cough is followed by great thoracic weakness and dyspnœa. The patient is worse from every little exposure.

It is stated, I think by Buchner, that *Phosphoric Acid* is useful for diphtheritic croup. I have given the remedy in diphtheria but once, and then, although it seemed nicely indicated, it gave no relief. The apathy, the drowsiness and the cough were all so marked, that had the case been one of typhoid I should have been astonished at the failure. It did not fail because I gave a high potency, for I used the 2x or 3x.

Phosphoric Acid is indicated in bone complaints, periostitis, caries, etc., when the only pain is as if the bone was being scraped with a knife. This symptom is generally worse at night, and is accompanied with weakness.

Phosphoric Acid is of use in typhoid types of fever, when the most marked symptoms are these: "Complete sensorial apathy; the patient is utterly regardless of his dangerous condition. He has but few wants. If you ask him any question he either does not reply to it or replies in the most laconic language. Very characteristic, too, is drowsiness; he goes readily into a deep sleep, but from this condition he is usually quite easily aroused, and then is clear-headed, but soon drops off again." Accompanying this mental state, are great debility, nosebleed which gives relief, dry tongue or tongue covered with sticky mucus. The abdomen is bloated, with rumbling of wind, with or without the diarrhœic stool which I mentioned to you a few moments ago.

There is another form of debility for which *Phosphoric Acid* is indicated; one from loss of animal fluids. Hence it is useful after protracted nursing, and after excessive venery. The debility is often accompanied by symptoms of great nervous exhaustion, shown by a tingling and formication, which no remedy is more likely to cause. It is also an excellent remedy when sexual excesses have taken all the tone out of the sexual organs, particularly in young men who are not suffering from any constitutional taint, and whose organs hang flabby, the penis refusing to become erect on any excitement. This condition *Phosphoric Acid,* given low, will remove, but *China* will not. *China* will be of use for the acute effects of loss of semen.

Before passing to one of the other remedies, I want to place before you some of the analogues of *Phosphoric Acid.* *Sweet Spirits of Nitre* runs close to the acid in this sensorial apathy of typhoid fever. Hahnemann was accustomed to give it when the patient lay like a log in this complete state of apathy. He has no wants and no complaints. He is simply dull and sleepy; arouse him and he looks like a man awaking from a drunken sleep. There are no marked organic changes going on in the abdomen. The whole burden of the poison seems to have been thrown upon the sensorium. Hahnemann used a few drops of the *Nitre* in water, given every few hours until relieved. His instruction was to give it when the drug was old enough not to redden the cork in the bottle.

The next remedy in this group is *Sulphuric Acid.* The hour is so nearly spent, I can but allude to it at present. This acid is much more irritating than the *Phosphoric.* It is a more violent corrosive poison.

First as to the mind. The *Sulphuric Acid* patient is usually rather hasty, nervous and restless in his disposition. He cannot do things fast enough to suit him. He lacks the stupidity of *Phosphoric Acid.* He suffers from neuralgic pains, which come gradually and leave suddenly. They are not like the *Belladonna* pains, which come suddenly, last awhile, and then leave as suddenly as they came. The face is apt to be pale. Sometimes the patient has a sensation as if the white of an egg was dried on the face.

This acid is a valuable remedy in diphtheria, especially in the naso-pharyngeal form. Of course, you will expect to find the acid debility and also fetid breath but the symptom which will lead you unerringly to this remedy is that there hang from the posterior nares strings of a sort of lemon-colored mucus. It is not the stringy, tough, fibrinous membrane of *Kali Bich.*, but is a thinner, yellow mucus. The "lemon color" is borrowed from the color of the diarrhœa of this remedy, a diarrhœa in which the movements have a lemon-yellow chopped-up appearance; or there is fecal matter mixed with shreds of lemon-yellow mucus. I remember once making a rapid cure of milk-crust guided by this sort of stool. An elder brother of my patient, similarly affected, gave its parents incessant worry for eight months before a cure was effected. The second child, which I was called to treat, started in with the same trouble, to the dismay of both father and mother. With the milk-crust on the face was a frequent, lemon-yellow, mucus diarrhœa. The child was cured by *Sulphuric Acid* 30 in three weeks, and remained well. Some physicians, remembering this symptom, transfered its ailments to the nasal mucous membrane, with the result of curing many cases of catarrh and diphtheria.

You will find *Sulphuric Acid* useful in certain cases of dyspepsia. The patients vomit everything they eat or drink. They have a craving for brandy or some other alcoholic stimulant after taking which they can retain food. This fact has led to the use of the acid for inebriates who cannot retain food and who are weak and trembling. Dr. Hering used to give *Sulphuric Acid* in the crude form, one drop in a tumblerful of water, a teaspoonful to be taken every few hours until symptoms were produced, such as diarrhœa. Aversion to liquor soon followed. If the diarrhœa becomes annoying, *Pulsatilla* modifies at once.

Sulphuric Acid cures a peculiar cough. We may say it involves the stomach. It ends in the belching of wind. *Ambra* has a simlar cough.

The essential debility of *Sulphuric Acid* is of a peculiar kind. It is accompanied by characteristic sore mouth with aphthæ in yellowish-white dots over the buccal mucous lining. You will be astonished to see how readily that condition is cured by *Sulphuric Acid,* especially if there is present a subjective trembling sensation of the body.

ON SEVERAL REMEDIES MORE OR LESS ANÆSTHETIC.

A WIDE field for study, and one scarcely yet trodden by the therapeutist, is that which gives us substances capable of causing and curing asphyxia. Want of oxygen in animal tissue invariably leads to a general disturbance, the central phenomena of which appear in respiratory and cardiac symptoms. The blood in the capillaries is retarded in its flow, and at length fails utterly to pass into the veins. Then the heart, which at first worked harder to overcome the resistance, beats more and more quickly, but at the same time more and more feebly, until it finally becomes paralyzed. Such a calamity follows, first, because the heart muscle is exhausted by its undue efforts, and secondly, because its blood, deprived of oxygen, fails to impart its essential stimulus.

The symptoms which more or less characterize asphyxia are: "Pectoral anxiety, dyspnœa, rapid feeble pulse, surface coldness, restlessness or stupor, with cold blue skin."

Among the possible remedies, which may be added to those already so well known, are the following:

Carbonous Oxide (CO) is one of the few substances which can, like oxygen, combine with, or unite itself to the red corpuscle. Hence its poisonous action depends principally upon the displacement of oxygen, with consequent suffocation. At first there is a notable increase in the blood pressure. There is flushed face, deep-red as from venous hyperæmia. A characteristic headache sets in, throbbing in the temporal arteries; lightness and constriction, worse about the temples; palpitation of heart. The patient soon feels stupid, confused or acts like one drunk. Respiration becomes stertorous and slow; the breath becomes cool, and complete unconsciousness, or trismus with convulsions, follows. The surface of the body, at first red, soon turns livid, cyanotic, and the temperature falls perceptibly. Death may close the scene, or partial recovery occur, with well-defined hemiplegia. Other cases end in perfect recovery.

This picture forcily reminds one of the effects of *Opium,* and doubtless *Carbonous Oxide* will compare with the latter remedy in practice. The suddenness of its symptoms, the cerebral hyperæmia, and subsequent hemiplegia, suggest its trial in apoplexy and also in embolism. As a remedy serviceable in asphyxia arising from pulmonary affections, it would seem to stand between *Carbo Veg.* and *Opium* having the hyperæmia of the latter with the coldness of the former. Cases of poisoning with the gas have developed pleurisy, bronchitis, emphysema, with bloody sputum, weakened vesicular murmur, and pneumonia. Its subjective symptoms are: "Anxiety in the chest, or feeling of a heavy load on the chest, etc." There are also recorded, rattling of mucous in the air-passages, bloody mucous raised from the bronchi, heat in chest, and abdomen, extremities cold.

Aniline ($C_6H_5NH_2$), though chemically different from carbon, containing hydrogen, nitrogen, etc., behaves like the carbons, and may be medicinally considered with them. *Aniline* is not an intense poison, but its effects are those of asphyxiation. The patients, after inhaling its fumes, is seized with giddiness, and may become insensible. Face and body become cold and blue, pulse slow or imperceptible, breathing heavy and labored. If conscious and able to speak, he complains of pain in head and chest. Compare *Hydrocyanic Acid.*

The *Sulphate of Aniline* has been proved and successfully administered by Dr. C. Wesselhœft. He has used it in diseases accompanied by excessive flatulence, loathing, disagreeable taste, and costiveness, common after too much fruit, cabbage, beans, etc. Compare with *Carbo Veg., Graphites,* etc.

Nitrobenzine ($C_{12}H_5NO_4$) is used in the preparation of perfumes, and also as a substitute for oil of bitter almonds. It is much more poisonous than its near relative, *Aniline.* When inhaled it causes a benumbed feeling in the head, anxiety, want of breath; increasing sensorial confusion, and convulsions or stupor follow. The pupils are dilated, the face purple or livid, breathing slow, difficult, and the pulse small, slow, accelerated, or irregular. Convulsions are tetanic, with trismus and spasms of the flexors, especially of the upper extremities, and are followed by coma. One can scarcely fail to see in this group of symptoms a marked resemblance to *Hydrocyanic Acid.*

Carboneum Chloratum (C_2CL_2) acts very much like *Chloroform,* but rather more slowly. The main characteristic is its depressing influence on the heart. The heart-beat falls to forty-eight per minute, with extreme lassitude and deep sleep. It may prove a remedy in cardiac affections, or in diseases with impending cardiac paralysis.

The *Bisulphate of Carbon* (CS_2) is of interest, as we may have to antidote its effects in workmen who prepare the caoutchouc for rubber toys, etc. Its first transient effect is one of exhilaration. The prover is disposed to laugh and chat like one under the stimulus of alcohol. But intermingled with this excitement is a depression, which eventually becomes persistent. A constant symptom is an intense oppressive headache, spreading from the root of the nose towards the temples, with a feeling of giddiness and intoxication. Muscular weakness is quite general, especially in the lower limbs, in some cases amounting to paresis. The mind becomes distressingly apathetic, with inability to find the words wanted. Speech is stammering, as from lingual paralysis. A noteworthy symptom of the nerves is a lancinating tearing pain, erratic and inconstant, associated with formication or anæthesia. In other instances it is associated with sour belching and borborygmi. The lower half of the body is icy cold. The senses are all diminished. Ringing in the ears seems to be a characteristic symptom. (Compare *Bromhydric Acid.*) Congestion of the lungs has been noticed and even tubercular deposit in rabbits. This circumstance together with dyspnœa and a very characteristic night fever, suggest the drug in pulmonary consumption.

As an anæsthetic it is far inferior to the others, and as a substance tending to produce asphyxia, it cannot compare with the previously mentioned drugs. It seems to act paralyzingly on the nervous centres very much as does *Chloroform*.

The nervous sensations, muscular debility, loss of sexual power, etc., suggest its applicability to diseases of the nervous centres, especially of the spine. Mayhap it may even find a place in the treatment of the neuralgia incident to locomotor ataxia.

Its gastric and enteric symptoms place it between *Sulphur* and *Carbo Veg.;* fetid eructations, heart-burn, pressing-stitching pains from pit of stomach to cardiac region, relieved by loud belching. Thin, yellow evacuations 5 A.M., etc.

Of the Ethers, with *Chloroform* and *Chloral,* not much is known therapeutically; yet in some cases their employment will prove satisfactory and highly advantageous.

As a general fact, it ought to be remembered, that the Ethers, especially *Chloric Ether,* cause a predominance of respiratory symptoms. (*Chloroform*)

Ether (especially *Chloric Ether,* with which these symptoms have been confirmed) may be given in convulsions, whether epileptic, hysterical, or puerperal. The characteristic symptom is intense dyspnœa. Hence it may be remedy in such cases as have what is termed convulsions from asphyxia.

This same characteristic belongs also to *Nitric Ether, Ethyl Nitrate,* etc.

Ethyl Nitrate, as contained in the *Sweet Spirits of Nitre* ($C_2H_5NO_2$), comes to us recommended by Hahnemann in typhoid conditions, with well-marked sensorial apathy. When aroused, the patient answers intelligently, but quickly relapses into his state of sleepiness and indifference. Here the drug rivals *Phosphoric Acid.* But there are other applications of the drug, particularly that which calls for its present recommendation: "Breathing slow and regular, but on walking a short distance, it becomes hurried, then quick, difficult, and painful, with a distressing sense of constriction under the sternum. On walking, the heart beats rapidly and tumultously. How suggestive this is of angina pectoris, or of hypertrophy of the heart! It is very similar to the well-confirmed characteristic of *Aurum Mur.*

The *Amyl Nitrite* ($C_5H_{11}NO_2$), causes constriction in the throat, which extends to the chest. There is, however, not much dyspnœa; but the circulation is wonderfully altered. The venous and arterial blood are said to become of the same hue. Oxygenation is lessened and with it the animal heat, the whole system becomes weakened and relaxed. The vascular phenomena are due to a paresis of the vaso-motor nerves: throbbing, bursting fulness in the head, protruding eyes, throbbing in the ears, flushed face, neck swollen, fulness of the chest, anxiety, with cardiac oppression and tumultuous heart-action, constriction and pain about the heart, general sweat. The constriction of the chest is evidently not a true dyspnœic symptom, but arises from hyperæmia.

This drug may often be called for in sudden derangements of the circulation; as blushing, flushing of the face at the climaxis, hysterical anomalies, etc. Also in heart affections, where it is similar to *Cactus* and *Glonoine.* Its application in epilepsy is not *Homoeopathic,* since it there acts only palliatingly by lessening spasm of the blood vessels. It is recommended in asphyxia from drowning, chloroform, etc.

Nitrous Oxide, (N_2O) is one of the few gases capable of sustaining life, at least for a while, after the withdrawal of oxygen. Under its effects, the experimenter seems to be in a sort of ecstasy. Fancies and thoughts are vivid, intense, and generally pleasant. The mind tries to grasp the marvellous and supernatural. The senses are all exquisitely acute. There is a feeling of muscular energy and often a strong inclination to laugh. This cheerfulnes and activity sometimes continue for several hours after the inhalation. The temperature of the body, while inhaling the gas, rises steadily and keeps pace with the mental exhilaration. The nerves experience a not unpleasant thrilling, vibratory sensation. In fact the prover is living too fast, crowding the work of days into a few moments. The symptoms thus far remind one of the extravagant hallucinations of *Cannabis Indica*.

When the gas, however, is inhaled in large quantities, or without the admixture of air, anæsthesia quickly follows. The mental ecstasy is but transient. But hearing remains acute much longer than the other senses.

Sometimes attacks of fainting occur, with a feeling of oppression of the chest. At other times, convulsions set in, resembling epilepsy or hysteria.

I can recall a case of a colored woman, who took the gas at the dentist's. For days afterwards she was subject to spells of semi-consciousness, which were preceded by a numb feeling in the head, spreading thence over the body. Then she would fall backwards to the ground.

In the open air, the attacks were often postponed, but were more severe when they did come. While at work, she was free from attacks, but while seated, or unoccupied, the seizures were frequent. She was conscious of feeling sick, but could not help herself. She often complained of a drawing in the neck, as from contraction of the skin.

With these suggestions, could not the laughing-gas be utilized as a medicine? Some of its symptoms remind one of the Ethers and their compounds. These semi-conscious spells are not uncommon in hysteria. Here *Nitrous Oxide* may serve as well as the frequently used *Moschus*.

A question presents itself, while considering the efficacy of Ethers and similar substances. Of what Homœopathic value are they in the treatment of that dread calamity, puerperal convulsions? There can be but one answer to any such query, and that is, their value depends upon their homœopathicity. But with this general answer ever in mind, may it not be asked, when are they indicated?

Certainly only when characteristic symptoms agree with the individual case under treatment.

Ether will help if there is opisthotonos, unconsciousness, violent convulsions, and especially intense dyspnœa.

Chloroform is antipathic, except for the intense precursory excitement; or, later, for deep coma, stertor and impending cardiac paralysis, with blue, cold surface. The order of the symptoms here, suggests a similarity to *Hyoscyamus;* and I believe Dr. Lippe has antidoted the effects of *Chloroform* with this drug.

The *Carbonous Oxide* must wait confirmatory evidence; but, as similar to *Opium*, it ought to receive attention.

Nitrous Oxide produces symptoms like hysteria, but should not be forgotten in the more alarming puerperal convulsions.

The mode of administration deserves a passing notice. I have no quarrel with him who prefers the crude preparations, but think, nevertheless, that more certain and abiding results will follow the use of potencies. Dr. Allen, in his valuable Encyclopædia, has taken the precaution to indicate the method of preparation as follows: *Chloroform* and *Ether,* in alcohol; *Carbonous Oxide* and *Nitrous Oxide,* in distilled water. Hahnemann gave the *Sweet Spirits of Nitre* dissolved in water; and suggests that it should be old enough not to redden the cork. *Amyl. Nitrite,* it is claimed, acts best by inhalation, although many symptoms have resulted from its use prepared in alcohol. The *Bisulphide of Carbon* has been employed by allopaths as a local application in neuralgia. The dangerous and awkward method is quite happily unnecessary, since its successful use in potencies is well attested.

REMARKS ON SEVERAL SUMMER REMEDIES INFREQUENTLY USED.

THE season has come which is so unrelentingly severe on the very young, the old, and the weak. Concerning the first class it behoves us to study well the remedies particularly adapted to their ailments, which are provoked or aggravated by heat. Prominent among such affections are bowel complaints.

Well-tried remedies, such as *Aconite, Bryonia, Sulphur, Ipecac, Arsenic, Carbo. Veg., Podophyl., Verat. Alb.*, etc., should be uppermost in our armamentarium, for they will be most frequently needed; but there are several newly added drugs which must not be forgotten in the limited number of cases calling for them. We subjoin a few.

Œnothera Biennis, or *the Evening Primrose* common in fields and waste places, is an invaluable remedy in exhausting, watery diarrhœa. It does not act, as has been suggested, as an astringent, by its tannic acid, but is a genuine Homœopathic remedy, producing and curing diarrhœa. The evacuations are without effort, and are accompanied by nervous exhaustion, and even with incipient hydrocephaloid.

Gnaphalium causes a watery, offensive, morning diarrhœa, which repeats itself often during the day. The provers were children, and well have they portrayed a very common group of cholera infantum symptoms. They had rumbling in the bowels, colicky pains, and were, at the same time, cross and irritable. The urine was scanty, and the appetite and taste were lost A writer in the "Homœopathy" used this drug very successfully last summer, and Dr. Hale refers to it in his Therapeutics.

Geranium Maculatum is also a successful baby's remedy. Dr. Hale devotes eight pages to *Geranium* and other astringents, dividing their actions according to his rule of primary and secondary symptoms, and deducing thence two propositions for use in practice. The provings, brief though they are, help us in the choice of the drug, *viz.,* "Constant desire to go to stool, with inability for some time to pass any fecal matter when the bowels move without pain or effort. Mouth dry, tip of tongue burning." Allopaths use it as an astringent.

Paullinia Sorbilis has been suggested for diarrhœa which is green and profuse, but odorless.

Opuntia comes to us recommended by so careful an observer,—Dr. Burdick—that although we have not used it, we do not hesitate to present it anew: "Nausea from stomach to bowels; feels as if the bowels were settled down into the lower abdomen." Confirmed in adults. In infants we may perhaps look to this drug when the lower part of the abdomen is the seat of disease, as this seems to be its characteristic seat of attack.

Nuphar Luteum causes a yellow diarrhœa, worse in the morning, either with colic or painless. It has been employed for diarrhœa during typhoid, and indeed seems to cause nervous weakness. Whether it will be of service for infants remains to be seen. We should look to it when *Gamboge, Chelidon.,* etc., fail and when exhaustion is a prominent attendant.

Kali Bromatum has been several times given successfully in cholera infantum when there were great prostration, cool surface, and symptoms of hydrocephaloid. Compare *Cinchona* (incipient hydrocephaloid, following prolonged or oft-repeated diarrhœic discharges), *Calc. Phos., Carbo Veg., Verat. Alb., Camph,,* etc.

Among dietic adjuvants, *Koumiss* and *Lactopeptin* are comparatively new.

A BRIEF REPERTORY OF MEDICINES AFFECTING THE POSTERIOR NARES, WITH COMMENTS AND SUGGESTIONS.

IT has become an approbrium of Homœopathic practice that postnasal and pharyngeal catarrhs are frequently not cured by internal medication. Specialists, treating nose, throat, and ear affections are daily receiving patients who have been dismissed by Homœopathic physicians as incurable, or who have become disgusted with the general practitioner. I grant that one who devotes his exclusive attention to a given subject should be better qualified therein than those engaged in common practice. But the question is not one of comparative success in the employment of internal medicine; it is one of contrast between local applications and legitimate Homœopathy. If the system of Hahnemann is universally true, that is, if it is founded upon law and does not constitute a mere rule, it must as assuredly remove a post-nasal catarrh as a sorethroat or a cold on the chest.

There are three modes of defence, one or another of which is invariably employed in defending Homœopathy against a charge of inefficiency; first, that if one can obtain the *similimum,* the cure or relief will follow; secondly, a local affection is always a part of a more or less latent constitutional dyscrasia, and therefore cannot be permanently cured until the latter is; thirdly, the failure is claimed to be due to errors in selection or in potency, in repetition or in the administering of drugs singly or in alternation.

To all such illogical proposition, I emphatically object. I believe that the *similimum* will help because I believe in the universality of the law, and consequently, I reject alternation of remedies. I accept the law because I think that it is logically deducible from revealed truth. If any one agrees with me here, my strictures do not apply to him. They apply to those who admit the truth of Homœopathy, because they have tested it and have been satisfied from experience; and this class includes the entire medical profession. Having proved Homœopathy, then, in the same manner as did Hahnemann, the only reasonable position is that the system is effective because it cures. When, therefore, it fails, a consistent defence is not paucity of material and knowledge, but an earnest, painstaking and persistent series of experiments instituted as a crucial test.

With all due deference to specialists, they have not carried out this plan. Failing with the means at hand, they have felt compelled to preserve their reputations by resorting to collateral measures; for more is expected of them by the public than of the general practitioner. Specialists should spare no pains to institute provings. There are many unproved or partially proved plants and minerals which are known to exert some sort of an influence upon the naso-pharyngeal passages. It is incumbent upon those most interested to thoroughly explore the subject and determine what this influence is in each drug. A few years ago we could not readily cure cases which now, since the introduction of *Sanguinaria Nitrate* and *Antimonium Auratum,* are easily relieved.

I propose to enumerate the remedies known to affect the posterior nares, and to offer some suggestions concerning a few not often employed.

The known drugs are:

Aconite.	Granatum.	Plumbum.
Æsculus Hip.	Hepar.	Psorinum.
Alumen.	Helianthus.	Phos. Acid.
Alumina.	Hydrastis.	Phytolacca.
Anacardium.	Iodine.	Penthorum.
Ant. Crud.	Iris Vers.	Physostigma.
Ant. Sulph. Auratum.	Kali Bich.	Phosphorous.
Argentum Nit.	Kali Jod.	Pæonia.
Ammon. Brom.	Kali Mur.	Rumex.
Baptisia.	Kreosote.	Rhus. Tox.
Bryonia.	Lycopodium.	Saponine.
Baryta.	Mercury.	Staphisagria.
Calcarea Ost.	Mer. Corr.	Sumbul.
Calcarea Sulph.	Mer. Cyan.	Sepia.
Carbo An.	Mer. Prot.	Sulphur.
Carbo Veg.	Mer. Bin. Iod.	Silica.
Cepa.	Mag. Carb.	Sinapis Nig.
Coral Rub.	Mag. Sulph.	Sang. Nit.
Coccus.	Mezereum.	Spigelia.
Cistus.	Natrum Ars.	Theridion.
Cinnabaris.	Nat. Carb.	Thuja.
Chlorine.	Nat. Phos.	Tellurium.
Digitalis.	Nat. Mur.	Ustilago.
Eriodictyon.	Nitric Acid.	Vinca Minor.
Euphrasia.	Nitrum.	Wyethia.
Fagopyrum.	Nux Mosch.	Yucca.
Fer. Phos.	Osmium.	Zinc.
Flouric Ac.	Oxalic Acid.	Zingiber.
Gallic Ac.	Petroleum.	

A BRIEF REPERTORY OF MEDICINES, ETC.   87

Of these eighty or more drugs, some are so rarely indicated as to be of little value to the general practitioner, several are useful only in acute catarrh, and but a few offer the usual symptoms of chronic catarrh of the posterior nares. These few are:

Alumina.	Hepar.	Psorinum.
Amm. Brom.	Hydrastis.	Sepia.
Ant. Auratum.	Kali Bich.	Sulphur.
Arg. Nit.	Kali Mur.	Silica.
Calcarea Ost.	Mer. Proto. Iod.	Sang. Nit.
Corallium	Mer. Bin. Iod.	Spigelia.
Cinnabaris.	Natrum Ars.	Thuja.
Fagopyrum.	Nitric Acid.	

The relative value of this group is indicated by the variety of type, reducing those of the highest value to the two *Mercuries, Sang. Nitrate,* and *Kali Bich.* and *Kali Mur.*—a very small armamentarium for so stubborn a disease. But the list could be enlarged if specialists would test known symptoms and publish the results.

For instance, *Phos., Natr. Mur., Cistus, Natr. Ars., Alumina,* have glazed or varnished appearance of the posterior wall of the pharynx. Why not use one or another of these when such a state of the membrane obtains higher up?

Alumina and **Nat. Mur.** affect the mucous membranes, causing scanty secretions, the latter drug being distinguished by smarting sensation. Why, then, may not *Alumina* be often used, especially as in addition it causes, scurf in the nose, plugging of the Eustachian tubes, snapping sound in the ears on swallowing or chewing, and dropping of mucus from the posterior nares.

Kali Mur. often relieves hawking of mucus from the posterior nares. Why not note carefully its effect upon the catarrh itself and report results at a future meeting? Compare also *Paeonia.*

When the pharyngeal walls are varicose, *Pulsatilla, Hamamelis, Vespa, Natr. Ars.,* and *Phytolacca,* may be consulted. The first two have relieved the catarrh, though I have been compelled to follow *Hamamelis* with some other drug to effect a cure.

Vespa, like **Natr. Ars.,** produces œdema and varicosis. The first caused purulent catarrh of the middle ear, and also recurrent tonsillitis, and ought to be used. The second, with thickening of the mucous membrane, lasting for months and hawking of a thick mucus from the posterior nares, offers a valuable remedy for winter catarrh.

Fagopyrum pictures a common and very annoying form of the disease, one in which exposure is sure to increase the catarrh with rawness and dryness, formation of dry crusts, granular appearance of the mucous membrane and an intolerable itching and burning.

Sensitiveness to inhaled air is not especially important in acute catarrh but is in chronic. It calls for *Arsenic, Natr. Ars., Corallium, Hydrastis, Lithium, Osmium, Kreosote,* and probably *Fagopyrum.*

Dryness of the posterior nares is not only in the latter remedy but also in *Alumina, Æsculus, Sinapis Nigra, Wyethia,* and a few others,

Æsculus, as well shown by Dr. T. F. Allen, suits colds extending from the posterior nares down the pharynx, with dryness, scraping and burning; at times secreted mucus drops low down and causes choking. Patients are weak, with soft pulse, backache, constipation and piles. Why should we neglect this and devote our attention to the more familiar *Nux? Æsculus* would relieve more promptly and more permanently.

Sinapis Nigra has cured dryness of the anterior nares, and has caused dry sensation in the choanæ and pharynx. Why not dry it when, in addition, there is the characteristic condition of the mucous membranes, *viz.,* dryness, with at most scanty chunks of tenacious mucus secreted?

Wyethia I have never used; it is claimed to have produced and cured pricking and dry sensation in the posterior nares. According to Hale it is useful in chronic pharyngitis, removing the granular appearance, and never failing to relieve dryness of the pharynx and burning of the epiglottis.

Penthorum Sedoides belongs to a class of plants that do not act very deeply. Still by reason of their acridity they produce catarrh, skin symptoms, and some of them, hæmorrhoids. The *Penthorum* ought to be tried when there is a continual feeling as if the nose were wet, but without coryza. Sense of fullness in nose and ears. Posterior nares feel raw as if denuded.

Osmium rivals the more commonly employed *Phosphorus.* It is highly irritating to mucous surfaces, provoking coryza, sneezing as from snuff; nose and larynx sensitive to the air. Small lumps of phlegm are easily loosened from the posterior nares and larynx.

Like **Phosphorus,** it attacks larynx and lungs. Characteristic severe pain in the larynx, worse when coughing or talking; hoarseness.

Ammonium Bromidum is said to be effective when the patient hawks down a stringy, bloody mucus. Here it resembles *Sanguin, Nitrate* and *Kali Mur.,* but is far inferior to either.

If the mucus is of a lemon-yellow color and not very fibrinous, *Sulphuric Acid* is almost sure to cure. It is only when it is tough and stringy that *Kali Bich.* claims precedence.

When hardened clinkers are hawked from the posterior nares *Kali Bich., Cinnabaris, Sepia* and

Teucrium are serviceable. The latter, suggested by Dr. Walter Williamson, Jr., is needed when very large and irregular masses are hawked down. *Cinnabar* for dirty yellow lumps.

Saponine causes tough tenacious mucus in the posterior nares, extending into the larynx.

Quillaia, one of the plants from which *Saponine* is derived, has been quite extensively used in California by homœopathists for a cold in the head, contracted during warm, damp weather. Here it rivals *Gelsemium,* both causing general lassitude and tiredness and weakness of the muscles—states of relaxation favoring colds.

Dr. August Korndoerfer has made some excellent cures with *Spigelia,* guided by Hahnemann's symptoms; "Profuse discharge of mucus through the posterior nares; nasal mucus passes off only through the posterior nares." I have not been very successful in using it.

But, after all, the majority of cases call for such remedies as *Mer. Iod., Sang. Nitrate, Antim Auratum* and *Pulsatilla.* And it is such accurately fitting remedies as these that I hope to see greatly increased in number by energetic provings, conducted by those whose ability to diagnose disease of the nose qualifies them for the work.

Sanguinaria Nitrate, given persistently—and nasal catarrh needs repeated doses—will often help when there are burning rawness and soreness in the posterior nares, and hawking of thick, yellow, sometimes bloody mucus.

Pulsatilla acts better if the mucus is thick, yellow-green and bland; and *Merc. Iod.* when there is swelling of the glands of the neck and yellow coating on the dorsum of the tongue.

Antim. Auratum, proved under the auspices of Dr. C. Neidhard, causes increased mucus secretion. In one prover it aggravated a chronic catarrh with increased discharge of a greenish-yellow mucus, more offensive than before. It is used by Dr. Hugh Pitcairn as a co-relative of the *Iodide of Mercury.*

Nitric Acid follows when dirty, bloody mucus flows; and *Mezereum* in mercurialized patients when there are scraping, burning and rawness posteriorly with thin, yellow and bloody discharge.

In conclusion, I desire to say that, as many nasal catarrhs have a specific origin, no remedy, not active in influencing the cause, can materially relieve the catarrh. In addition to *Sulphur, Kali Iod, Aurum.,* etc., we should consider *Theridion,* confirmed by Dr. Korndoerfer as an introductory drug in scrofulous cases—*Thuja,* well-known in sycosis, and invaluable when the discharge is thick, green or bloody and green —and *Psorinum,* despised by some, but fully appreciated by others as often superior to *Sulphur.*

For convenience I add a brief repertory, confining myself to the limited region under consideration.

Nature of the Discharge:

Yellow, Thick: *Arg. Nit., Aur., Natr. Ars., Hyd., Calc. C., Berb., Cinnab.* (dirty lumps), *Kali Bi., Sulph. Ac., Nit. Ac., Puls., Spig., Sulph., Ant. Aur., Sang. Nit., Therid., Nat. C., Hep., Lyc., Phos., Kali Sulph., Alumina, Rumex, Cal. Sulph., Sumbul, Mez.* (thin).

Green: *Berb., Puls., Thuja, Kali Bi., Nat. C., Phos., Sep., Merc.*

Plugs, Clinkers, etc.: *Teucrium, Kali Bi., Sepia, Cinn., Lyc., Mang.* (yellow or green lumps), *Mer. Iod.* (blood-tinged), *Nat. Ars.*

Like Tallow: *Coral. Rub.*

Irritating, Corrosive: *Ars., Ars. Iod., Cepa., Kreos., Carb. Acid.*

Brown: *Kali Bich.* (bloody and offensive).

Bloody: *Canth,* (and tough), *Arg. Nit.* (yellow mixed with clots), *Hyd., Nit. Ac., Sepia* (with yellow-green shreds), *Sang. Nit., Kaolin, Kali Bi., Lach.* (bloody pus), *Phos.* (in streaks), *Sulphur* (in threads), *Mez.*

Offensive: *Aur., Graph., Mer.* (trickling mucus), *Sulph., Thuja, Nit. Ac., Nat. C., Elaps.* (relieved a case for me marked by disproportionate fetor), *Therid, Asaf., Lach., Kreos.* (old people), *Tell.* (herring brine), *Ant. Aur?*

Stringy: *Amm. Brom. Sulph. Ac., Kali Bi., Cinnab., Hyd., Coccus Cac., Yucca* (and greasy-looking).

Scanty Tenacious: *Sinapis, Alum., Osmium* (large lumps), *Nat. Mur., Phos. Saponin* (tough, tenacious), *Phyt.*

Membrane Dark:

Lach., Phyt., Amm. Brom., Yucca.
——Red: *Arg. Nit.*

Scales, Ulcers:

Arg. Nit. (with yellow scales), *Kali Bi.* (punched), *Alum., Calc. C., Graph., Lyc., Puls., Sepia, Silica, Zinc, Psorin, Thuja, Therid., Lach.,* (bloody), *Baryta* (and behind uvula), *Kali Carb.* (foul crusts), *Fagop.*

Choanæ:

Too dry: *Silica, Sepia, Fagop., Rumex, Sticta, Wyethia, Æsc. Hip., Alum., Sinapis, Zinc, Sang.*

As if too open: *Flour. Ac., Iod., Nat. Mur.*

Obstructed:

Anac., Cal. Sulph., Hyd., Iris. Ver., Kali Iod.

Ears Affected:

Mer., Vespa, Phyt., Gels. (itching in Eustachian tube, also pain in ears), *Nux* and *Silica* (both itching in Eustachian tubes), *Kali Bi., Rum.* (ear feels stopped, voice sounds strange—relief in one, but not cure), *Alum.* (Eustachian tube stopped with mucus) *Graph.* (Eustachian tube stopped up), *Iod.* (Catarrh of the Eustachian tube), *Lith. Carb.*

Crackling Sound on Swallowing:

Graph., Hep.
Nitr. Ac. (Eustachian obstruction), *Petrol.* (passages dry, whizzing in ears).

Sensitive to Inhaled Air:

Ars., Nat. Ars., Ars. Iod., Coral., Hyd., Lith. Carb., Osmium, Fagop., Kreos., Fer. Phos.

Nose Feels Wet:

Penthorum.

Rawness, Scraping, Soreness:

Æsc. Hip., Mer., Mer. Iod., Mez., Nux Vom., Sang. Nit., Nit. Ac., Chlor., Kreos., Iris V., Nat. Ars., Ars., Ars. Iod., Fer. Phos. (on inspiration), *Mag. Carb., Oxalic Ac., Phos., Phos. Ac., Osmium, Carbo Veg.* (on coughing or swallowing, soreness), *Gallic Ac., Penth., Sepia, Nitrum.*

Burning:

Æsc. Hip., Arg. Nit., Phos., Osmium, Ars., Ars. Iod., Nat. Ars., Fagop.

Like a Fine Leaf:

Baryta Carb.

Like Something Hanging:

Yucca.

DRUGS AFFECTING THE OCCIPITAL REIGON

(*Confirmed symptoms are marked* *; *merely clinical,* º; *>means amelioration;* > > *entire relief;* < *signifies aggravation;* < < *marked aggravation.*

Aconite. Occiput: as if injected; jerking, tearing; shooting. Head drawn backwards.

Useful in congestion; neuralgia; convulsions.

Actæa Spicata. Hammering pain in occiput; rheumatic patients.

Æsculus Hippocastanum. Heavy feeling, pressure; bruised feeling with lameness in back of neck; dull pain to ears; lancinating at base of brain, as if too full. Dull pain, flushes of heat in integument.

Useful in congestion, especially in persons suffering from piles, suppressed hæmorrhoidal flow; or from the characteristic spinal weakness.

Æthusa Cynapium. Distressing pains in occiput and nape of neck, extending down spine; feels as if stretching stiffly backwards would relieve; sticking and beating in upper part of right side of occiput. A tearing in right occiput, shoots through the whole head and extends to the right side. Tearing stitches from occiput forwards.

Doubts have been thrown upon the validity of the toxic symptoms of *Æthusa*. The above, however, are unquestioned and suggest the drug in irritation of the brain and spine. Crampy, constrictive and band-like pains, so common in this drug, shows its spinal action. These symptoms seem to be reflex from gastro-enteric irritation, for nausea, vomiting, tendency to diarrhœa, and a sense of a lump or load in the stomach attend or precede them; while excessive prostration, shrinking and dryness of the skin, peaked face and coldness, show how damaging the drug is to nutrition, and warrant our common use of it in cholera-infantum, dentition, etc.

It seems that the distress in the occiput and the desire to bend back as in opisthotonos, tally well with the toxical cases, which claim cerebral congestion and effusion, and intestinal inflammation. I should then consider it.

Useful when the occipital pains are accompanied by the gastro-enteric characteristics, or even by convulsions, with colic, green stools, tenesmus, distended abdomen; clenched thumbs, up-turned eyeballs.

Agaricus Muscarius. Boring, burrowing, pressive, drawing, tension, sense of heaviness; tearing, stiches; creaking; stiffness.

Useful in chorea, cerbro-spinal irritation from abuse of alcohol. It has been given successfully for irritation in back of brain and in spine, with rolling head in pillow.

Ailanthus. Electric thrill from brain to extremities. Darting through temples and back of head, with confusion of ideas. Pain in occiput, dizzy, ringing pain in forehead; left side of face swollen, face erysipelatous; patient heavy, sleepy, nauseted at times. Beating in occipital arteries.

Useful in the course of scarlatina, erysipelas and typhoid states, when occiput pains, mind is dull and face of a dark, livid or mahogany color.

Alcohol. Sensation of fullness at crown and back of head. Apopletic congestion, with snoring, usually dilated pupils, suffused, dark face and paralytic trembling and weakness. Muscles of neck and back give out..

Employed more for general cerebral congestions especially with evidences of organic lesions of brain; but may be useful in the progress of typhoid states, when congestion of brain and spine obtain, with above symptoms. It compares here with *Bellad, Opium, Agaricus,* and particularly ABSINTHIUM.

Allium Cepa. *Headache in occiput, then in right side over eye. Headache on both sides of occiput, afterwards in two large round places in upper posterior part of head; later, a general humming of part as if asleep; seems to be in the bone rather than in the scalp; also with confusion in the occiput; better in open air, worse in warm room.

Useful in "catarrhal patients," who suffer from headache if they study or work in a warm room.

Allium Sativum. Dull pain in occiput in morning while lying on back.

Aloes. Congestion to occiput; sense of dull pressure in whole head when walking, shaking as if brain was loose, worse in fresh, cold air, also on lying head down; then and a while after rising, beating, thumbing pain, like pulsating, especially in occiput. In the occiput and abdomen, beating at night when lying down; stiches when stooping; external soreness.

Useful for passive hyperæmia accompanying or rather depending upon abdominal congestion. Hæmorrhoidal and abdominal symptoms must decide, though if the occipital symptoms are accompanied with dull pain over eyes, lids feel heavy and draws eyelids together for relief, *Aloes* will remove all. Compare *Ailanthus,* but particularly *Sulphur.*

Sometimes the *Aloes* headache alternates with pains in the lumbar region.

Alumina. Pressure on occiput and forehead as from a tight hat. Short-lasting, dull pain in occiput.

Headache in occiput as if bruised; passes of on lying down. Pain in head and nape of neck; increases on going to bed, ceases in the morning on rising.

Ambra Grisea. Pressive drawing from nape through head, and over root of nose, considerable pressure remaining in lower part of occiput. Confusion of occiput. Tearing and pressure up as far as top and forehead.

Useful in nervous patients, hurried manner, anxious; when conversion unduly fatigues, causing heaviness of head, oppression of chest, tremor and weakness. Limbs go to sleep easily; loss of sensation in feet. Comprehension slow; memory weak; nervous vertigo, especially in old persons.

Ammoniacum. Pains pressive, $<$ supra-orbital and occipital regions; confused, intellectual labor interfered with.

Useful for those who are subject to catarrhal asthma, violent action of the heart, ebullitions of blood; or, for those whose eyes become easily strained when taxed; bright sparks or mists before eyes.

Ammonicum Muriatium. Occiput feels as if in a vise; later, in sides of head, with excessive ill humor.

Amyl Nitrate. Throbbing and fullness of head to bursting, even becomes unconscious; face livid. Throbbing in occiput; not here distinctive, but only a local manifestation of the general action of the drug upon the blood vessels.

Anacardium. Constrictive, *band-like,* headache; feeling as of a tense band from nape to ears; must lie down.

Dull Pressure as from a Plug.

Characteristic, is the peculiar pressure. *Anacard.* is especially called for when the occipital headache is accompanied by a contractive stiffness of neck, felt at rest and not usually worse from motion, though it may be. (Compare *Rhus Rad.*)

Augustura. Pressure in occiput, afternoon. Drawing at sides of occiput. Tension and drawing in muscles of neck. Drawing in occiput, sides of head, fingers, etc.

The occipital pain is merely a part of the general tension caused by the drug—an action that has led to its use in tetanus, and this, too, since the discovery that there are two sorts of *Angustura;* one the *Vera.;* the other, a variety of strychnos *Nux Vom.*

Antimonium Tartaricum. Occiput becomes heavy, with an anxious, oppressive sensation. On stooping, sense as if something in occiput fell forwards. Raging or throbbing pain on right side of occiput.

Probably useful in chest and stomach affections, when the occipital heaviness indicated a congestive state of the medulla and base of brain, with consequent involvement of the pneumogastrics. Antimony has an affinity for the base and medulla. Heart symptoms, dyspnœa, drowsiness, nausea—one or all will be present.

Apis. Aching, increased by shaking head. Headache with fullness and heaviness in occiput. Pressure. Tension from the back of the neck. Violent drawing from back of neck over left half of head.

The well known value of *Apis* in meningitis leads us to infer that the above may very readily indicate irritation, congestion, etc., within the cranium.

Argentum Metallicum. * Pressing pain in forehead with stupor, and drawing pressure in occiput. Nape of neck feels stiff; there seems to be something foreign in the occiput, a sort of drawing and pressing.

The silver headache is neurotic, seemingly in the brain substance and outgoing nerves. It reaches its culmination, raging as if a nerve were being torn into, and then suddenly ceases. Sometimes the occipito-frontalis muscle twitches spasmodically. There is also painful tension on both sides of the foramen magnum.

Argentum Nitricum. Digging, cutting motion through left hemisphere from occiput to frontal protuberance; increasing and decreasing rapidly. Band-like strips, traction, from occiput into middle of brain. * Digging and tumultuous raging in right hemisphere until he loses his senses; if pain abates in forehead, it increases in sides of head and towards occiput, extending thence down the neck.

Arnica. Pressive headache, now more in forehead, now in occiput. * Pressive as if head were being distended; pain seemingly from something soft in vertex, with drawing in occiput. Violent sticking in forehead and occiput on waking in morning. Pain in occiput, as from electric shocks.

Headaches in general are accompanied with confusion, fullness, heaviness, with dizziness; * burning in brain, the body being cool. Occipital pains are not characteristic.

Arsenicum. * Headache in occiput; tearing.

Arum Italicum. Damp weather causes persistent headache, worse at the occiput.

Arum Triphyllum. Shooting pain in occiput when turning eyes upwards in morning.

Asafœtida. Aching in occiput, gradually extending over the head as if the brain was compressed by a cloth thrown over it. Drawing. Pressure.

Asarum Europoeum. Feels arteries in occiput, then all over. * Tension of whole scalp.

Asclepias Tuberosa. Headache presses deeply upon base of brain and is like that of *Ipecac*.

Asterias Rubens. Pains more severe at back of head than at the forehead. Dull occipital headache, comes and goes suddenly.

The *Asterias* headache is congestive and neuralgic.

Arum. * Fine tearing from the right side of occiput through the brain to the forehead; worse during motion.

Aurum Mur. Natronatum. Heaviness and heat in occiput. Boring in left side of occiput. Drawing in bones.

Aurum Sulphuratum. Lancinations in occiput.

The prover of *Aurum Met.,* who furnishes the pains in the limbs, back and joints and even in the teeth, (above confirmed symptoms), describes similar tearing with swollen gums. It is a fair inference that the tearing is periosteal.

Baptisia. Dull feeling, especially in the occiput, where there is slight pain and fullness. Dull pressure.

Baryta Acetica. Pressing-asunder stitch, traverses left side of occiput, ends in the cervical vertebræ. Heavy sensation in whole occiput, $<$ close to neck, with tension in same not $<$ motion. Sudden sensation of drawing from the occiput over the right ear and lower jaw. Dull pressive pain in occipital bone, from cervical vertebræ behind right ear, obliquely to parietal bone.

Baryta Carbonica. * Rheumatic pains in occiput; cervical and occipital glands swollen. Throbbing, extending to frontal eminence.

Baryta Sulphurica. º Throbbing in the occiput or in whole head.

Baryta irritates the nerves slightly, and then causes muscular weakness, paresis and even paralysis. It is useful in neuralgia and in rheumatism from exposure, especially to damp. The CARBONATE cures, particularly when stiff neck, rheumatic pains and swollen glands

DRUGS AFFECTING THE OCCIPITAL REGION

obtain. The *Acetica* deserves a trial for its well-defined pains. Accompaniments may be, in either remedy, tension of the face as from cobwebs, general tenseness of skin, which is as dry as parchment. Scrofulous persons, who take cold very easily, have large, hard abdomens, and mentally are dejected, irresolute, slow in comprehension. Also in old, infirm, persons, whose blood-vessels are undergoing senile changes, who are threatened with apoplexy and who readily catch cold on the least exposure.

Belladonna. * Jerking headache, worse when walking quickly or going upstairs, and when at every step there is a jolt downwards as if a weight were in the occiput. Throbbing pressure, left side of occiput. Cutting in head to left occipital protuberance. Severe, rapid stabs in occiput behind. * Sensation of weight, with violent pressing in the occiput. * Head drawn backwards and bored deeply into pillows.

The occiput may participate in the general congestive and inflammatory action of this remedy, and in some cases, may be the chief point of attack. Then the patient cannot lie down on the back or incline the head backwards. Inflammation at the base of the brain causes boring in the pillow, and if this extends into the spine; also opisthotonos.

Benzinum. Severe darting in occiput from below upwards, recurring in paroxyms, < from motion, and especially rising after sitting.

Berberis. Pressive, tearing pain in occiput, as if scalp was too small and brain too large. Tearing in left occipital region. Tearing, sticking in left side of neck and posteriorly in slow jerks upwards to occiput.

These are the well-known pains of *Berberis*, and indicate the remedy in neuralgia of neck and occiput, especially if the patient is weak from defective assimilation and tissue-oxidation, the urine depositing a copious loamy sediment.

Bismuthum Oxidum. Dull cutting in brain, begins above the right orbit and extends to the occiput. Pressure and sensation of heaviness, < on motion. Twitching, tearing whole left side of occipital bone, < close to parietal.

This oxide, which however, is probably the subnitrate, is of eminent service in pains of head, eyes and spine, when reflex from gastric origin. The tongue is white, the taste bitter, and there are nausea, burning, pressure and distress in stomach through to the back, *with a sore, burning spot in the spine.* Prostration is excessive, while the face is often indicative of poor nutrition and of abdominal distress; earthy face, blue rings around the eyes, features changed as if he had been sick.

Trousseau used the drug for eructations non-fœtid, diarrhœa worse when child is weaned, also when continuing after dentition; stools cadaverous; excessive exhaustion, but surface remains warm.

Borax. Throbbing in occiput as if it would suppurate, shivering all over. Pulsating rush of blood into occiput.

Bovista. After walking in open air, violent pressive headache, heavy feeling < occiput, > night and in room. Confusion and heaviness, lids inclined to fall, eyes feel as if they would be drawn backwards, especially in a bright light in evening; anxiety and uneasiness of body. Dull pain with tension in temples. Pressive pain, extending over vertex to forehead. Feeling in occiput as if everything would protrude. As if a wedge was being pressed in occiput. Violent sticking and tearing in left side of occiput. Dull boring; pressive stitches in occiput to forehead and over left eye, in warm room. Tearing in occiput and in lower jaw. Violent fine stitches in left side of occiput.

Bovista affects the brain so as to cause anæsthesia and symptoms of asphyxia. It has, therefore, been used for the ill-effects of the fumes of burning charcoal. It should be thought of in occipital headaches of weak persons, who have cerebral hyperæmia, tendency to ptosis, drowsiness, etc. A sense as if the head were enormously large is an excellent characteristic.

The drug here resembles *Gelsemium.* In a clear case, however, the *Bovista* cutaneous symptoms will be present.

Bromine. Heat in occiput. Toward evening in rather damp weather. Pains in bones of head, mostly in forehead and occiput.

Bone pains are less characteristic of *Brom.* than are congestion to chest and head, croup, pneumonia, etc. They come usually after these other symptoms. As they were rather worse in damp weather, and as we know clinically that *Bromine* has aggravation from dampness, etc., we may essay the remedy in rheumatic, scrofulous patients with pains in occipital bones, etc. Compare *Baryta, Aurum, Dulc., Merc.*

Bryonia. Awoke with headache, < over left eye, after rising, pain extended towards vertex and occiput, and there disappeared. Slight headache left side of forehead and in occiput, with slight tension below mastoid. Drawing, distending headache, left half of forehead and occiput while walking. Slight drawing in forehead and pressure in occiput. * Pressive pain above left eye, followed by dull pressive pain in occipital protuberances, whence it spreaded over the whole body; pain so severe on quick motion and after eating that it seemed like a distinct pulsation within the head. Hollow throbbing in forehead and occiput. Pressing together in temporal muscles alternating frequently with drawing pains in occipital protuberances. Sensible beating in vertex with same and fullness within cranium in region of cerebellum. Numb sensation, occiput feels enlarged. Dull pain. * Headache in occiput to shoulders, like heaviness on sore spot, morning in bed after waking while lying on back. Painfulness in lower portion of left side of occiput, < by touch. Dull pressure. * Pressive pain with drawing down into neck, > towards noon. Sharp pain in left occipital protuberance, coming and going suddenly.

The direction of pains, from before backwards, is very characteristic of the *Bryonia* headache. Few drugs act so prominently as this upon the occiput. Its symptoms, some of which have been confirmed, show it to be useful in gastric, bilious, congestive, neuralgic and rheumatic occipital headaches. In rheumatic cases, stiff neck is a common accompaniment. Although in typhoid *Bryonia* has generally been given in frontal headache, its occipital pains must not be neglected. Compare here, however, *Rhus Rad.* (*q. v.*).

Bufo. Hammering from eyebrows to cerebellum. Lancinations in cerebellum, making head fall backwards; loss of consciousness, falls down, tonic and clonic spasms, face turgid and distorted, bloody saliva, involuntary urine, repeated shocks through body, legs in more violent motion than arms, face bathed in sweat. Pains in head make nape of neck feel as if compressed.

Some of these indications are doubtful because derived from the experiments of Houat, but we know enough of *Bufo* to be certain that it affects the region we are investigating. It should be remembered in epileptics who suffer from occipital compression and stiff neck before paroxysms.

Cactus Grand. Heaviness and pain in posterior of brain, < lying on back. Constant dull pain in cerebellum. Pain and drawing < moving head. Pressure > by quick exercise or mental activity.

Cereus Bonplandii. Head as if suspended under skull and base of brain. Head felt drawn backward. Pain through forehead, left side, to occiput. Disagreeable feeling in back of head, seeming to pass down neck and end in a disagreeable sensation approaching qualmishness at the stomach. Sense of a board bound to back of head, < left side. Occipital headache. Pain running through to cerebrum. Drawing. Pressing sensation, left side of occiput, immediately afterwards counter pains on left side of forehead. Forcing inwards in occiput on line with sagittal suture, on walking and descending one or two steps. Pain in upper spine and medulla oblongata, up through brain < stooping or bending head forward.

Cereus Serpentinus. Back of brain feels detached and as if rotten.

The cactus plants seem to exert considerable influence upon the circulation in the occiput. This with the well-known constrictive, band-like sensation—a sensation varying from the iron grip at the heart to mere pressure, heaviness or drawing—constitute the chief characteristic of these remedies.

In one prover, *Cactus Grand.* caused some incoordination of cerebral origin; difficulty in fixing the attention, slight reeling gait, muscles obey inaccurately, occiput sore to touch, pressure there, which quick exercise or mental activity relieves. This last modality proves that there is an undue fullness of the transverse sinus and probably, too, of the veins in and about the cerebellum, which exercise causes to move heartward.

Calcarea Acetica. Drawing pain right of forehead above eye and in occiput on exerting the mind. Drawing, pressive, tearing, headache, now in forehead, now in occiput, now in temples > pressure or exerting mind. Feels as if occiput would be pressed asunder. Pressive pain, suddenly shooting through the occiput. Jerk-like pressing outwards left side of occiput, extends down into neck. Drawing, pressive headache in left of occiput, stiff neck. Sore pain in occiput when touched, as if place was suppurating.

Calcarea Carbonica. Violent dull headache, first in forehead, then in occiput. Cracking, audible in occiput, followed by warmth in neck. Heaviness, pressure. Headache in occiput whenever she ties anything tightly about the head. Drawing always towards side he moves head, > after sneezing. Gnawing. Tensive pressure. Cutting in occiput and forehead < walking and from pressure. Stitches in right side of occiput.

Calcarea Caustica. Confused, dull pressure in forehead extending to occiput, could scarcely attend to business. Dull rheumatic pain; neck stiff. Pressive pain.

Calcarea Phosphorica. Staggering, dizzy when walking, with drawing in nape of neck, and confusion of head. Headache on top of head, behind ears, and drawing in muscles of neck to nape of neck and back of head. Muscles of neck hurt up to occiput. A slight draft is followed by rheumatic pain in neck, stiffness and dullness of head. * Crawling, running over top of head as if ice were lying on upper part of occiput; head is hot, with smarting of roots of hair. Aching, drawing around lateral protuberances. Dull, sleepy, oppressive pain of whole head, < in cerebellum.

It is in rheumatic headache of the occiput and neck that the *Calcarea Salts* are most effective. Still, in headaches even congestive, when the peculiar ice-like feeling is present, CALC. CARB. and PHOS. are both useful.

DRUGS AFFECTING THE OCCIPITAL REGION   107

Camphor. Headache, front to occiput. * Contractive pain at base of brain, especially in occiput and above root of nose; < stooping low, lying down and from pressure; with cold hands and feet, hot forehead and coma vigil. Fine tearing in left side of forehead and of occiput. Pressure. Uneasy feeling. Cutting pressure from left side of occiput towards forehead. * Throbing in the cerebellum. (See *Glonoine*.)

Cannabis Indica. Vertigo on rising, with stunning pain in back part of head, he falls. Vertigo head inclines backwards. Dull heavy throbbing pain through head, with sense of heavy blow on back of head and neck. Jerking in right side of forehead towards interior and back part of head. Headache in occiput and temples. Fullness in right of cerebellum. Dull pain, < shaking head. Sense of pressure at back of head, before convulsive movements, changing to an unpleasant feeling of heat, then of cold; he carries hands automatically to the spot; they are held there as if it were difficult to detach them. Feeling of surging from posterior of head towards forehead. Surging up neck into head, seeming to press it forward. Peculiar feeling as if a stream of warm water, gradually stealing up back into brain. Sense of a redhot iron rod passed up from sacrum to atlas, around the occiput over eyes from right, stooping at left ear, leaving a feeling as if charred.

A very precious remedy is this hashish, serving well in uræmic headaches, congestions of brain and spine, meningitis, abuse of alcohol, etc. Characteristics are errors of space and time, perception of both being extravagantly overestimated.

Cannabis Sativa. * Pressure beneath frontal eminence, deep through brain to occiput. Heaviness. Heat. Tension in occiput, then in forehead, lastly in temples. Drawing to occiput. Pressive pain right side of occiput.

Cantharis. Twitching in right occipital bone, then in left knee. Sticking pressing pain. Stitching in left side of occiput. Stitching tearing from both sides inward. Stitches deep into brain on right occipital bone. Dull violent stitches in succession in occiput, extended into forehead, deep internally. Tearing from left side into left forehead, with vertigo lasting longer than pain. Tearing in nape of neck and stitching in right cervical muscles on moving head, when it extends into upper part of head.

The deeply penetrating stitches extending towards forehead, occured in same prover who had deep soreness and heaviness in forehead, head feels as if being pressed forward.

Carbo Animalis. Heaviness, especially in occiput and left temple with confusion. Pressive headache. Pressive pain in small spot. Stitches and throbbing. Twitching tearings shoot back and forth in left occiput. Painful tearing sticking in right.

Carbo Vegetabilis. Dizziness as after intoxication spreading from occiput, < walking. Severe headache, on stooping it presses out in forehead and occiput. Drawing all over head from occiput. Sticking headache extending into occiput. Tearing through whole head, starting from small spot in occiput. Crackling in occiput while sitting. Confusion in occiput as after intoxication. Confusion like a tension from within. Much severe pain in occiput and boring in forehead, with sweat, pale, cold face, trembling hands, nausea. Drawing, tearing left side of occiput. * Dull headache in occiput. * Violent pressive pain in and on the occiput, in the lower portion. Pressure < after supper. Pressive headache in upper part of right side of occiput, pressure in eyes. Pressive headache, first in neck then in forehead, then lachrymation with closure of lids. Burning-sticking in a small spot. Tearing here and there, in left side of occiput, face, shoulder, thigh, etc., with severe pressure in arms and legs. Throbbing headache violent in occiput as if suppurating. * Drawing in nape up into head, with nausea and rush of water from mouth.

These two forms of carbon are characterised by headaches with a feeling of weight or heavy pressure, the mind is dull and confused, as after a debauch. Very important in *Carbo Veg.* is headache from occiput forward, with nausea, dizziness, etc., particularly in old offenders in debauchery, or in old dyspeptics with an abundance of flatus in the abdomen, causing distension, dyspnœa, headache.

Carbo. A. has relieved heaviness in cerebellum, < in cold air, > after dinner; feet weary.

Carboneum Sulphuratum. Compressing, band-like pains in occiput and temples.

In these days of the menthol craze one is reminded of the carbon sulphide, which ought to relieve terrible headache with cerebral intoxication or with paralytic weakness. *Phosporus* antidotes.

Castoreum. Pain in occiput as if head would be drawn backwards.

Pressure and throbbing in left side of occiput externally in small spot, internally widely extended; pressing spot relieves pain, but sensitiveness retained and she felt stupefied, during dinner. Throbbing, as from an ulcer; with sticking and tearing in right side of occiput. Tearing and sticking right side of occiput like shootings, while standing.

To be thought of for nervous women, after exhausting disease, when they remain weak; relief from pressing spot is very important.

Causticum. Occipital bone feels numb, pithy or dead. Drawing pain. Tensive headache arising from nape. Sudden pain in occipital bone while sitting, as if something in muscles had been displaced. Throbbing pain right side of occiput; on rubbing it extends towards vertex, where it continues for a long time as if beaten. Drawing pressure in right side of occiput and muscles of neck, < on rapid walking, arising in the open air.

This drug should be remembered in rheumatic or neuralgic patients especially when they suffer from every exposure to cold winds, or pains are accompanied with paralytic weakness.

Cedron. Dull pains in head, but very sharp in occiput and in nerves of face and eye; sharp, flying pains all over on getting warm in bed. Bending head backwards, with pressure on occipital and parietal regions, as if they would burst. Headache deep in orbits extending to occiput; must shut the eyes; with shuddering of body; hands, feet and nose cold; heat of face. Pain in occiput and forehead.

Excellent in neuralgia, periodic or not, malarial or not, provided only the patient is nervous, excitable, with cold hands, feet and nose, and congestion to head.

Chamomilla. Sense of confusion, heaviness, pressure and fullness; inclination to bend head backward. Dull stitches, desire to bend head backward. Excited disposition.

Chelidonium. *Heaviness, as if could not raise head from pillow; or, feels as if head is lifted when he arose but occiput remained lying, held firmly by the neck. Pain in occiput with sensation as though head would be drawn backward. *Tensive sensation right side of back of head. Drawing, with anxiety in chest. Pressive drawing left side of occiput. *Drawing, pressing-like stitches from left side of occiput to forehead. Heaviness and tension in muscles of nape and in occiput. Violent pains back and forth from vertex to neck, shoulders thereby drawn up.

These symptoms seem to be a part of the spinal irritation caused by *Chelidonium*. They are not necessarily connected with hepatic symptoms. Clinically the drug has: º cold sensation in occiput and nape.

China. Drawing, painful; drawing in left side of occiput or in articulation of occipital bone and atlas, > bending head backward. Severe pressure as if cerebellum would be pressed out. Drawing headache from occiput to forehead as if latter was drawn together, ending in throbbing in temples, > walking and pressure of hand, < when sitting. * Violent pressive headache deep in brain, constricted sensation, < right side of forehead and in occiput, < walking.

Chininum Sulphuricum. Headache in forehead, extending to occiput.

Cimicifuga Racemosa. Pain from right eyeball through to right side of occiput, slightly affecting the ear, at night. * Pain in head seems to extend over and through whole brain, producing distinct sense of soreness in occipital region, << by motion. Pain in forehead over vertex to occiput; dizzy; yawns.

Cinnabaris. Drawing pain from crown to occiput. Fullness, pressure in occiput and back of neck after rising from bed, > at noon. Rush of blood to back of head; violent itching and heat extending to each ear; lumps formed behind left ear. Pain in back part of neck when head is thrown back, extending to occiput. Constant pain in right side of head; from temples pain goes to occiput.

Clematis. Pain in occiput in morning, < in open air.

Coca. Pressive headache on right side and in occiput. Pain in lowest part of occiput when yawning, sometimes preventing its completion. Drawing in occiput while reading, extending to temples. Headache, in fresh air, changed to occiput as if it was held from ear to ear in a vise. When head is bent forward while he is writing, transient giddiness seemingly from occiput forwards.

Coca acts more on the forehead than on the back. still, in some cases of brain-fag, the occiput becomes affected.

Cocculus. In an epidemic of cerebro-spinal meningitis, Dr. James was very successful with this drug, when there was present a sensation as if the occiput opened and shut.

Coccus Cacti. Pressive pain in right side of forehead, sometimes to occiput. Violent raging pain in right eye along squamous portion of temporal bone on inner side to occiput; as if fluid injected paroxysmally into a small blood vessel. Sense of a hot constricting band from mastoid to mastoid, across occiput, finally, the whole scalp seemed drawn. Dull boring towards left ear. Pressing pain, scalp as if swollen.

Colchicum. Sharp, painful drawing, tearing in left half of head, commencing in eyeball and extending towards occiput. Headache from forehead towards occiput. Dull drawing from nape across occiput to ears. Pressure deep in cerebellum from the slightest literary work. Oppressive heaviness in occiput, < on motion or on bending a little forward. Tearing in a small spot left side of occiput.

Excellent for overtaxed brains; if the patient loses any rest, he becomes mentally tired, and suffers with nausea, bitter taste, etc. He is irritable and intolerant of even slight pain.

Colocynthinum. Heaviness, pain. Cerebellum sensitive on turning head. Stitches traverse occiput, when he treads heavily; or dart through cerebellum like lighting on coughing.

Colocynthis. Boring in right side of occiput. Violent, long continued pressure in lateral occipital protuberances. Pressure, tension, < at inferior lateral protuberances. Pressing, boring,—drawing in muscles of neck, on different parts of occiput, < right side. Sensation in neck, extending towards occipital protuberance, as if a heavy weight lay there transversely.

Useful in rheumatic and neuralgic patients. Motion aggravates, but firm pressure often relieves.

Comocladia. Violent pain from posterior of right eye to occipital protuberance; eyeball sore, profuse lachrymation, eye feels as large as two. Sharp pain in occiput down the neck. Aching in right temporal bone, thence to occiput; whole base of head painful on moving head.

Conium. Heavy sensation, < sitting bent, when erect. Fullness and confusion. Pressure on left side of occiput; or in right side like a plug. * Pain at every pulse as if pierced with a knife. Tearing while walking. Tearing in occiput, nape, and especially orbits with constant nausea so that must lie in bed. Pressure in forehead, then heaviness; later, same in occiput. Headache from forehead to occiput, as if something were loose on shaking head.

Copaiva. Dull pain. Lancinating pressure in occipital protuberance. Pulsating, deep-seated stitches. Stitches in left occipital protuberance, with occasional shocks in whole head.

Crotalus Horridus. Sudden vertigo; nearly falls off of chair; full, congested feeling in front of brain;

aching over left eye, with sharp pain small spot in centre of left occiput. Cerebellum, post mortem, found injected. Pain as from a blow, lying down again after rising.

Croton Tiglium. Confusion of left or whole of occiput. Pressive headache. Sticking pain between nape and occiput.

Cuprum Arsenicosum. Dull, heavy aching back of head. Dull soreness in right occipital bone, < pressure.

Digitalinum. Confused, < forehead with pulsating pain in occiput, > walking in open air. Confusion in occiput. Dull pain. Violent boring in left side of occiput. Drawing, as if occiput and vertex were rising; afterward pressure in occiput.

Digitalis. Violent pressure in left half of occiput. Sensation of pressure in occiput, right to left; from occiput to vertex, confusion and incipient vertigo. Violent sticking pain, < occiput and vertex, less the forehead.

Dioscrorea. Severe pain, > pressure. Sharp, twisting pain, > rubbing. Pulling pain, causing stupid sensation. Dull pain. Severe pain in back of neck to back of head and both shoulders.

Dirca Palustris. Pain in head low in occiput, thence over top of head to forehead, there a strong congestive headache with throbbing of carotids. Pains all through head, vertex and occiput extending down into spine. Headache in left half of head, throbs and beats, < coughing or moving < touching back of head, > when hair was down or high on head.

Dulcamara. Whole head heavy as if scalp were tense < in nape, where it becomes a crawling. Occiput heavy. Occiput feels enlarged. Pressive, stupefying pain in occiput, rising from nape. Slow sticking as from a needle drawn in and out.

Elaps. Pain seems in the right side of cerebellum. Pressive pain in nape as if from sinking down of the cerebellum.

Equisetum. Slight boring changing from side to side in occipital region. Dull drawing back of head and neck. Very sharp and quick pains near left superior curved line of occipital bone. Pains change from frontal to occipital region and dart from left to right there.

Eryngium Aquaticum. Dull dragging pain in occiput, neck and shoulders. Pain extends forward into eye with blurring, < exercise or least excitement.

This drug causes a headache that is worse in frontal region, < over left eye, < thinking intently, lowering head, etc.—Sitting stooped it passes into neck and along muscles of shoulder. Dimness of sight is a valuable accompaniment. The eyes burn and are congested, with purulent, fluid, profuse discharge. The symptoms are very suggestive of headache of optic region.

Eriodyctyon. Aching in base of cranium. Sense of outward pressure on all sides of head, < at cerebellum upwards. Pressure outward, < back of head. Intense, dull, heavy, pain in back of head and over eyes. Burning pain.

In asthmatic colds, with supra-orbital and occipital headache, this herb will prove very serviceable.

Eupatorium Perfoliatum. Pain from forehead to left occiput, < left side.

Eupatorium Purpureum. Hard thumping pain in occipital bone.

Eurhorbium. Pressive pain. Bruised pain, left side, cannot lie on it.

Euphrasia. Sharp tearing stitches left side of occiput.

Eupion. Clawing in left side of occiput; sticking, drawing in occiput, drawing along left cervical muscles to back of chest, also in middle of chest with every breath; when these are gone, teeth as if loose when pressed. Stitches right side of occiput.

Fagopyrum. Back of head tired. Pain in occiput and weary feeling in back of neck. Sharp, sticking pain. Sharp darting very persistent pain left occipital region radiating to left side. Pain in temples and back of head on rising, > bending head back, < stooping. Pain through whole head and occiput to back of neck, > pressure and gentle motion, especially in cool air. Pressing out, < in occiput. Dull pain from back of eyes through head and occiput.

Headache to occiput, dull pain in eyes, with aching, tired, neck, ought to be characteristic.

Ferrum. *Drawing from nape up into head, in which there is then shooting, roaring and humming. Oppressive, somewhat acute pain in back of head and neck, gradually extending to forehead. Weight from ear to ear. Beating, almost insupportable, pain in back of head and neck, gradually extending to sides and forehead << moving or stooping. *Pain in back of head when coughing.

Excellent in congestive headache with hammering, beating, must lie down. It is usually < in temples, but as with *Phosphorus,* etc., it may seemingly come up the neck, commencing with drawing, etc. Often the feet are cold, the fingers stiff and the mind confused.

Fluoric Acid. Feeling of a warm breath from nape to occiput. Pressure on both side of occiput. Pressure and compression, < towards right. Dullness of occiput only. Cramp-like pain in lowest part of occiput towards left.

Gelsemium. * Dull aching in occiput occasionally extending into *os frontis*. Aching < stooping. Dull heavy pain, on rising, also slight throbbing on right side of head. Pressive pain < temples, at time in occiput, at others all over head. When writing headache in vertex, then in left occipital region, then both sides and in upper cervical region and again on vertex; finally settled, dull ache < in occiput, mastoid and upper cervical region, extending to shoulders, > sitting, reclining head on high pillow. Drawing on right side, on crown towards occiput. Pains over top of head to occiput, dizzy, disagreeable painful sensation in whole head. Pain over occiput, crown as if lifted off in two pieces. Persistent and distressing numbness in occipital region lasting some hours after consciousness returned.

Very important are all of these. First in the headache beginning in the cervical spinal vertebræ and extending over head, with bursting pain in forehead and eyeballs, < 10 A.M., with nausea, vomiting cold sweat, etc. Next, is the fullness to bursting in the medulla oblongata before spasms. Then we note vertigo and confusion spreading from occiput, with dim-sight,, large pupils, etc., < from summer heat. Then come the various neuralgic pains showing the action of the drug on the occipital nerves.

Geranium Maculatum. Slight pain low down in occipital region.

Ginseng. Dizzy, with pains in nape; large pupils. Reeling sensation in the occiput, gray spots before eyes: Ground seems to waver. Sensation in occiput as if head was swaying to one side. Drawing, he involuntarily bends head backward. Pressure, with sense of impending vertigo. Pressure as if in sinuses of cerebellum. Sudden blow on occiput, followed by severe bruised pain.

This famous Chinese nerve remedy seems to be worthy of our consideration in vertigo of occipital origin, with consequent incoordination. Right side of body is weakest. Gait is unsteady and difficult; and generally there is dull rumbling in abdomen.

Glonoine. Affects occiput and neck more than any other part. Subdued sensation as if something was moving in nerves from back of neck to head. Pain up from back of neck to occiput, and then spreads upward. Pain in occiput, then in vertex. Pain in occiput towards crown, <shaking head backward and forward. Pains in occiput and slight in forehead when moving head. After fullness in occiput, pain to forehead growing more violent. * Severe pain in occiput, to eyes and temples. On shaking head great pain in spot in right side of occiput (where he habitually suffered from headache). Thumping fullness in occiput, when sitting down, < after shaking head. * Such intense congestion in occiput, like pressure, seems as if must lose reason. Violent tensive pain in occiput, up and down and towards both ears; also from time to time, tension above right eye. Constant gnawing. Pressure from occiput to crown. Sore pain, constant inclination to bend head backward. Dull pressive pain, < in occiput and region of ears, same in nape, as if in medulla oblongata, < moving head or twisting neck, neck stiff. Headache in glabella, spread up and back, at last to occiput; throbbing from below up and from front back. Paroxysms of beating and throbbing in vertex, temples and occiput.

Characteristics of this remedy are; upward surging, as if blood was forcing itself through the constricted neck; this congestion is as marked in the area of the vertebral arteries as in that of the carotids. Shaking

DRUGS AFFECTING THE OCCIPITAL REGION 119

the head aggravates intensely, as do also wine, sun's heat, and artificial heat. Motion increases the dreadful throbbing, though gentle exercise in the open air, relieves. The throbbing from the neck and occiput upward in and over head, is very characteristic. *Glonoine,* then, as an "occipital" remedy is to be remembered as one causing congestion there, spreading the blood thence directly to the back of the brain. Here it excels *Belladonna.* Like *Aconite* and *Gelsemium,* it has increase of urine with the headache.

Glonoine should be thought of in apoplectic congestion when stiff neck and a feeling (*worse at the back of the neck*) as if clothing were tight, shows the direction of the hyperæmia. This is a genuine symptom.

In the effects of exposure to the sun, *Glonoine* is inimitable; though if there is pulsation and constriction in cerebellum *Camphor* is needed; if anxiety, fever, or coldness and weak quick pulse, *Aconite.*

Graphites. Violent, but dull pain in occiput, with heaviness of head, tension, stiffness of neck; pain intolerable on walking, not noticed lying, $>$ in night. Pressive headache in occiput. Much pressure in occiput and nape. Severe tensive headache on waking, $<$ on surface of brain, $<<$ in occiput, without impeding thought; neck painfully stiff; the more he tries to fall asleep, the worse the pain. * Pain, as if constricted especially in occiput, extending to nape, which pains as if broken when he looks up; afterwards pain extends down back to chest. o Pain as if constricted with a cord, $<$ in occiput.

In fat, but anæmic patients, who suffer from spinal irritation, especially in women, *Graphites* is very useful for a nervous headache *with stiff neck, spine sensitive,* $<$ *at vertebra prominens; tension* on nape, shoulders and head.

Guarea. Constriction and hammering, in occiput.

Guaiacum. Dull pressive pain obliquely upward from left side of neck to vertex, ending in a stitch. Tearing right side of occiput. Drawing, tearing, in occiput and forehead.

Hamamelis. Dull throbbing pain in back and top of head.

Helleborus Niger. * Pain in occiput. Headache from nape to vertex. Pressure. Pressive pain extending towards nape, as if bruised in occiput, < stooping. Violent pressive headache, with great heaviness in occiput, on waking. Brain feels too large in front and occiput empty; afterwards reverse in forehead, occiput feels as if would fall forward; wants to lie down and roll head from side to side; feels helpless as an infant, etc.

Helonias. When reading, feeling of fullness, pressure outwards in vertex and occiput; scalp burns, > > concentrating mind.

Hepar. * Pressive pain externally right of occiput, gradually extending to nape, throat and shoulder-blades. Severe stitches in occiput and temples, as if a plug or nail was being driven in.

Hura. Headache from occiput to vertex, with throbbing and sharp pains. Constriction. Pain behind head and in neck, to left gums.

Hydrastis. Dull, heavy, pain in left occiput, with pale face, much heat in head and pressing from within out in region of temporal fossa, > pressure of cool hand and cool, open air. Aching pain in cerebellum right, then left.

Hydrocotyle. Intense pain with some tumefaction in posterior portion of skull. Constriction. Occiput acutely sensitive, especially to touch.

Hydrocyanic Acid. Violent pressure in occiput and forehead, < right side; pressure soon leaves, *but confusion lasts*. Pressure from vertex towards forehead on both sides and to orbits where it became fixed, while from occiput it extended down nape of neck; it caused *confusion* of head. Sudden feeling as though every thing about him moved slowly; dizzy without reeling; slight pressure left side of occiput over left half of head to frontal region.

Confusion, weakening of pulse, are valuable accompaniments of this powerful agent. (See *Laurocerasus* below).

Hydrophobinum. Throbbing headache in forehead, vertex and occiput, down to the neck.

Hypericum. Pressive pain on motion; also with drawing stitches. Tearing. Back of head feels "Bothered". Severe scalp headache left side of occiput. Shooting of dull pain up the left occipital nerve. After breakfast severe scalp headache on left side of occiput sharp, at other times dull.

Ignatia. Pain in occiput just above mastoid process at times involving the auditory apparatus, then hearing seems blunted. Pressure and pressive pain in occiput, right half, till he falls asleep. Pain as if occipital bone was pressed inwards. Head heavy as if filled with blood, as after stooping too low, with tearing pains in occiput, > lying on back, < sitting erect, >> bending head low forward while sitting. Vertigo changing to pain in right half of occiput. Confusion of head. Pains in right side, < in occiput, < thinking and also speaking.

It is not locality so much as universal effects that distinguishes *Ignatia*.

Indigo. Painful raging in bones of left side of occiput. Dull headache like a heaviness in occiput.

Warmth and rushing like boiling water. Heat in occiput, afterwards, < in middle of brain. Pain in left side of occiput, lancinating, shooting, through head to occiput. Violent stitches. Throbbing, with painful stitches in occiput.

Ipecacuanha. Painfulness of occiput and nape from moving head. Tensive, pressive headache in occiput and nape, extending into shoulders.

Iris Versicolor. Pain shoots like an electric shock, from right temple to left side of occiput; depression of spirits, debility. Slight dull pain at situation of posterior fontanelle. Severe stitch in interior of occiput.

Jaborandi. Aching in lower part of occiput. Dull pain in lower part of occiput over left side of head to forehead; weak; palpitation of heart, stitches in chest.

Kali Bichromicum. After nasal discharge ceases, pain from occiput to forehead. Pressive headache, < forehead and occiput, waking in morning. Pressive headache with transient violent stitches now in vertex, now in temples or occiput. Tearing sticking over whole head, < in right temporal and occipital region. On waking A.M., pain in forehead and vertex, after rising changes to occiput. Violent tearing from temporal region to occipital of either side. Sticking in right side side of head and whole occipital region. Pressure. Biting.

Kali Carbonicum. Heaviness, like confusion; or like lead, head falls backward, with stiffness of nape extending to between shoulder-blades. Aching and heaviness, < swallowing. Pressure and burning low down in occiput, heaviness of head even to falling. Violent pressure in occiput with rush of blood in head and feeling of heaviness, while standing.

Stitches from nape to occiput. Stitches in occiput on stepping or stooping, as if on surface of brain. Tearing now in right, now in left side of occiput and now in forehead. Throbbing, tearing in right side of occiput close to nape. On stooping, sensation as if something was sinking from occiput towards forehead.

In anæmic patients, who suffer from headache with stiff neck and spinal irritation, *Kali Carb.* is very useful.

Kali Chroricum. Confusion in occiput with peculiar sensation in muscles of nape. Pain in occiput extending into both jaws.

Kali Cyanatum. Slight, dull pain in back of head just before going to sleep. Head drawn backwards.

Kali Iodatum. Pressive heaviness. Tension as if in bone, with stitches.

Kali Nitricum. Violent compression, everything stiff, afterwards pain in nape like pulling on hairs, extending into shoulders, with tension and stitches over face and neck, impairment of swallowing, anxiety, arrest of breathing from eleven A.M. to four P.M. Headache in occiput > binding up hair. Drawing, tearing, could not move head, neck stiff; two hours afterwards drawing and tearing in scapulæ, weakness, can scarcely lift feet. Pressure, heaviness. Pressive pain towards occiput, gradually changes into stitches < by touch, seem like rhythmical sticking. Violent pressive pain, mingled with beating in occiput. Violent stitch in left side of occiput during menses. Burning, throbbing on left side of occiput. Jerking as if in bone; later in hip-bone also; and at last alternate with tension behind right ear. A certain coldness in occiput always with the pains in the head. Pain right side of forehead, suddenly, walking; soon towards top of head and thence into occiput and both temples; seemingly in scalp. Painful pulsation in occiput and temples. Skin of forehead feels bruised.

Kalmia. Pain in back of head and neck. Dull pain around back part of head, frequent sharp, darting in right side of head. Headache in occiput and pain in neck. Dull in occiput and temples. Shooting from nape up into head. Dull headache one place and another, < in back of head, and especially those parts back of forehead. Pains shoot from temples to occiput.

In rheumatic patients, the shooting upward is important.

Kreosotum. Whole occiput full, heavy, feels as if he would fall backward. Pain as from suppuration below left side of occipital bone.

Lachesis. *Heavy as lead; morning, waking, with vertigo, tensive pain in right side of occiput extends to orbits and down into nasal bones. Rush of blood to head on stooping, with headache on right side, extending towards occiput.

Lactic Acid. Pain at base of occiput and over eyes. Slight pain from occiput to vertex, with rough and constricted throat. Dull, weighty pain in occiput; on lying down, pain left and went to forehead, tendency to close eyes; later, pain back to occiput, the eyes still heavy; on again lying pain went to forehead. Severe headache in left mastoid, extending obliquely across by way of occiput to over the right ear. Light darting pains from centre of brain in straight lines to centre of occipital protuberance, < motion.

Lactuca Virosa. Heaviness, pressure. Dull pain. Pressive, tense feeling, with heat in forehead and cold hands. Compressive pain. Pressive, heavy feeling.

This pressive, tense feeling is very important. It is a similar tightness in the chest that makes Lactuca so invaluable in dyspnœa of spasmodic origin.

Lamium Album. Pain in occiput as if lying on a stone, and as if bed was too hard when lying on either side.

Laurocraeasus. As if tendons too short and head would be drawn backward, like painful heaviness with cessation of pain in forehead. Feeling of tension in right side of occiput as from taking hold of a lock of hair. Drawing deep in right side of occiput. Twinging pain, with sleepiness. Painful pressure on left side of occiput to neck. Painful pressure from within outward, beneath left side of occipital bone; thought vanishes. Transient stitches in occiput or forehead. Throbbing in left side. Headache alternately in forehead and occiput, pressive; pulse diminished. (see *Hydrocyanic Acid*.)

Lilium Superbum. Pain in right occipital protuberance.

Lilium Tigrinum. Headache in occiput and over eyes. Screwing pain in left occipital protuberance, with drawing pain on left side of nucha. Dull pressing-aching from left temple, over ear to occiput, in paroxyms, with steady, dull frontal headache, over left eye. Dull heavy pressive pain from forehead and temples to occipital protuberances.

Lobelia Inflata. Dull feeling. Tension in occiput, in region of lambdoidal suture, only when paying strict attention to anything. Pressure, after removing head covering. Pressive pain in occiput in open air.

Lycopersicum Esculentum. Boring in left of occiput.

Lycopodium. Heaviness. Dull heavy feeling in occiput, with confused pain in forehead, < motion. Burning pain in both occipital eminences. Pain as if scalp was inflamed. Occiput fills with blood after he stoops. Pinching pain in head behind ear. Pressure in right half of occiput, extending towards ear. Pressive pain. Sticking pain. Sticking and throbbing at night. Stitches at times in occiput, with almost excessively joyous mood. Constant stitches with slow pulse. Tearing. Pressive tearing in left side of occiput, in small spot near nape. Throbbing and pressure. Violent shock from back up towards vertex, obliged to hold on to head, while sitting (after eating to satiety). Nausea affects head, which pains as if compressed and confused as far as nape. Fine stitches in both occiput. Stitches in vertex and occiput. Jerking headache from occiput to vertex. Violent throbbing in forehead, afterwards tensive, and extending across occiput to nape. Drawing pain in right side of head to nape. * Tensive pain in nape and occiput while writing.

Lycopus. Pain from cerebellum transferred to temples, more acute. Congestive pain in occiput without mitigation of temporal aching. Severe aching, with cessation of cardiac pain. Aching at superior curved line, one inch to left of occipital protuberance, passing to corresponding spot on right side. Distressed feeling in cerebellum. Pain of temples transferred to cerebellum, seemingly congestive. Fronto-occipital headache, with toothache; or succeeded by labored cardiac action. Frontal headache, extending afterward through to occiput, succeeded by cardiac depression. Frontal, then occipital aching and subacute pain in fifth right interspace, each quickly abating, succeeded by return of aching pain in temples.

Suggestive of fronto-occipital pains with cardiac labored action or with the depression.

Magnesia Carbonica. Deep dull stitch through brain from vertex to right side of occiput. Heaviness in forehead, with pain as from suppuration in left side of occiput. Tearing in forehead and drawing backwards in nape, disappearing in bed. Fine stitches in right side of vertex, cease there and on her moving her head towards left, tearing in right side of occiput. Tension and drawing in occiput as if head would be drawn backward during and after swallowing; < standing, > sitting. Violent stitches.

Magnesia Muriatica. Sharp stitches in left side of head and in occiput. Much pressure, also sharp and pinching < on vertex and in occiput. Heaviness; also dizzy feeling as if in danger of falling. Pressure. Sharp stitch in right side of occiput, then burning there. Two sharp stitches in right occipital protuberance. Tearing also throbbing tearing from occiput to vertex. Tearing and throbbing in occiput, at last involves whole head after entering the house; >> sitting. Painful jerking, tearing in right side of occiput. On rising from stooping, throbbing in occiput, soon involving whole head. During menses, throbbing pain in occiput, with feeling of heaviness, morning, after rising.

Magnesia Sulphurica. Pressive pain, morning, >> in open air. Must lie down with pressive pain in occiput from both sides. Occiput very senstitve; on stooping, feels in forehead as if something would fall forward; pain, < lying, he dared not cough on account of the shock. Headache in occiput renewed by carrying heavy weight on shoulders.

An excellent remedy in neuralgic cases.

Mancinella. Hammering pain in head and nape, inability to bend head down when writing. Pain in nape and forehead when stooping.

Manganum. Dull, pressive headache, with feeling of emptiness, taking away his senses, > applying hand.

Beating, throbbing in right side of occiput, like suppuration, during rest and motion. Needle-like stitches externally on right side of occipital bone, morning in bed, thence down to fifth cervical vertebra, < turning neck. Drawing pain in occiput, orbits and forehead, where it is < stooping, >> on pressure with hand. Burning, pressive pain in sides of head and in occiput, > going into open air.

Manganum Muriaticum. Tearing in right side of occipital bone.

Marum Verum Teucurium. Sticking in occiput and even in whole head. Painful pressive sensation in whole occiput.

Melilotus. On talking, headache leaves forehead and settles in occiput, returning to forehead on stooping.

The headaches are congestive, severe enough to cause delirium; nose bleed may relieve. The headache that affected the occiput was < in left supra-orbital region.

Menlispermum. Headache through temples extending to occiput. Headache in temples and occiput.

Mephitis. Feeling of heaviness; dull pressure, < in occiput, as if pressed with a finger.

Mercurius Corrosivus. Whirling vertigo, almost loss of hearing, < 9 P.M., lying down, seldom in day, with tearing pains in occiput. Sudden, dull, aching in forehead and vertex, < stooping or shaking head, > cold hand to forehead, extends to centre of cerebellum, when it felt like a bone-ache, five P.M., feels rather low-spirited; suddenly leaves.

Mercurius Iodatus Flavus. Numbness of occiput and nape; stiff neck. Sharp pain in occiput after rising in morning.

Mercurius Iodatus Ruber. Dull pressure in cerebellum below the occipital protuberance, a while after pressure over eyes. Pains in bones of head, < occiput.

Mercurius Precipitatus Ruber. º Leaden heaviness in occiput with diarrhœa.

Mercurius Solubilis. Constrictive headache, as if screwed in, now in sinciput, now in occiput, now in left side with watering of the eyes. Violent tearing from occiput to forehead, where it is a pressure. Pressive. Boring. Tearing, lower portion.

Mercurius Vivus. Frontal headache, with fullness, soon passing to occiput, with vertigo.

In syphilitic, rheumatic or scrofulous patients, the *Mercuries* suit for a tearing headache, that arises from the periosteum, the bones, or the nerves. General symptoms must be present but the *Proto-Iodide* will cure if the tongue is coated thick yellow on base; the *Red Precipitate*, if there is present leaden heaviness; the *Corrosive Sublimate* in bone pains, scalp very sore; the *Bin-Iodide*, when there is also hot vertex.

Clinical use for *Solublis* is tearing in (left) side of head and temple, extending from neck, insupportable heat and sweat; < at night and in heat of bed, > towards morning and while lying quiet.

Mezereum. Heavy sensation. * Boring in occipital bones. Acute drawing right side of occiput. Pressive pain, < entering house; also occiput and nape, < moving head. Tearing back and forth in bones of occiput. Tearing, throbbing in one spot above nape. Stupefaction in sinciput and occiput.

In periosteal and bone pains, especially after mercury.

Millefolium. Transient drawing after eating. Sticking in left side of occiput. Painful stitch in right side of occiput. Dull headache < in occiput.

Mitchella Repens. Dull, heavy aching in cerebellum. Throbbing in occipital region on inside of skull. Whole brain feels dull < in the cerebellum, morning.

Moschus. Pressive painful sensation in cerebellum. Throbbing, beating in occiput. Headache as of something beating in occiput, thence spreading to forehead. Painful drawing in head from occiput to ears and from ears into teeth, < right side. Pressive and boring through whole head at one time, at another behind ears, at another in forehead, at another in vertex and then in occiput. Slight pain in forehead alternating with pain in occiput.

Murex. Pain. Tightness, involuntarily raises her hand to part affected, when tightness goes from left to right; bending head backwards seems to relax nerves of occiput and neck. Sharp, transient pains above cerebellum.

Suggestive of uterine and kindred affections and so probably of use only when accompanied by the depression, acute diagonal pain from the right side of the uterus to the left breast, profuse menses, etc.

Muriatic Acid. Heavy sensation, with drawing stitches extending towards nape; cervical glands swollen and painful to touch; head heavy, dizzy, eyes dim. Heavy as if head would sink backwards as if from weak cervical muscles. Pain in left occipital protuberance from walking in wind. Tension, sticking. Violent tearing and sticking. Shock like paroxysmal tearing in side of occiput, extending into forehead. Pressive, tensive headache from occipital bone through brain to forehead.

This acid acts on the occiput in the highest degree. Especially characteristic is the heaviness with obscure sight, said to be worse by any effort to see.

Myrica Cerifera. Heaviness in back of head. Pain, right side.

Nabalus. Occipital pains, probably muscular, with pain and feeling of stiffness in nucha and in trapezoid regions, < turning head.

Naja Tripud. Dull pain shooting up the occiput.

Fronto-temporal headaches are characteristic of this remedy; but the prover who exeperienced the above occipital pains, also had tired feeling in cervical and dorsal vertebræ with the peculiar burning of exhaustion. The two, then, may belong to spinal irritation.

Natrum Arsen. Feeling of pressure over each side of posterior and inferior part of occiput as from a photographer's head-rest.

Natrum Carbonicum. Painful sense of emptiness in occiput, with weakness and hoarseness of voice. Pain from occiput to vertex. Tension. Dull pain. Drawing and tension in right side of occiput as if they would draw the head back. Long continued pressure in right side of occiput. Dull pressure; also from occiput to nape with drawing pain, at last extending to forehead, with vertigo, eructations and dim vision. Headache at noon, < low down in occiput. Headache and tension in nape before menses.

Natrum Muriaticum. Head dull, with throbbing in occiput. Heaviness and pressure. Heaviness in occiput with pulsation and stiffness in nape, a feeling of constriction in occiput behind ear, with stitches in head. Pressure; also in nape. * Stitches as with knives in the occiput. Transient stitch from nape into occiput. Throbbing. Lying on back, feels drawing from forehead to occiput, feels almost as if losing her senses. Sticking, from forehead to occiput, taking away appetite. Stitches between right occipital protuberance and styloid process.

Natrum Sulphuratum. Wandering pains in occiput and head, afterwards in zygomata. Boring pain. Drawing and pressive pain in occiput with feeling of heat and heaviness in it. Pressive or squeezing pain in whole occiput. Pressing from both sides of occiput followed by quiet night; in morning returned, and then extended all over right side of face. Tearing and pressure in right side of occiput. Tearing in occiput, soon afterwards in forehead.

Clinical for *Natrum Mur.* is heaviness in back of head, it draws eyes together; < morning, warmth, motion; > sitting, lying, or perspiring.

Niccolum. Heaviness. Painful boring and gnawing, < left side. Feeling of fullness and heaviness in head, feels as if cut to pieces, on stooping; in occiput sensation as if beaten and sore, and a stupefied feeling in head generally.

Nitri Spiritus Dulcis. Heat. Pressure. Heaviness with heat.

Nitric Acid. Violent sticking pain in right side of head and in occiput, even sore to touch. Transient headache in occiput after slight exertion, especially in thinking. Pressive bruised pain. Pain like that from mercury. Stitches in both occipital protuberances to lower jaw. Violent stitches in left side of occiput during breakfast, so that head is drawn back and respiration impeded. Violent stitches suddenly in right side of occiput evening; afterwards another kind of violent headache, both > > on going to sleep. Throbbing.

Neuralgia, periosteal and bone pains, mercurial or syphilitic, need this acid; especially when in addition to above there are sensitiveness to rattling of wagons, to touch or to pressure of hat. Bones of skull feeling constricted by a tape.

Nitro-muriatic Acid. On rising, 7 A.M., feels as if brain was all in occiput, making it feel heavy; food slow in digesting.

To be remembered in dyspepsia.

Nitrogenium Oxygenatum. Headache and aching along spine, as if they were asleep. Numb feeling in head and all over, followed by semi-consciousness; she falls backwards; open air postpones spells.

An observation I made several years ago. I think the drug should be tried in hysterical fainting and perhaps in *la petit mal*.

Nux Moschata. Pressure between vertex and occiput. Pressure in left side of occiput towards nape. Pressure in right side of head, in part above ear, in part at right angle of occiput as from pressure inward on bone.

Nux Vomica. * Aching pain in occiput, morning, just after rising. Headache in occiput at time of menses as from ulcer in brain and as if suppurating; < lying down. Drawing posteriorly as if chilly. Pressure in occiput outward from both sides as if skull there was forced asunder, with heat in brain, > momentarily by pressure of hands. * Violent jerking or dull stitches in left hemisphere of brain from orbits towards parietal bone and occiput, soon after eating. * Drawing pain, first in temples, then in forehead, then in occiput. Pain in occiput as if brain was knocked forwards.

Clinically: o Intense occipital headache; dizzy; pains in eyes; stomach deranged. o Sensation as from a bruise in back part of head.

Characteristics are the starred symptoms; and also sensation as if skull would burst. The integuments are intensely sore as if bruised. Hair on occiput seems painful.

Oleander. Sharp pressive pain externally in left side of occiput. Dull pressure in a small spot in occiput. Tensive stitch in occipital bone.

Oleum Animale. Pressure from vertex towards occiput. Tearing and sticking in upper part of right side of head, leaves and goes to right side of occiput. Tension of occipital muscles. Blood seems to rush into occiput on going into house. Pressure from occiput forward, one hour after dinner. Pressure in left side of occiput, must hold head forward, continues even on moving head, lasting from one hour after dinner till 6 P.M. Gnawing pain in occipital region less on left side. Boring pain in small spot on left side of occiput. Sharp stitches.

Opium. Occiput feels like lead, head falls backward. Dullness and confusion becoming pressive sensation extending forward over orbit and backward to nape. Pressive, at times, throbbing headache from behind forward along median line. Pain, pressing outward in right frontal eminence, preventing writing; later felt in occiput; $>>$ rubbing with hand and pressure. Very painful headache, involving occiput.

Occipital pains, etc., are not very distinctive of *Opium* and its alkaloids.

Osmium. Fullness and aching at upper and back of head, $<$ throwing head back (second day). Occipital headache continued (sixth day).

Oxalic Acid. Cutting from right side of forehead, behind ear, down to insertion of sterno-mastoid.

Pain along base of occipital bone. Pain pressing invariably between vertex and occiput on a spot.

This pain in a "spot" is very characteristic. It is more often noticed in forehead.

Pæonia. Heaviness. Pressure. Pressive pain in occiput and nape.

Paris Quadrifolia. Pressure. Intermitent drawing in muscles of right side of occiput. Tension in skin of forehead and occiput as if adherent. Meninges and brain feel tense, with tensive sensation in occiput as if skin was thicker and could not be wrinkled. Sensation as if dura mater were drawn tight, < in occiput.

Two conditions are characteristic: sensation as if head was very large, and, this tightly drawn feeling. Most marked is the latter through eye to mid-brain, but it also occurs in the occiput.

Petroleum. * Heaviness like lead. * Pressure and sticking pressure, morning. * Pinching. * Pulsation when lying upon it. Pressing, stinging, in cerebellum.

Clinically determined: ºOccipital headache, spasms, screaming; loss of appetite, constipation. ºPain from occiput over head to forehead and eyes; blindness, losses consciousness.

Throbbing and pulsating in occiput is most characteristic, indicating the remedy in many ailments.

Phellandrium. Distressing, intermitting pressure. Burning, constrictive sensation. Pressive dullness. Dull headache, < in occiput. Painful tearing. Slight burrowing in left occiput. Sharp stitches in right side of occiput. Sensation of heaviness as if head would be drawn backwards to nape. Hot orgasm from occiput to vertex and slight dull stitch left side of vertex, a quarter of an hour after dinner.

Headache "like a heavy weight on vertex, with aching and burning in temples and above eyes, pain in eyes, congested conjuctivæ," has yielded to this plant. Quite like it will be useful when, as in the symptom, the heaviness weighs occiput-ward.

Phosphoric Acid. Pinching, tearing pressure in occiput, < noise or least motion. Painful pressure outward in right side of occiput. Tearing in vertex and occiput. Pressure as if lying on something hard; as from hard body, > rubbing. Pressive pain in occiput in part extending forward, < pressure and turning head. Heaviness and pressing forward in occiput on bending forward, >> bending back. Headache in occiput, must lie down. Drawing in occipital bones. Bruised pain at insertion of cervical muscles. Digging boring right of occiput. Hard pressure above left temple, to occiput; dread of motion.

Clinically: º Occipital headache and pain in nape from nerve exhaustion.

Phosphorus. Dull pain, fever and flushed face. Pain in back of head and left side of head. Heaviness in occiput and nape; also with pressive pain in occiput. Occiput and nape stiff and painful. Transient pressive pain, as if in bone in side of occiput. Sticking, then pressure followed by throbbing in forehead. Stitches. Pulsation in occiput on rising. Throbbing in occiput and in vertex. Stitches, at times burning, in frontal region, in vertex, sides extending into left side of occiput; sense as if pulled by hair. Neuralgic pain, 10 A.M. as if head was drawn forward by a weight, face feels full as if too full of blood, as after intense study; with drawing in left side of occiput.

I have cured with this remedy, º rush of blood to head, seeming to come up the spine and thence into head. It suits long-standing congestions, with stinging in occiput and pulsations there and in whole head; < mental work, brain fag, etc. It has also relieved o cold sensation in cerebellum; brain feels stiff.

Physostigma. Tired sensation in cerebellum. Shooting pains through right side of head down into back part of neck, < rising or walking. Severe pain in mastoids.

Phytolacca. Severe general headache, but < part of time in temples, with slight vertigo, and part of time, < in occiput; < walking or riding. Dull bruised pain.

Pimpinella. Rushing in head, < down back part with pressure, that is increased by the rushing. Pressive and pushing from temples to occiput and into nape. Headache, < in occiput and nape. Sensation of coldness in occiput as from sharp draft, in a closed room. Sensation of tension and pressive pain in occiput into nape. Constant dull, pressive pain. Pain < reading so that thought is difficult. Acute stitches in occiput, concentrated about protuberances. Tension and sticking in nape of neck and occiput.

Piper Methysticum. Dullness, fullness and pressure in forehead. Vertigo on elevating or moving head to either side; after dinner, pain shifted to lateral and occipital regions, and on lying increased, though not enough to constitute real pain; was apprehensive of pain by rapid movement but none followed, felt impelled to move cautiously, as if something there that would not admit of rapid movement. Front of head as if solid with pain, this gradually moves to base of brain and along medulla oblongata; > slight motion; < active motion; slight mental effort, passing from topic to topic relieves, though sustained effort increases pain; lying with head elevated resting bend forward on cushion, frontal pain better but occipital pain. < Vessels of neck and base of brain full as if circulation had been cut off by a cord, back of head and cerebellum and neck felt congested to the brain and cord-centre, sore inside and tender outside to pressure; all these parts felt double or treble their size. After business anxieties, evening, pain along under forehead outward to sides, after retiring, passed to posterior of brain, medulla, cerebellum, etc., as if compressed by an even pressure, especially from front to back; constriction extended to chest and stomach; nervous system in high tension; > while moving.

The essential characteristic here seems to be that the pains are relieved by temporarily turning the mind to another light topic.

Picric Acid. Dull pain in right side of lower occipital region, comes and goes gradually; also with sensation as of a band along right parietal eminence. Dull, heavy, throbbing and burning pains from occiput forward to supra-orbital foramen and thence to eyes, which throb and feel sore to touch. Pain in lower right occipital region as if cerebellum was loose, keeps throbbing, < walking, > sitting quiet. Heavy pain in occipital region down neck and spine. Fullness and heaviness of head, developing into intense throbbing pain in left side of head, < eyeball and forehead, extending back to occipital region; > keeping quiet, < motion, << going upstairs. Fullness and heaviness of head, disinclined to mental or physical work, becoming throbbing headache, < left eye and occipital region, << going upstairs, which causes intense throbbing in eyeball.

Zincum Picricum. Dull, heavy, drawing, occipital headache. Periodic.

These two remedies are invaluable in serious cerebral and spinal affections. They cure headache from brain-fag, from sexual excesses. The latter especially relieves headache accompanying morbus Brightii.

Plantago Major. Dull boring. Dull pain, passing off quickly. Headache morning, < back of head. Pain all around back of head, cannot rest head five minutes in one place. Dull stupefying pain in sinciput, finally extending to each side of occiput. While walking and driving in cool air, pain in left side of head from over left eye back toward occiput. Twinges now in right temple extending backward, then through occiput from ear to ear, then in other parts of head.

Both the major and minor are good in neuralgia. The major is excellent when either ears or teeth are involved; back head particularly with ear pains, caused by catching cold.

Plectranthus Fructicosus. Drawing pain in right frontal eminence, returning on walking out of doors, < pressure of hand, afterwards it suddenly disappears and reappears as a drawing in occiput towards nape, > > here going into open air. Pressive pain and tension in occiput, nape and cervical muscles, across scapulæ and down arms. Pressive pain in occiput, < lying on back, must often change position, 4 A.M. on waking. Pain at 6-40 A.M. on waking extended to sinciput and from eyebrows into upper lids, which are raised with difficulty; drawing pain in occiput so bad in evening that it disturbs work; must get up and walk about the room, which affords transient relief. Drawing < out doors, > > in house.

Plumbum. Sense of heaviness in occiput, as if its weight was increased. Violent headache in occiput to ears and temples; dull pressive pain commencing while asleep; often arose and walked about holding the head until relieved. Headache in occiput extending to forehead. Dull pain in occiput from spine upwards. Pressure forward and feeling as if eyes would close from heaviness, >> on standing up. Violent stitches. Severe pain in head, especially in occiput.

Invaluable in chronic headaches, congestive, with occipital heaviness; or, violent, agonising from behind forward, > walking and pressure of hands.

Prunus Spinosa. *Shooting like lightning through brain from right side of forehead coming out at occiput. Violent nervous pain in left side of occiput takes away thought. Pressive pain outwards. Pressive sore pain in occiput forward into some of the teeth.

Crushing and sharp pain are very characteristic.

Psorinum. Like a cord tied firmly around skin, < about occiput, which feels as if pressed outward. Pressing pain, right side of occiput as if strained.

Clicinally: ○ Pain in occiput as if a piece of wood was lying there.

Ptelea Trifoliata. Headache in occiput, passing to frontal region over eyes. Heaviness in occiput with gloomy feeling in forehead. Headache seems more in cerebellum. Severe pains in forehead and occiput.

Pulsatilla Nuttalliana. Hot, full, feeling in cerebellum.

Pulsatilla Pratensis. Drawing headache above nape in morning. Pressive, tearing, pain in left side of occiput, morning. Pressive pain in occiput, with frequent heat of body and constant sweat. Rhythmical throbbing in occiput. Tearing in left side of occiput. Stitches from occiput through ears; also < lying down, >> on rising. Violent pulsation in the left side of occiput, externally.

Excellent in congestive occipital headaches, with throbbing, > pressure. Pains of gastric origin or in conjunction with spinal congestion I cured promptly with this drug. º Throbbing in occiput, in a patient who had chills suppressed by quinine.

Its occipital headache extending into ears is similar to Plantago.

Ranunculus Bulbosus. Pain in occiput after slight chagrin, morning. Drawing sticking. Violent tearing in evening in left side of occiput as far as nape, afterwards along lower jaw from behind forward. Transitory (beating?) pain while sitting, in left side of occiput, with general debility. Subdued, soft beats, not like pulsations, but at long intervals in the left side of occiput. Violent tearing in the right temple, preceded by vertigo in occiput when walking, as if he would fall. On entering a room from open air, suddenly there is aching in temples and in nape; with this there is vertigo apparently from deep in brain.

Ranunculus Scleratus. Dull pain in occiput, the whole head feeling painful externally. Pressing pain in both inferior tuberc. ossis capitis, >> when pressed upon.

The bulbosus affects the circulation in the occiput causing vertigo. Mental emotions such as chagrin, cause pain in occiput, and also trembling of limbs. He has turns of weakness, seemingly from the head, feels as if senses would vanish. Vitality is lowered by this drug. It is useful, too, for inebriates.

Further, it is indicated, in rheumatic patients, who are < in every change of temperature.

Raphanus. Dull pain in occiput, > throwing head back. Headache, morning and evening < in occiput. Head easily fatigued. Headache, morning, < in occiput; when she presses hand on occiput pain become general. Finger upon middle of occiput causes shudderings in back, chest and arms with loss of thought; there is sensation as if a sheet of water was before the eyes. Pain in occiput causing an uneasiness or fatigue. Drawing pain behind head and in neck. Gnawing followed by numbness. Violent headache in the forehead and occiput in the morning.

Ratanhia. Tearing from occiput up to vertex. Violent tearing in nape while walking, extending forward into forehead. Heaviness in the head.

Tension as if skin was tight here and there seems important.

Rheum. Pressive headache, then tearing, extending into occiput.

Rhododendron. Aching sore pain in right hemisphere and in cerebellum while sitting. Dull pain early in morning. Aching deep in right occiput, with paroxysmal drawing from below upwards. Dull pressure deep in the occiput in evening. Pain in right side of occiput as if a foreign body was forced in. Contusive pain in a small place on right side of occiput with alternate drawing in the direction of ear.

Rhus Radicans. Pain at the right hemisphere of cerebellum after intellectual labour, 11-30 A.M.; same place and over right eye at eye-brow. Dull pain in right side of occiput, with constipation: also awaking, morning. Pressive pain in left side of occiput. * Pain in head and nape. * Pain in occiput and neck. Feeling of crowding upward at occiput. Pain in occiput on awaking. Semi-lateral pain at right side of occiput. Dull pain in occiput and neck, $<$ bending head forward. Headache in occiput, with feeling of weakness in head and inability to exert much the body or the mind.

Rhus Toxicodendron. On opening eyes after sleep sudden violent headache in the forehead behind eyes as if brain was torn to pieces; as after intoxication by brandy; < moving eyes, then in occiput as if cerebellum was bruised, with a pressing outward in temples. * Headache in occiput disappearing on bending backward. Single jerks in occiput. Drawing in occiput and temples with pressure in eyes, driving him from bed. Burning pain, at times in occiput and at times in forehead.

Rhus Venenata. Tearing in right temple, from forehead up to left half of head, in bone; thence to left side of occiput and down the nape. Throbbing and tearing from each temple back to the occiput and down neck to the shoulders, with flushes of heat. Jerk-like headache in the occiput.

Clinically, *Rhus Radicans* leads the list, followed in importance by the *Rhus Toxico*. *Rhus Glabra* also has cured occipital headache.

Clinically: º *Rhus Tox.* presents terrible headaches from the occiput forward; must move about continually, which relieves somewhat.

Rhus Tox. cures occipital headaches after mind and body are worn out with hard work, in typhoid states, etc. But *Rhus Radicans* is more certain to relieve pains in this region, even, as has been shown by Drs. Korndoerfer and Middleton, in typhoid. The pains º commence in back of neck; and spread up and over the entire head or remain in occiput. The muscles are sore to touch. In rheumatic cases, particularly, the pains are worse during rest and in cold and are better in warmth and from motion.

Closely allied is *Juglans Cathartica* proved and confirmed by Dr. Jacob Jeanes; there are terrible pains in the occipital region. A single dose is all that is usually needed to effect relief.

Rumex Crispus. Dull aching pain low in occiput, which comes and goes. Pungent tingling pain in left side of occiput; headache in forehead; similar pain in left nostril and a feeling as if coryza would ensue. Headache until he sleeps, returning on waking, < in temples. Pain is felt in occiput.

Ruta Graveolens. Pressure. Heaviness and tension. Beating and pressive pain.

Sabadilla. Pressure in occiput from behind forward with reeling sensation. Headache as if something was thrust from upper part of occiput through brain to forehead. Pain in left side of occiput as if a wound was violently pressed. Headache as if a thread had been drawn from middle of forehead to occiput above temples, leaving a burning sensation. Hard pressure from both temples towards vertex and thence to lowest part of occiput.

The reeling sensation and the thread-like feeling are the characteristics. *Croton Tiglium* has something similar: º Feeling as of a string pulling from eyes to back of head.

Sabina. Heaviness of occiput and nape down to small of back. Pressive heaviness in occiput, painful < by strong pressure upon hard cushion. Sensation as if a sharp wind penetrated the left side of occiput. Pressive, tearing pain externally in left side of occipital bone in a curve, as far as left side of frontal, < when touched. Tearing in the whole of the right hemisphere from occiput to forehead. Drawing first in forehead and afterwards in occiput.

Sambucus Nigra. Tearing stitch through left of occiput, with dull sensation in same place.

Sanguinaria. Moderate pain in back of head and neck, gradually down to renal region, where it is very severe, dull and heavy.

Clinically, º the sick headache begins in the occiput and spreads over the head, < over right eye.

Saponium. Dull heavy sensation in head, < over left eye; eyeball aches and feels sore; spreads thence running back to occiput; great heat in frontal region, > by cold and by pressure, < stooping.

Sarsaparilla. Stinging pain in left side of occiput. Twitching in left side of occiput. Pressing in forehead and occiput. Strong pressure in right temple, with drawing stitches from occiput to forehead.

Clinically, º pain from occiput, darting forward to eyes. This is a clear deduction from the symptoms. Dr. Neidhard has confirmed this. Here it compares with *Spigelia, Puls.* and *Sep.*

Secale Cornutum. Dull headache in occiput. Severe pain. Pressive pain. Lightning like pain in occiput down nape.

Selenium. Great heaviness, at times waving in brain, fluttering in ears, twitches and pressure in eyeballs. Pressure in occiput and vertigo on standing. Drawing in occiput, with ringing in ears and stoppage.

Senecio Aureus. Giddy, like a wave from occiput to sinciput. Suddenly dizzy while walking in street, feeling like a wave from occiput to sinciput.

Senega. Pain in occiput afterwards to temples and finally affecting whole head. Aching, stupefying pains in occiput. *Aching in head, in sinciput and occiput; < sitting in warm room; accompanied with pressure in eyes, which will not bear touch; it comes daily.

This last is interesting in connection with the well-known eye symptoms.

Sepia. Stitching pain in head, coming up the back at every step. *Occasionally pains from left eye over side of head towards occiput, > after meals, < mental labour. * Drawing pain externally on forehead back to occiput. Severe pain, head feeling like a soft bladder; intensely hot and covered with wheals. Pain involves the occiput; causing nearly raving or loathing of life. Stitches in left side of head in the afternoon, and in occiput in evening. Heaviness, < in the morning. Dullness of the left side of the occiput. Awoke with a dull feeling in the back of head, down spine, passed off an hour after rising. Headache comes on with heat and gets better with it, but does not leave; it is as if occiput was opening and shutting, > by cold water and open air, < bending head down. Pressive pain as if on something sore. Drawing pain, when touched feels like subcutaneous ulceration. Tearing. Pains run down back of head. Pain in occiput < at night and when lying on it, as if hollow and ulcerated, > pressure with hand. Severe stitches extending towards vertex.

Clinically, °pulsating pain in the cerebellum, beginning in the morning, lasting till noon or evening; < least motion, when turning eyes, or when lying on back: >lying on side, when closing eyes, at rest and in dark.

Serpentaria. Pain in frontal region and in right side of occiput. Sticking in forehead extending to base of brain.

Silicea. * Pressive pain in occiput, > warm wrapping of head. * Pressure soon followed by stitches in forehead, with chillness in nape and back. Tearing in right side of head from occiput upward and forward. Tearing in right temple, after half an hour, in occiput. * Tearing in whole head from occipital protuberance forward and upward over both sides of head. * Headache as if from neck rising up to vertex. Pains alternating in different parts of head, for an hour in sinciput, then in whole head; tearing in right temple also in occiput, later in left temple. Cold kind of headache from nape to vertex. * Attacks of vertigo seem to rise painfully from back through nape to head; inclined to fall forward; knows not where she is.

Two symptoms are markedly characteristic: the direction of the vertigo and of the headache, and the relief from wrapping up the head warmly. Useful for over-worked brains, for nervous persons who are made worse by even normal and ordinary stimulation of functions.

Spigelia. Occiput heavy, drags like a weight. Pain as from a blow. As though an artery was beating against an obstacle. Cannot lie on occiput, it is painful; painful as if ulcerated, with, at times, dull sticking, jerking, penetrating deeply. Violent pains in occiput and nape, 3 or 4 A.M., seems stiff, in the morning could not move head till after he was up and dressed. Boring in occiput and vertex, as if drawing head back. * Burrowing and burrowing-tearing pain in occiput, left side of vertex and in forehead, $<$ on motion, from loud sounds, opening mouth even slightly; most tolerable loud sounds, opening mouth even slightly; most tolerable while lying. * Violent jerks in occiput and then in temples, on every step, while walking in open air. Violent pressure inward left side of occiput, unless presses hand hard on spot. Intolerable bubbling pain in occiput, $<<$ at first on walking, afterwards $<<$ by slightest motion, $>$ while leaning back sitting, $<$ lying horizontally. Intermittent drawing in cervical muscles and in occiput.

Invaluable in neuralgia from occiput forward, especially on left side of head over and into left eyeball. Pains may be boring, tearing, burning, stitching, stabbing, or throbbing.

Spongia Tosta. Painful heaviness as if a lead were in it while walking; paroxysmal. Heaviness and stitch in the afternoon, when turning head; face, hands and feet hot, rest of body chilly; inclined to coryza; body weak, mouth bitter; shaking chill in evening, then heat, except in thighs, which are numb and chilly. Pressing pain in left side of occiput, as if it would burst. Fine pressive stitches, now in forehead, now in occiput only on motion, with sensation of burning heat from behind ear over occiput to nape.

Its characteristics are heaviness and numbness in the thighs.

Scilla. Sudden transient drawing pain in occiput from left to right. Tearing pain. Long-lasting drawing and sticking while sitting.

Stannum. General heaviness $<$ in the occiput. Painful pressing in brain towards vertex and occiput, in evening, also after lying down. Painful, almost constant sense of weight on occiput; also heaviness with boring in occipital bones. Pressure outward in left side of occiput. Pressive tearing in left of occipital bone. Constrictive pain in right of occiput. Transient tearing, in forehead, top of head and occiput, afterwards shifting, generally $<$ in forehead.

Excellent in debilitated persons, who get tired easily when talking; empty feeling in chest; occiput feels heavy, not from compression but from occipital fullness and outward pressure. Very important is: Pains increase slowly, and as slowly decrease.

Staphisagria. Occiput feels as if compressed internally and externally. Heavy, pressing-asunder pain in occiput while walking in open air. Painful drawing on and beneath occiput persistent on every motion of the head. Transient burning stitches in occiput, right to left later below upward. Heaviness in head and weakness in cervical muscles, must lean head to side or backwards. Pressure in head, < in occiput, towards bones of skull, before going to bed, continuing after lying down. A tense pain in left side of neck and occiput, only at night; waking him; can lie on either side.

Clinically, º occiput feels as if hollow or as if brain was not large enough for the space.

Most characteristic of *Staphisagria* is the sensation of a heavy ball in forehead; but in some cases it is needed when there is heaviness and weakness in muscles referable to occiput and neck, or compression in occiput, caused or aggravated by sexual abuse, over-use of mercury or during convalescence, particularly too, if the peevishness of the remedy is present.

Stillingia. Sharp drawing pain in right occipital protuberance. Constant flowing pain, from median line of forehead to occipital process and left of cerebellum. Sharp darting in sinciput extending to occiput.

Suggestive of pains in mercurio-syphilitic cases, especially of bone pains.

Stramonium. Pain in occiput, during sudden pain over left eye. Occasional, sometimes throbbing, pains right or left side of occiput.

Strontium Carbonicum. Dull pain. Pressive pain. Violent compressing pain in middle of occiput. Violent boring pain in small spot in right side of occiput. Tearing in right side of occiput. Thrusts like stitches in vertex and occiput. Back and small of back as if beaten, < stooping, < removing back from sun-heat; pain extended from small of back over hips; as this disappeared, there are pressive headache, now in sinciput, now in occiput.

Suggestive are the back and head pains. The drug also causes violent palpitation and suffocation at night; must spring up out of bed. Diarrhœa.

Strychninum. Dull pains in back of head and temples. Pressure, with nausea. Constant pain in occiput and nape. Boring. Pains in occiput and down whole length of spine. Sharp pains extending to left eye and to back of right ear. Sharp pains in back of head and in glands of neck. Darting in back, and top of head. Head jerked backwards. Violent pains through head from back to front. Violent pains in head and in muscles of back of neck in the morning.

When the back is almost tetanically stiff, and there are darting, violent pains from occiput forward, *Strychnine* is more sure to relieve.

Sulphur. Weight and hot feeling in the morning. Aching, heavy feeling in the morning, after getting up, extending into nape. Sudden, aching, tension in left side of occiput. Stupefying pain or tingling in occiput, from noon on; must sit quietly. * Pain as from congestion on left side of occiput, after waking. Aching, drawing in forenoon; in occiput and nape. Drawing in occiput, violent while chewing. * Pressive pain, at night. Burning aching as if beneath the occipital bone. * Pulsating in left side of occiput, changing to jerking. Awoke, 5 A.M., aching throbbing in right side of occiput, pain in left side of small of back. Aching in vertex, and slight drawing in occiput after dinner, > open air; most aching is in vertex.

Clinically, º empty sensation in occiput, < in open air and after talking.

One of the best remedies in congestive headaches, general symptoms agreeing. Also in debility from loss of animal fluids, severe study, etc.

Sulphuric Acid. Compressive pain in sides of occiput > even holding hands towards head. Pressure, sticking in left side of occiput. Sticking, now in forehead and now in occiput.

Sumbul. Uneasiness, in cerebellum, painful, with stiffness of adjoining muscles, on moving head; uneasiness, heat, lightness, ebullitions of blood, chiefly in forehead and cerebellum. Occasional shooting from left cerebellum to left forehead. Uneasiness, dizziness, fullness and heat in cerebellum, extending to cord, < in sunbeams. Oppression in forehead and dull constriction over head, < from forehead to occiput.

Suggestive in ebullitions of blood and pains, especially in nervous persons who have violent, strong beating of the heart.

Tabacum. Stitches from forehead to occiput, >> lying down and pressure.

Taraxacum. * Pressure and heaviness in occiput after lying down. * Tearing pain, while walking. Heaviness, > stooping, < errect.

Clinically, °violent tearing in occiput in typhoid. Very useful in "bilious dyspeptics," bitter taste, nausea as after fat, mapped tongue, and pains in legs, > moving.

Tarantula Hispanica. Pain to posterior part of head. Pains as if hammer blows in occiput to temples. Intense pain, burning thirst. Pain in occiput as from a nail driven in. Compressive pains in posterior part of head, extending towards neck (relieved by *Acon.*). Headache, deep, restless, must change place often, pain flies to forehead and to occiput, photophobia. Pains in occiput, < inclining head backwards.

Characteristic is headache in occiput, compelling to rest head against pillow; restless, anxious, hysterical. Compare *Agaricus* and *Ignatia*.

Tellurium. Confusion, < towards occiput. Numb sensation in occiput and nape.

Thea. Tensive pain, almost as low as nape. Neuralgic pain and feeling of damp coldness in occiput; sharp, electric shocks in right occipital protuberance; thence slowly to nape, right shoulder and arm, > warm cloth or hand.. Neuralgic pain in nape; both sides of base of cerebellum like a cold flat-iron, pains extending up over cranium and down forehead to eyes, with excruciating suffering.

Characteristics are sick headaches in nervous, delicate women; palpitation; nausea. Pains in left ovary (like *Naja*).

Thuja. Sensation of heaviness in occiput. Spot near left occipital protuberance feels painful when lying on it, or even hair is painful. Drawing tension. Fullness and pressure when walking in open air. Tension in occiput, painful, from ear to ear. Jerking, tearing, < in right side of occiput. Tearing in occipital protuberance and in petrous portion of temporal bone for six weeks. Stitches in occiput. Stitches in brain from occipital foramen upwards. Painful stitch through occiput from above downward. Drawing pain, < left frontal eminence thence to posterior of left eyeball, thence at times to occiput. Drawing from head over nape to sacral region. Dull stitches from eyeball to occiput. Violent tearing stitch through right side of brain from occiput to forehead. Bruised and tearing sensation from forehead to occiput on waking from sleep, disappearing after sleeping again. Pressing headache on vertex and occiput, with sensation of lead in it, < false step, moving head; brain feels loose.

It is interesting to note that clavus occurs in the *Thuja* provings almost in all localities, save only the occiput. Practically *Thuja* is the best drug we have for neuralgia going from before backwards; thus the converse of *Spigelia*, which it in other respects resembles.

Theridion. °Violent frontal headache, with throbbing extending into the occiput. Its concomitants are nausea, worse from the sun, and a peculiar sensitiveness to noises; they make the nausea worse, and penetrate through the teeth.

Tilia Europea. Heaviness as from an in-seated weight; when head inclined forward weight seems to sink lower down in nape. Peculiar aching in occiput extending upwards towards back of head, after dinner. Pressure outward at mastoid process. Pressure and burrowing pain. Drawing in occiput into head and into forehead where it becomes a pressure.

Tongo. Confusion < occiput, somnolence and a sort of intoxication. Sharp dartings in the upper part of right parietal through head, coming out below occiput. Compressive headache, external sensitiveness, morning. Tearing from right side of occiput through head to a frequently painful tooth.

Upas. Boring in the frontal eminence and in the left occipital protuberance. Painful heaviness, with throbbing synchronous with pulse. Pressing inward pain in occiput.

Uranium Nitrate. Aching at the occipital protuberance. Occipital and frontal headache. Occipital headache when he awoke.

Valeriana. Pressure and drawing penetrating into side of occiput (from vapor). As from hammering internally in occiput, so intolerable he forcibly turns head to and fro.

Veratrum Album. Tension in occiput and forehead; also with sticking pain deep in occiput.

Veratrum Viride. Frontal headache back on left side to occiput, < lying, < < lying on occiput. On waking, indescribable sensation rising from forehead towards crown and grasping as it were vertex and occiput.

Clinical: ° Headache from nape, with vertigo, dim vision, dilated pupils. ° Congestion of brain and spine. ° Cerebrospinal meningitis. ° Muscles of neck contracted drawing head backwards; violent convulsions.

Viburnum Opulus. Neck stiff, with pain in occiput. Dull headache, < over eyes at times goes to occiput, < when delayed menses should appear.

Zincum. Acute heaviness. Pressing asunder pain in right of occiput. Drawing in occiput, with gnawing in forehead. Painful gnawing on right occipital protuberance as from a mouse. Bruised pain. Beating as of waves, feeling of heat in a spot on right side of occiput up to vertex. Tearing, with dull stitches on top of head. Tearing in right side of occiput when laughing. Boring in right side of head, < in occiput. * Vertigo in whole brain, < in occiput as if he would fall over, or to the left while walking.

Zincum Phosphoratum. Severe frontal headache, stabs of pain from before to occiput, but intracranial.

Clinical: *Zincum;* ° Internal, semilateral, headaches. There are pain in sinciput or in occiput, < from wine, in warm room, and after eating.

Zinc is a precious remedy in chronic headaches, deep-seated, maddening pains, with trembling hands or

DRUGS AFFECTING THE OCCIPITAL REGION 155

with fidgety feet. It is also useful in anæmia of brain and spine from over-work, loss of fluids, undeveloped or imperfectly cured exanthemata, etc. The characteristic vertigo is present, as may be, also, tearing pains. Wine aggravates.

The *Phosphide of Zinc* has a short proving, but even this justifies the clinical use of the drug in occipital headaches of a neuralgic character, but of evident central origin: stabs from before to occiput. (See also *Picrate of Zinc*, above.)

Zizia Aurea. Dull pains in occiput down muscles of neck.

A single symptom, but as it is in a prover who developed the characteristic choreic symptoms, it may be of value.

Symptoms characteristic, clinical or deductive are arranged in the form of a Repertory.

Congestion, etc.: ACONITE, head drawn back. *Æsculus Hip.*, spine weak, hæmorrhoidal hyperæmia. Æthusa wants to bend back; colic, green stools, spasms; vomiting. *Agaricus*, chorea or cerebro-spinal irritation; boring head in pillow. *Ailanth.*, confused dizzy; beating in occipital arteries. Alcohol, apoplectic fullness, face dark red, muscles of neck give out. ALOES pulsating; with abdominal plethora. Amyl Nitrite. *Ant. Tart.*, heaviness, difficult breathing, drowsiness, nausea. Apis, Asterias, º Baryta Sul., BELLAD., < bending back or lying. Borax, throbbing; rush of blood. *Bovista*, ptosis, drowsy, head feels very large. *Bryonia*, forehead to occiput, < motion. CACTUS GRANDIFLORUS, with band-like compression; with inco-ordination and sore pressure, > from mental or bodily exercise. CALC. C., chronic. *Calc. Phos.*, school girls. CAMPHOR, throbbing, < sun. CANN. INDICA, surging, throbbing; stunning pain, he feels, uræmic case, convulsions; errors in recognition of time and space, both are magnified; delirium. CARBO AN., throbbing; heaviness, confusion, < cold, > after dinner; feels weary. Cedron. CIMIC. *Conium,* pain with every pulse as if pierced. *Crotalus,. Digitalin,* confusion, pulsation, > walking in the open air. Dirca Palustris. FERRUM, hammering, coming up neck; feet cold, fingers stiff; mind confused. GELSEM., occiput over head; sight dim; drowsy; face suffused. GLONOINE. Hamam., dull throb. Indigo, throb, stitches; melancholy. Kali C., Laches., *Lycop.,* after stoops. Lycopus, fronto-occipital pains, congestion; heart-symptoms. Mancinella, hammering head and nape < stooping. Mitchella. Melilotus, *Natr. Mur.,* NUX VOM., hæmorrhoidal, abdominal plethora, < in the morning, skull bones as if would burst. Oleum Animale, Opium, PETROLEUM, pulsations, º even spasms; accompaniment of scrofulous ophthalmia, eczema, diarrhœa, etc., etc., PHOSPH., rush of blood up spine into head, < sun, < summer. *Piper Methysticum,* > light mental work or *diversion of mind.* PICRIC ACID, throbbing, << going upstairs. ZINCUM PICRIC. *Plumb.,* chronic, agonising pains from behind forward, > walking and pressure of hand. PULSAT., throbbing, caused by gastric or uterine derangement, <º after quinine. Ran. Bulb., RHUS TOX., RHUS RAD., SEPIA, º pulsation, < motion, etc. SULPHUR, abdominal plethora, chronic cases. Sumbul, ebullitions; violent heart-beat. º Theridion. Upas. º *Verat. Viride.*

Ice-like sensation: CALC. CARB., CALC. PHOS.

Coldness: ºChelid., Kali Nitric., ºPhos. (brain stiff), Pimpinella, Silicea.

Feeling of damp coldness: Thea.

Crawling: * *Cal. Phos.,* Dulcam.

DRUGS AFFECTING THE OCCIPITAL REGION

Heaviness: Weight: Feeling of lead: Agaric., Aurum Mur. Natro., Bryonia, Bar. Acetica, * *Bellad.,* Bism., Bovista, *Calc. Carb., Cactus,* CARBO. A., CARBO. VEG. (confused as after debauch), *Cham.,* CHELID., *Colch., Coloc.,* Con., Dulc., Graphites, Helleb., Kali C., Kali Iod., Kreos., * LACHES. (leaden), LACTUCA (but more tensive heaviness), Lauroc., *Lycop.,* Mag. Mur., Mephitis, Mitchella, MUR. AC. (obscure sight), Myrica, *Natr. Mur.* (draws eyes together), Niccol., Nitr. Spiri. Dulcis, Nitro-Muriatic Ac. (as if brain all in occiput; slow digestion), NUX VOM., Opium, Pæonia, * PETROLEUM, Phellandrium (vertex weighing down), Phos., *Phos. Ac.,* PICRIC AC., ZINC. PIC., *Plumb.,* * Psorin. (like wood there), Ptelea, Ruta, Rhus Tox., Sabina Saponin, Selen. *Sepia,* Spigelia, Spong, Stan, SULPH., * *Tarax.*, *Thuja,* Tilia, Upas, Zinc.

Mental overwork: Brain Fag: *Coca,* COLCHIC. (nausea, bitter taste, etc.), PHOS ACID (ºoccipital headache, pain in the nape), CALC. PHOS., PHOSPH., PICRIC ACID, Piper Methysti. (busines anxieties, pressure and congestion front to back), ZINC. PICRIC., *Natr. Mur.,* Raphanus, *Rhus Rad., Rhus Tox.,* * SEPIA, Silicea, SULPH., *Zinc., Zinc. Phos.*

Better concentrating mind: Helon.

Thinking: Writing: Reading, etc.: Nitric Ac., Pimpinella, Piper Meth. (intently or steadily), RHUS RAD. (occiput aches, weak, unable to exert mind or body), *Rhus Tox.*

Inco-ordination: Cactus, Ginseng.

Pains come and go suddenly: Asterias, *Argen. Nitr.,* BELLAD., Merc. Corros. (go suddenly).

Pains come and go gradually: Picric Ac., STANN.

Occiput seems to open and shut: º*Coccul.,* Sepia.

Anæmia: Graph. (neck stiff, spine sensitive < seventh cervical vertebra), Cimic., Ferrum, Kali Carb. (stiff neck < swallowing food), *Mangan.,* Zinc.

Rheumatism: Actæa Spicata, Cimic., * *Baryta C.* (glands swollen) Calc. Carb., Calc. Phos., Caust. (< cold, dry air), Dulc., Kali Bich., Lycop., Nux V., Ran. Bulb. (< changes of temperature), Rhus Rad., Rhus Tox.

Summer Heat: Sun <; Acon., *Camph.,* Bellad., Bryon., *Gelsem.,* Glon., *Theridion.*

Damp Weather: Dulc., *Brom.* (bone pains), Bar. C., Calc. Carb., Calc. Phos.

Touch > : Dirca Palustris.

Tight Bandage < : Calc. Carb.

Jarring: º Ferrum < coughing, * Glonoin., Mag. Sul. (dare not cough), * Nitr. Ac.

Pressure >: Diosc., *Bry.,* * Castoreum, Hydras, Nux Vom., *Plumb.,* Ran. Scele., Sabina.

Rubbing > : Phos. Ac., Tarent.

Vertigo from occiput: Calc. Phos., Coca, Cann., Ind., Carbo Veg., Cimic., Digit., Gelsemin, Ginseng, Hydroc. Ac., Mag. Mur., Ran Bulb., Sabadilla, Senecio, * Silicea, Zinc, Merc. Corros. (with tearing in occiput), º *Nux Vom.* (dizzy, intense occipital headache, eyes pain, stomach deranged), Selenium (pressure in occiput and vertigo on standing), º Verat V.

Head drawn back: Acon., Æthus., * Belladonna, Cereus Bon., Castoreum (as if would be; *better pressing spot*), Ginseng (bends back involuntarily), * Glon., Kali Cyan., Lactuca Virosa (as if would be) Mag. Carb., Natr. Car. (as if would be), Nitric Ac. (with stitches in left side of occiput), *Phellandrium,* Nux Vom., Strychnine, º *Verat. V.*

Head falls back: Bufo, Kali C., *Mur. Ac.* (from heaviness), Staphis.

Semi-conscious, etc.: Oxygen. Nitrogen., head and spine numb, falls backwards; hysteria.

As if would lose senses: Natr. Mur., Ran. Bulb.

Confusion, etc.: Ambra, Ailanth. (dull heavy), Ammoniac., Calc. Phos., *Carbo Veg.* (as after intoxication), Carb. Sulph. (intoxication), Digitalin, Digit., º Ferrum, *Hydroc. Ac.,* Kali Chloric., Lycop.

Pain takes away thought: Prunus.

Pains, Neuralgia, Bone and Periosteal Pains.

Tearing: Acon., *Ars.,* * *Aurum,* Berber., Bovista (and in lower jaw), Colchic. (Eyeballs to occiput), *Kali* Nitric., Magnesia Mur., MERCURIES in general (see Periosteum); Ranun. Bulbo. (preceded by vertigo in occiput), Rhus Ven. (from each temple back to occiput and down neck to shoulders), Sabina (pressive tearing), * Silicea (occiput forward), * *Spigelia* (burrowing-tearing), * *Tarax* (< in typhoid fever).

Sharp: Flying: Stitching: Neuralgic: ACON., CIMIC., BELL., BRY., *Cedron* (periodic, but even if not in ague, nervous persons, etc.) CHAM. (excitable, pains unbearable), * *Chelid.* (violent, back and forth, vertex to neck), CHINA (ague; < least touch, > pressure, unbearable), *Chin. Sulph.* (periodic), * *Conium* (pain at every pulse as if pierced with a knife), Diosc. (sharp, twisting pain > rubbing) * GELSEM. (sharp, occiput over head, pupils large, face suffused, ptosis), *Mag. Mur., Mag. Phos.,* Mangan., Naja (dull shoots up the occiput, spinal irritation), *Natr. Mur.* (* stitches as with knives in the occiput), *Phosph., Plantago Maj.*

(especially when there is toothache or earache), *Prunus Spinosa* (shooting, lighting-like forehead through to occiput), * Juglans Cathartica (severe pains in occiput), Sang. (º occiput to over right eye, nausea, vomiting, etc), * Sepia (shoot up < noise, > sleep), º Thuja (converse direction to Spig., which latter goes from behind forward).

Boring: Agaric., * *Coloc.* (> pressure), Equisetum, * *Mezer.*, Moschus (here and there in head), Natrum Sulph., Oleum An., Phos. Ac., Plantago Maj., Stann., Stron., Strychnine, Upas.

Burrowing: * Spigelia.

Digging: * Arg. Nitr.

Empty sensation in occiput: Helleb., Mangan., Natr. Carb., º Staphis (feels hollow), º Sulph.

Occiput as if loose: Picric Ac.

Jerking: * *Bell.*, Cann. Ind., Kali Nitric., * Nux-Vom. (orbit towards occiput), * Spigelia (occiput and then in temples), * Sulph.

Spasms: Bufo, Absinth., Acon., Bell., *Cann. Ind.* (even Uræmic), º Caust., º Gelsem., º *Petrol.* (and occipital headache), º *Verat. V.*

Pressure: Pressive. Alum. Ambra, Angus., * Arg. Met. (Arn.) Baryta Acetica (pressing asunder), Bell. Bism., Bovista, * *Bry.*, Can. Indi. (before convulsions), * Carbo Veg., Caust., Cham., * *China* (deep in brain), Coca, *Colchic.* (deep in cerebellum from least literary work), Conium, Digit., Hydroc. Acidum (with confusion), Lycop., Natr. Carb. (occiput to nape, at last to forehead, vertigo, eructations, dim vision), Nux. Vom. (* < morning; also as if skull was bursting), *Oxalic. Acid* (inward on * small spot), * Petrol., Phos. Ac. (outward; also as if on hard board, > rubbing), Pimpinella (and pushing temples to occiput and nape), Piper Methysticum, Ran.Scele. (>> pressing), Selen. (and vertigo), * SILICEA (> warm wrapping), Stann. (heaviness and outward pressure in occiput), * Sulph., * Tarax.

Sinking down sensation in cerebellum, etc.: Elaps, Tilia.

Pressure. Compression: Band; Tape: Tightness: Constriction: Like a Vise: Amm. Mur., ANAC. (also pressure as from a plug), Arg. N., Asafœt., CACT., Cereus (band, etc.), * Camph. (contractive pain in occiput and root of nose), Carb. Sulph. (band-like compression; terrible headache, intoxication or paralytic weakness), Coca (ear to ear in vise), Coccus (band from mastoid to mastoid), * GRAPH. (as if constricted in occiput), Kali Nitricum, Lactuca Virosa, Mercur. Sol. (constrictive), Natr. Sul. (pressive, squeezing in whole occiput).

Stiffness: Rigidity: Agar., Argen. Met., * GLON. (stiff neck as if clothing tight), GRAPH., Kali Nitric., Spigelia.

Drawing: Agaric., Ambra, Ammoniac., * Carbo Veg. (from nape into head then hammering, mind confused), Caust., * Chelid., Equiset., * Ferrum (nape to head, >> pressure of hand, then hammering, mind confused), Mangan. (pressure of hand), Moschus (occiput to ears, then to teeth), Natr. Mur. (forehead to occiput), Puls., * Sepia.

Tension: Angus., Asarum (* scalp), * Chelid., * Lycop. (nape and occiput while writing), Murex (tightness, > bending head back), Nat. Carb., Paris (as if in skin and in meninges), Pimpinella, Ratanhia (tension here and there as if skin was too tight), Thea, Thuja (from ear to ear).

Eyes affected: Cimicif., Eryngium Aquat, GELS., Lactic Ac. (tendency to close eyes), ALOES (must close eyes, heavy), MUR. ACID, *Natr. Mur.*, Senega, Bovista (lids inclined to fall), Eryngium Aquat. (blurring), Fagop. (eyes pain), Ginseng (gray spots, dizzy in occiput), Lactic Ac., Merc. Sol. (eyes water), Natr. Carb., Raphanus (like sheet of water before eyes; occiput feels fatigued), Saponin. (left eye feels sore), Selen., Tarent. (photophobia), ºVerat. V. (dim vision).

Pulse slow: *Hydrocyanic Ac.,* Lauroc., Lycopod., Gelsem., Opium.

Dragging: Eryngium.

Bones: Periosteum: *Merc. Iod., Mer. Bin. Iod., Merc. Corros., Merc. Sol., Merc. Praec. Ruber* (all these mercuries; *Merc. Iod.* with coated base of tongue; *Merc. Corros.* scalp very sore, pains leave suddenly; *Merc. Sol.,* º tearing from side of head to temple, < night in heat of bed, sweat, and no relief; *Merc. Praec. Rub.* ºleaden heaviness in occiput). * MEZER. (boring < night, < abuse of mercury), NITRIC AC. (mercurial syphilitic, <least jar, as rattling of wagons, also pressure of hat; bones as if constricted with nape), Stillingia (ºmercurio-syphilitic cases).

Extending from neck to occiput: Nat. Mur., Kali C., Kalmia (up into head), Diosc. (back of neck to back of head and to occiput and to shoulders), Dulc., * *Ferrum,* Flour. Ac. * GLONOINE, Helleb. (nape to vertex).

From the whole head to occiput: Fagopyrum (dull pain in eyes, aching, tired neck), * *Piper Meth.* (> diverting mind).

From above eyes to occiput: Bism., Cimic., Colchic., * NUX VOM. (orbit to occiput), * *Sepia,* * THUJA (excellent in neuralgia).

DRUGS AFFECTING THE OCCIPITAL REGION

From temples to occiput: Cinnab., Iris Vers., Kali Bich., Lycopus. (cardiac depression), Rhus Ven.

From the forehead to occiput: BRY., * Cann. Sat., Cantharis (deep stitches), Cimic., Chin. Sul., Coccus, Equiset., Eup. Perf., Lilium Tig., * Nux Vom. (temples, then forehead, then occiput), Plantago Maj., Prunus, Sabad. (like thread from forehead to occiput), Sabina (drawing), * Sepia, o Theridion.

From front over head to occiput: * CIMIC.

From vertex to neck: * Chelid. (and vice versa), Gelsem.

From crown to occiput: Cinnab.

From sacrum to occiput: Cann. Ind. (hot iron).

From neck to shoulders: Kali Nitric.

From nape to vertex: * Silicea (headache; also cold headache).

Extending from Occiput.

To forehead: China, Merc. Sol., Moschus T. Conium, Bovista, Mur. Ac., * Carbo Veg., Dirca, Kali Bich. (after nasal discharge, Jaborandi, * GELS., Kali C. (like something sinking), Mur. Ac., Sabadilla through brain to forehead; reeling sensation), Sabina, o SARS., Senecio, Tarent.

To Temple: Menisperm., Coca. (reading), * Spig.

To Vertex: Mag. Mur., Natr. Carb., Digit., Lactic Acid, Lycop. (shock), Phellandrium, Ratan.

To Head: Merc. Sol.

To Jaw: Kali Chlor., Bar. Acet., Nitric Acid.

To Nape of Neck: * Bry, Kali C., Kali Nit. Lauroc., Mur. Ac., Pimpinella, Ran. Bulb. (then along jaw forward), Sabina (and down the whole spine).

Down Neck: Arg. Nit., Comoclad., Hydroc. Ac., Mangan (to fifth vertebra), Tarent.

To shoulders: *Bry., Diosc., Gelsem., Ipecac., Kali C., Kali Nit.

Down Spine: Æthusa, Sang (to renal region and there <), Sepia, Strychin., Thuja.

To Ears: Colchic., Puls., Plantago, Strychnine.

To Eyes: Eryngium. Aquati., * Spigelia (< over and in left eye), Strychnine.

Forward: Oleum An., º Rhus Tox. (must move about continually, which relieves), º Rhus Radi. (< cold, > motion).

* Pain in head and nape, or in occiput and nape: Rhus Rad.

DISCUSSION.

Dr. Van Artsdalen: For vertigo in the occipital region I have found *Baptisia* to cover almost the same symptoms as those given for *Petroleum.* If the pain runs from occiput through to the eyes, *Agaricus* is the remedy. *Bovista* has drowsiness, reflex from the stomach, and transverse half sightedness. In brain-fag, *Phosphoric Acid* is useful.

Dr. Guernsey: I think with Dr. Martin that cases of poisoning by matches should not be included in our provings of *Phosphorous,* for we must, in such cases, get a combination of *Sulphur* with the *Phosphorus.* I am glad that the repertory of remedies for occipital pain has been prepared, for we have long needed it. I would mention the use of *Coca* for brain-fag, taken as a drink. It is given to athletes to enable them to withstand fatigue, and its use is not followed by depression. It is also used as an antidote to alcohol. I believe that we do get symptoms from the provings of higher potencies and that we get the finer shades of the provings without any of the effects of the crude drugs.

Dr. James: I have had some experience with *Coca*. In one case of a lady suffering from nervous depression I gave a malt preparation, but it only served to increase her sufferings. I then obtained the fluid extract of *Coca* and putting ten or twenty drops in a half glass of water, let her sip it as she would a glass of water. I brought her up much better than alcoholic stimulants had ever done, and it had no bad effects. I have used it after cases of exhausting diseases, as typhoid fever, etc., and find it much better than alcohol.

Dr. J. B. McClelland: There was a remedy mentioned by Prof. Farrington in his Lectures on Materia Medica, for the occipital headache, that I have not heard spoken of to-day, and that is *Juglans Cinerea*.

Dr. Farrington: That was mentioned as *Juglans Cathartica,* which is the same thing. Dr. Guernsey is right in regard to *Coca*. Dr. Van Artsdalen spoke of some remedies that are included in the paper. As I only gave an abstract of the paper, I have not mentioned all the remedies given.

REMEDIES IN NEURASTHENIA AFFECTING THE LUMBO-SACRAL REGION

IT is quite natural that neurasthenia should manifest itself in those portions of the nervous system that are most vulnerable. And since the lumbo-sacral region is less fully supplied with blood than other parts, it suffers more from the consequence of nervous exhaustion.

Another reason why the small of the back is subject to numerous symptoms of disease, is because of its relation to several important organs, as well as to the functions of the lower extremities. Abdominal plethora, with consequent hæmorrhoidal fullness, favours passive congestion of the lower spinal vessels; and a similar vascular relaxation often accompanies affections of the female genital organs. Sexual excess very naturally exhausts, first of all, those spinal centres which have to do with the genitals. And long or severe exercise of the legs induces backache and weakness in the lumbar region.

Still another factor in the interesting symptomatology of this region is fatigue from strain; as after lifting heavy loads, after violent gymnastic exercise, etc. The ligaments and muscles are overtaxed, and with them often the spinal cord itself. From this factor arise many symptoms common in scrofulous children, who suffer from spinal curvature. It also accounts for the prevalence of lumbago in persons of a weak nervous system.

Symptoms of the lumbo-sacral region may be considered under various heads, according to the particular nerves affected. The *filum terminale* ends at the first or second lumbar vertebra; below this point nerves go to the various tissues from the lower part of the gluteal region to the feet. Hence, here is included nervous control of the flexors, and extensors, and abductors and adductors of the lower limbs, of the anal and vesical sphincters, and of the genitalia.

We will take *Nux Vomica* as a typical remedy, and consider others in connection with it.

Nux Vom. is eminently suited to backache accompanying abdominal plethora, with piles, constipation and urging to urinate. Pain as if beaten or bruised. Pains worse at night; the patient must sit up in order to turn over from side to side. Back worse at 3 or 4 P.M.

Allopathic physicians hesitate to employ *Nux* if there is any spinal congestion, since they believe it may cause irreparable mischief (Hammond). But if the universal characteristic of the drug is present, we, who depend solely upon molecular action, can administer the remedy regardless of the status of the blood vessels.

This universal characteristic is in harmonious action with the various functions of the body.

If we apply this to the symptoms accompanying lumbar neurasthenia, we find: Stiffness of the legs, with tottering gait; trembling to the limbs, with sudden sensation of loss of power. Tension in the calves. Convulsive jerks of the legs. Ineffectual urging to micturition and to defecation not from atony, but from irregular, inco-ordinate action or from spasmodic constriction. If paralysis obtains, it is ever associated with evidences of irritation, such as violent jerks, great debility, but with over-sensitiveness to external impressions. All this arises from the well-known fact that *Strychnine* increases reflex excitability.

Phosphorus, in many respects, is very similar to *Nux Vom.,* but increases impressionability. Both cause spinal anæmia. But *Phosphorous* tends to a complete paralysis. *Nux* generally to an incomplete paralysis, depending upon exhaustion, though both have proved useful in spinal softening.

Phosphorus causes: Nervous sensitiveness with weakness, most severe in the lower portion of the spine, in the region of the last lumber vertebra and in the sacrum (very common seats of neurasthenia).

Every trifling fatigue, or the carrying of even a light bundle, causes pains in the back. Pain at the union of the sacrum and last vertebra; worse while standing, with numbness of the feet when pressing on the last two lumbar vertebræ. Small of the back weak and as if asleep. Burning also, in small spots; better from rubbing. Back pains as if broken.

Legs feel weak; feel as heavy as lead, with numbness, trembling and coldness. Numbness increased by every exertion. Awkward, stumbling gait, not from clumsiness, but from sheer weakness.

Urination involuntary; passes during coughing or if the inclination is not immediately attended to. A similar weakness of the anal sphincter; stool involuntary the moment fæcal matter enters the rectum. Involuntary passages on the least motion, as though the anus stood open.

Sphincter weakness is not a common accompaniment of neurasthenia, but in some cases it exists, and is manifested by slight prolapsus recti during stool, and by some dribbling after micturition. *Phosphorus*, then, stands as it were in the border-line between spinal weakness and organic spinal disease. Dr. Hammond has observed involuntary urination as a precursor of locomotor ataxia, manifesting the disease long before the appearance of any of the ataxic symptoms. It behoves us to remember this clinical fact, and to strive to cure all sphincter relaxations with the hope that we may be warding off incurable organic lesions.

Dribbling after micturition is found under: *Agaricus, Selen., Helon., Graph., Silica, Calc. Car., Natrum Mur., Picric Acid, Petroleum, Conium, Kali Carb., Cannab. Indica, Arg. Nitr., Staphisagria.*

Selenium is suitable to neurasthenia from sexual excess, with dribbling of prostatic fluid and also of semen, both at stool, the latter also during sleep.

Helonias applies excellently to neurasthenia when the lumbo-sacral region is weak and feels tired. Burning and aching. Feeling of numbness in the legs; numb feet while sitting. Feels tired all over, but better from motion or when the mind is occupied.

Graphites is neglected in spinal disease. It is applicable to both sexes, to the male with impotence, to the female who, though obese, is really anæmic, with profuse leucorrhoea and weak back, and with delayed, scanty menses. The limbs go to sleep readily, and walking is difficult from muscular weakness. Sudden sinking of strength. Throbbing of the blood vessels; rush of blood to the chest and head, but not from true plethora. The blood is watery and contains a relative preponderance of white corpuscles. Vertigo to falling, and faintness, in the morning. Spinal anæmia, with pain, mostly noticed in the cervical region, but also noticeable in the lumbar region. The patient is cold from want of animal heat, and suffers from flatulency, as under all the carbons, and also from a herpetic, rough, rhagadic skin; eruptions oozing a sticky moisture.

Natrum Muriaticum, in its first effect stimulates the nervous system, causing muscular contractions very much like those induced by galvanism. It also increases the red-corpuscles, glandular secretion, digestion, etc. It is from this stimulating action that salt is so effective when applied locally with friction to weak muscles, etc. Later, however, *Natrum Mur.* exhausts the nerves, diminishes glandular activity, and develops asthenia and anæmia with emaciation. The skin is dry, harsh and sallow; mucous membranes are dry, cracked and glazed, with smarting and rawness, or with scanty, corroding discharges. Great complaints are made that the mouth is dry, when in reality the annoyance arises from the stickiness of the secretions; they are not normally fluid.

Now, from this atonic effect of salt, we observe spinal neurasthenia. The small of the back feels paralyzed, especially in the morning, on arising. Back feels as if broken. Legs weak, trembling; worse in the morning. Feet heavy as lead. With all this, it may readily occur that the bladder becomes weak: troublesome dribbling of urine after a normal stool. And we may admit this vesical symptom as a concomitant of spinal weakness, even though the prover had no such association, because such a combination is quite in keeping with the genius of the remedy. We may regard both spinal and cystic atony as a part of a general tendency in salt to produce exhaustion, hence not as a symptom of paralysis, but rather of neurasthenia.

Picric Acid is a new claimant for recognition in spinal affections. Studied in its relation to the localities we are considering we find that it causes heavy, dull pain in the small of the back; aching, extending into the legs; dragging sensation; tiredness; weak feeling in lumbar and sacral regions with excessive languor. Then, too, the legs are weak and heavy.

The prover who recorded dribbling of urine after micturition, suffered from a general tiredness from the least exertion; the mind was dull, so that he could read but little; mental work prostrated him. He suffered from occipital headache, throbbing in the cerebellum. In fact nearly all his head symptoms were occipital. He refers to morning erection, recurring on four successive days. His symptoms, then are just what we would expect from congestion of the spine; and they constitute a group worthy of consideration in the precursory stage of locomotor ataxia to which Dr. Hammond refers. The tendency of the *Picric Acid* disease is rather to softening than to sclerosis. But if, as Dr. Hammond surmises, the involuntary micturition which precedes tabes is due to congestion, why should not *Picric Acid* act in such a contingency?

Pulsatilla is neglected in neurasthenia of men. It causes sensation in the back as if it was tightly bandaged—a very characteristic symptom, which may be mistaken for the girdle of myelitis. It means simply an irritation of the posterior nerves, not inflammation. There is, too, in the *Pulsatilla* case, a peculiar sensation, aptly compared to a sense of subcutaneous ulceration. It is a sort of smarting.

Accompanying the backache is a general fatigue with heavy, tired aching, not relieved by repose. The patient feels weary in the morning, vying with *Nux*. Such a condition of the nervous system may be produced by dyspepsia, or by excess in venery.

The general condition of the patient is one of relaxation, with poor blood, defective animal heat and diminished motility. *Pulsatilla,* in large doses, at first excites the heart and circulation and then weakens the cardiac walls and relaxes the veins. Engorgements and varicosities follow; and hence the patient, despite his chilliness, is oppressed in a warm room. Autopsies on poisoned animals showed hyperæmia of the spinal meninges—not an active congestion but a passive fullness of lax vessels. Hence arise numbness, crawling, going to sleep of the limbs, feeble heart's action, etc.

As a "venous remedy", *Pulsatilla* is nearly related to *Hamamelis*—a drug much abused by the laity and much neglected by the profession. It causes dull backache, weakness of the limbs, with going to sleep of various parts of the body, and great languor. Seminal emissions give rise to dull pains in the loins and increase the weariness. If there are present, enlarged veins or soreness in the course of the bloodvessels, the choice of *Hamamelis* is certain.

Sepia is another drug resembling *Pulsatilla*. It relaxes the tissues and favours stasis. The patient complains of aching in the lumbar region. Sense of subcutaneous ulceration. Soreness and pain in the sacral region. Dull heavy aching from sacrum to thighs. Weakness in the small of the back. Limbs go to sleep. Numbness after manual labour (like *Phosphorus*). Sensation as if drops came from the bladder after urinating. Atony of rectum of bladder, urging even for papescent stool; urine is tardy in beginning to flow.

And here we may mention *Sulphur,* which has caused paraplegia from spinal congestion. It produces violent bruised pain in the small of the back, down to the coccyx; weakness formication; legs weak, numb, paralytic. Sudden violent jerks of the limbs as the patient falls off to sleep—a symptom of organic spinal affections, but also present in so-called functional disease. Abdominal plethora, hæmorrhoids, etc., very much like *Nux* and *Sepia*.

But in pure nervous weakness, we may expect good results from such remedies as the following:—

Dioscorea, excellent when weak back and weak knees follow seminal loss. *Calcarea* follows well. And

Kobalt is a good substitute if the backache is markedly worse while the patient is sitting.

Nymphæa Odorata claims attention for weak lumbar region with weak bladder and weak legs.

Zinc has backache worse when sitting and from long walks. Legs weak, trembling; hungry at 11 A.M. with increase of spinal weakness. Small of the back weak while walking. Muscular twitchings. Wine increases the pains and the nervous weakness. Violent pain in the small of the back when walking, steadily relieved by continuing to walk. Drawing in the back.

Æsculus Glabra and **Æsculus Hippocastanum**, both cause paralytic weakness. The latter induces hyperæmia, with numbness, prickling, tingling, great sacro-lumbar pain; and especially a paralytic weakness of the symphyses, making locomotion difficult or impossible. It may be that the *Æsculus* patient must display also irritation of the mucous membranes, catarrh, gastric disturbances and symptoms of piles. But nervous symptoms, in Dr. Burt's provings at least, were the first to appear.

This symptom of the symphysis calls to mind a much profounder remedy than *Æsculus*. We refer to *Argentum Nitri*. Silver Nitrate impresses the nervous system most profoundly. At first, it irritates the sensory nerves and increases reflex excitability somewhat like *Strychnia;* but soon paretic symptoms appear, characterized by vertigo, unsteady gait, trembling, headache, etc. His legs feel weak as after a long journey. The legs jerk during sleep. Pains in the small of the back, relieved when standing or walking. The lumbar region feels rigid, as if put on the stretch; paralytic heaviness. Sacral region so painful that blowing or sneezing makes him start. Backache on rising but not on walking. Symphyses weak, loose, as if they would give way.

Inco-ordination is present, even in non-tabetic cases. In a restless, nervous state, he fails to judge of distances, and dodges projecting signs, etc. This is due in part also to the dizziness, which is constant. He staggers in the dark or when the eyes are closed. He is depressed in mind, gloomy, even to thoughts of suicide. He suffers from dull frontal headache, with nausea, irritations and burning in the stomach, with great prostration and restlessness. The heart beats irregularly with a faint feeling in the præcordia. Emotions increase the palpitation.

In other cases, somewhat akin to those suggesting silver, *Arsenic* is the remedy. We must not neglect *Arsenic* in neuroses. Its irritating effects are noticed in nervous as well as in other tissues. There are loss of strength in the small of the back; pain as if bruised; aching. Starting of the limbs when falling asleep. Legs uneasy, he cannot lie still, reminding us of the fidgetiness of *Zinc*. Legs weak. Feet feel fuzzy, numb and cold; Distressing general weakness disproportionately severe. *Arsenic* affects especially the lower portion of the spine.

This fuzziness suggests another drug, *Alumina*. Pain through the lower vertebræ as from the thrust of a hot iron. Bruised pain. Legs heavy, he can scarcely drag them; when walking he staggers. Nates go to sleep while sitting. Tension in legs. Numbness of the heel on stepping upon the foot. Heaviness of the feet. Soles pain, when stepping upon them, as though they were soft and swollen.

Rectum inactive as if paralyzed. Urine passes when urging to stool—a very unphysiological condition, but very characteristic of the remedy.

Bonninghausen cured several cases of undoubted locomotor ataxia with *Aluminium*. But the drug is also applicable to neurasthenia. Dr. T. F. Allen records cures with *Alumina*. His patients were tired, drowsy, with unconquerable disposition to lie down. Impaired co-ordination. Loss of contractile power of the bowel, with lack of secretion and tendency to rupture of the hæmorrhoidal vessels. Weak bladder. Fulminatory pains. Sudden jerks and starts from sleep.

Cocculus Indicus causes paralytic pain in the small of the back, with spasmodic drawing across the hips, preventing walking. Knees sink under him from weakness. The soles of the feet go to sleep while he sits, with sticking as from pins. Attacks of paralytic weakness, with pains in the back.

There is in *Cocculus* a peculiar combination of convulsive irritability with paralytic weakness, eminently qualifying the remedy for neurasthenia. Like *Strychnine* its active principle *Pictrotoxine,* causes tetanic spasms. But respiration is accelerated by the latter, not from spasm of the respiratory muscles only, but by spasm of the glottis and there is not the same over-susceptibility to touch in the two poisons. In the *Cocculus,* spasms tend more directly to paralysis than in *Strychnine;* and we observe a speedily developed relaxation of tissues as shown in the the empty, gone feeling in all the splanchnic cavities.

We find *Cocculus* needed, then, when any loss of sleep, any drain on the mental powers, or any loss of fluids, leads to speedy nervous exhaustion, combined with irritability. Thus, though sleepy, he is so nervous and weak that he cannot calm his brain. Though very tired, he is too restless to keep still.

Gelsemium is a priceless boon, the introduction of which is mainly due to the provings made by Dr. J. C. Morgan.

It causes dull pain in the lumbar and sacral regions. Weak back. Loss of muscular control, ending in complete motor paralysis. Every little exertion causes fatigue of the legs, with muscular soreness. The patient is languid, listless and drowsy.

In protracted sleeplessness from nervous exhaustion, it disputes the honors with *Cocculus*.

The various preparations of *Peruvian Bark*, though almost universally abused, nevertheless are of inestimable value in anæmia with spinal irritation or exhaustion. No remedy equals *China* in weak back from loss of animal fluids, especially in rapid or excessive loss. With the weakness are usually evidences of over-sensitiveness; excessive tenderness of the surface, making the least touch unendurable; senses morbidly acute; restless and fidgety despite the tiredness and exhaustion.

Chininum Arsenicosum caused a pressure in the "solar plexus" (usually felt only after eating tough meat or hard nuts, of which, however, the prover had not eaten) extending to the back, where it changed to a pinching sensation; spine painfully sensitive to touch at this point. Heart as if it had stopped; no perception of its beating. Legs weary.

This "solar pressure" compares with the well-known *China* pressure, and seems like a genuine symptom. The weak heart is a very common accompaniment of neurasthenia.

Chininum Sulphuricum, according to the confirmed provings of Otto Piper, causes as excellent picture of neurasthenia: Despondency. Aversion to mental labour. Mental confusion. Lustreless eyes; dim vision; sensitive to the glare of light. Noises in the ears. Sickly expression. Oppression of the epigastrium from flatus; abbdomen distended. Difficult stool from inertia. Urine contained phosphates. Sexual depression. Oppression of the chest with tenderness of third dorsal vertebra. Sticking in the apex of the heart. Sensitiveness of the last cervical and first dorsal vertebræ; dorsal most sensitive during the chill; limbs weak, feel bruised, feel numb and trembling on slight exertion. Sensation during stool as if drops of fluid passed from right hand to shoulder. Emaciation. Weak and dull after a siesta. Excessive general sensitiveness of the body. Sleep unrefreshing. Sleepless. Chill, with tender dorsal spine. Heat of the face.

The only evidence that the drug causes sensitiveness of the lumbar vertebræ is contained in the remark by the prover that during chill the dorsal vertebræ are more sensitive than either the cervical or the lumbar.

Finally, the sort of pain experienced is some times of importance. The pains of neurasthenia simulate those of ataxia, but are transient, usually less severe, and referred to the lumbo-sacral region only. *Ipomoea* helps, especially when they provoke nausea; *Sulphur* when there are transverse stitches; *Natrum Mur.* with cutting through the back; *Zinc,* cutting down into the legs; *Sepia* pains go around like *Pulsatilla, Berberis,* etc., or down the thighs; *Gelsemium* when there is severe pain extending into the hips. Bruised sensation is common to nearly all. Tension is marked in *Zinc, Nux Vom., Sulphur, Natrum Mur.* and *Valerian;* while sensation of a band is very characteristic of *Pulsatilla.*

The lumbar spine is sensitive in *Phosphorus, Agaricus, Bryonia, Lycopod., Pulsatilla, Sepia, Arsenic, Aluminia.*

Those who suffer from lumbar weakness should avoid tea, as it tends to increase the disease.

ANTIPSORICS IN THE ATROPHY OF INFANTS

THE following collection of symptoms is the result of a protracted study of a case which cost the writer many anxious hours. Failing by carefully selected remedies to even relieve the patient, it was determined to sift our materia medica as thoroughly as time and other engagements would permit, in order to find whether any antipsoric or deep-acting drug could be found suitable to the case.

This fact will explain the lack of complete system in the paper, and also the defective relation existing between the first and second parts, the latter containing some symptoms and additional drugs not found in the former. These defects there was not time to correct.

In arranging the symptoms the writer has not restricted himself to the pathogenesis of genuine atrophy, the tabes mesenterica, which is essentially tubercular, but has included symptoms of rachitis, scrofula, and simple indigestion, with attending marasmus.

In several instances, however, especially in the repertory, mention is made of symptoms known to be characteristic of some one or other of the diseases included under the general term atrophy. But in so doing the writer by no means wishes it to be inferred that he would teach that therapeutics is dependent upon pathology. The latter helps him in obtaining his "totatilty", abridges his phraseology (as, for example, when he writes scorbutic sore mouth—*Mercurius*—meaning thereby all the well-known buccal symptoms of that remedy), and acquaints him with the unmodified course of disease. But when he has his case well-understood, the symptoms, subjective and objective, must be submitted to the rules of Homœopathy, not to the restrictions of so general a science as that of pathology.

If omissions are noticed, let it be the pleasure of each one to mention them. If the paper does but call forth a healthy criticism, it will fulfil a useful purpose, and save some one hours of labour, and mayhap a mother her darling child.

PART I.

ANTIPSORICS IN THE TREATMENT OF ATROPHY OF INFANTS

Sulphur is characterized by emaciation; the skin is dry, harsh and wrinkled, giving the child an "old-man" look. The body has an offensive odor, not removable by washing. Eruptions are chiefly eczema capitis, generally dry, easily bleeding; itching more at night; scratching relieves, but causes bleeding; excoriations; intertrigo, especially at the anus.

Glands swollen, particularly the cervical, axillary and inguinal.

Appetite voracious; child eagerly grasps at everything within reach and thrusts it into its mouth.

Abdomen distended and hard. Constipation or diarrhœa; the stools are slimy, green, watery and changeable; worse at night; sudden urging awakens him in the morning followed by copious watery stools.

If hydrocephaloid sets in, the child lies in a stupor, its face pale, lower jaw dropped, eyes half-open, and forehead covered with cold sweat. The urine is suppressed and there are frequent muscular twitches.

In less severe cases the child is restless at night; sleeps in "cat-naps"; awakens often screaming, or on going to sleep is annoyed by sudden jerking up of the limbs. At other times an almost unbroken fever obtains, the skin for days remaining dry and hot.

The child is cross, obstinate; cannot bear to be washed or bathed. Its face is pale, sunken, with deep and hollow eyes. Dentition is slow; muscles and bones develop very tardily, so that a year-old child looks scarcely larger than a new-born babe. Complains of fatigue every little while; sits bent forward, refuses to stand long, but crawls or runs about.

Calcarea Carbonica is very similar. The emaciation is more marked in other than adipose tissue. There are atrophy of muscle, soft bones, retarded teeth, all evidences of defective nutrition, and yet an excess of fat gives a deceptive appearance of plump health. When wasting shows itself in fat too, the body dwindles, the pale skin hangs in folds, but the abdomen seems to remain disproportionately enlarged. Partial sweats are more prominent than in *Sulph*. The scalp is covered with a cold sweat; the knees are clammy; the feet feel damp and cold. The eruptions, especially crusta lactea, develop on the face, or quickly spread thence; crusts are dry or yield a mild thick pus. At times they appear isolated and look like chalky masses. Again the eruption forms in rings or spreads like ringworm. The child's scalp seems thin, blue veins show distinctly, and the little one scratches its head on awakening.

The glands are engorged, particularly the mesenteric.

Appetite is voracious, yet emaciation persists. Morbid appetite for indigestible articles of food. The child is thirsty and feverish every afternoon. The stools are green, watery, sour, or pungent, or clay-like, and worse in the afternoon; or again creamy, fetid, frequent; urine strong, fetid, clear.

If hydrocephaloid sets in, the child is hot and dry or bathed in cold sweat. The fontanelles are open and sunken, the face is pale and pinched, the child frequently scratches at its head; cries as if hurt when lifted from the cradle. The stools are white and slimy, and the urine is clear, but very strong-smelling, fetid, and is passed with difficulty.

Vomiting is very marked in both remedies, but in the *Lime* it is principally sour food or lumps of curdled milk; in the *Sulphur* it is sour, watery, fetid. The differences are only in degree, curdled milk more frequently calling for the Lime.

The child is obstinate, self-willed, cross before stool and faint after. Its face is pale, bloated or sunken and emaciated, looking like a tiny doll. At other times it is more like *Sulph.*, old and wrinkled and cold. Growth is retarded; the child, though old enough, will not put its feet to the ground. Spine seems weak, it sits stooped. The legs are often curved, and the bones can be bent quite readily. While the *Sulphur* child dreads washing, the *Calcarea* patient has less dread, but is made worse by bathing.

Calcarea Phos. has numerous similarities with both the foregoing. It is distinguished by the following:

complexion is sallow; the whole child is emaciated and poorly developed; the posterior fontanelle is also very large, showing greater nutritive defect than in the Carbonate. The abdomen is shrunken and flabby. The stool is watery, hot; or green, slimy; passed with much offensive flatus. The child is attacked with pain so soon as it eats. When lifted, breathes short, has an anxious look.

If hydrocephaloid ensues, the child is exhausted and limp, its slender neck refuses to support the head, while the fingers are all skin and bones. The child craves food, is greedy, like *Sulph.,* and *Calc. C.,* but while the latter longs for eggs, the *Calc. Phos.* craves salt meat, bacon, etc.

Calcarea Iod. is to be preferred to other lime salts when the child, though looking plump and healthy, shows well defined scrofulosis, with thick scabby eruptions, otorrhœa and engorged glands and enlarged tonsils.

Hepar necessarily resembles both *Sulphur* and *Lime.* Under an apparent plumpness, the attentive physician detects that the flesh is flabby, the muscles withered and digestion weak. The child is intolerant of pressure about the stomach after eating. Food seems to temporarily relieve the debility. If the child were old enough, he would describe the feelings as one of invigoration, like a stimulant in the stomach. The stools are green, watery, undigested, or white, sour-smelling and painless, and worse during the day.

There is but little tendency to cerebral symptoms. The glands are swollen, and the child is subject to catarrhs from the least draught of cool air. In dry, cold, windy weather, croup develops. It has eczema, which is worse in the morning, when it itches, burns and smarts.

Silicea again changes the picture. The whole body is wasted, while the head is exceedingly large. The face is earthy or waxy-pale and the bones are diseased. Pain in the sternum and lumbar spine; rachitis. The eruptions are prone to ulcerate or suppurate. Small pricks or cuts fester. The toe-nails fester and grow into the flesh. The crusta lactea is moist, oozing, and is worse from scratching. The appetite is often lost, with an especial aversion to the mother's milk, which, even if taken, is at once vomited. The stools are watery and offensive, or the child is costive. In hydrocephaloid there are rolling of the head, suppressed urine and great weakness. Electric changes, as an approaching thunderstorm, depress the child and cause extreme prostration.

The child is nervous, irritable, susceptible to mental impressions, however sluggish may be its scrofulous symptoms. It is susceptible and timid. The whole head is covered with a sweat and the forehead often becomes cold. This, however, is quickly relieved by wrapping the head warmly. Like *Sulph., Calc.* and *Hepar,* the skin readily ulcerates and refuses to heal. *Hepar* is distinguished by the soreness and tenderness of its ulcers and eruptions.

Phosphorus exhibits emaciation combined with nervous debility. Brain and spine have suffered severely. The child is over-tall but is slender, emaciated but big-bellied; face pale, almost waxen. Delicate eyelashes, soft hair, and rapid breathing, indicate what belongs to the sequel. Even thus early the diarrhœa is associated with dry cough, The child, however, shows well-marked nervous excitability. He is irascible, vehement, which results in tremor and weakness; he is susceptible to external impressions and so also to electric changes in the atmosphere.

Glandular swelings, suppurations and caries are similar to those in *Silicea*. The appetite is good; he craves cold food, cries when he sees ice cream, etc. often awakens at night, hot and restless, and will drop off at once to sleep if fed. The stools are green, watery, bright-yellow, undigested, hot, involuntary, coming out with force, worse mornings. Stools often contain little particles looking like tallow, Vomiting accompanies the diarrhœa; longs for cold water, but ejects it so soon as it becomes warm in the stomach.

Hydrocephaloid may ensue. The face is hippocratic, with sunken eyes, surrounded by blue rings. The tongue is dry; the pulse thready; breathing quick; the child lies half comatose.

Petroleum stands btween *Sulph.* and *Phosph.* on the one hand and the *Carbons* on the other. It has emaciation, irritability; the child is vehement, susceptible to electric changes (like *Phos.*) sudden urging in the morning, followed by profuse watery stool (like *Sulphur*) and eczema, excoriations, cracked, bleeding rhagades (like *Graph., Carb. Veg.,* etc.). Its individuality, however, is maintained by the periodicity of the diarrhœa, stools only during the day, and by the colic arising from sleep in the morning, relieved by bending double. Hunger after stool. Its gushing stool and eruption make it a concordant of *Croton Tiglium.*

Iodium causes rapid emaciation, even though the appetite is inordinate. The child is restless and continually desires to change position. The face is yellow or brownish and shrunken.

It is especially useful in enlarged mesenteric glands, with the above symptoms and with intolerable irritability; the child will be approached by no one. Glands are swollen and painless; goitre.

Lycopodium produces emaciation. The abdomen is bloated while the limbs are wasted. The face is earthy, with blue rings around the eyes. At other times it is wrinkled. Eruptions are well described. The crusta lactea is thick, cracks and bleeds, and emits a mousy smell. TENDENCY to capillary bronchitis. The appetite is inordinate, but food soon produces a fulsome feeling, so the child begins hungry enough, but soon desists, and the abdomen seems distended, with much rumbling of wind, especially in the left hypochondrium. The child belches and is soon hungry again. The region of the stomach is distended and intolerant of any pressure, especially after nursing. The urine deposits a red sediment, or is suppressed. Sleep is disturbed by frequent awaking. The child springs up in bed, seemingly frightened, knows no one, pushes every one away angrily. The *Lycopodium* patient is weak, with well-developed head, but puny, sickly body. When sick, the child is irritable, nervous and unmanageable. After sleep he is cross, kicks or scratches at any one who approaches him.

Psorinum stands forth as an ally of *Sulphur*. There are great debility and sweat from any exertion. The skin has the same irremovable odor that so distinguishes *Sulphur*. The eruptions are well described. Crusta lactea forms on face and scalp, appearing prominently down over either ear and cheek. It exfoliates numerous scales, or cracks and discharges a yellow fetid humour. Boils form on the scalp, which looks dirty and emits an offensive odor. The body itches intolerably at night, worse in the warmth of the bed.

The child is pale, sickly, emaciated; nervous, crying out at night as from bad dreams; all medicines fail to relieve. The stool is distinctive, watery, brown or black, horribly offensive, worse by night. The child is worse when the weather changes.

The *Antimonies* have place here by reason of their resemblance to *Sulphur,* and because they are well adapted to scrofula, diarrhœa, etc. The child may look fleshy and well, but is subject to gastric catarrh. The eruptions are pustular, (especially in the *Tartrate*); or develop thick horny crusts, (*Crudum*). In the latter drug we find the nostrils and corners of the mouth covered with crusts, which crack and bleed.

The tongue in *Antim. Crud.* is white; the babe vomits sour curdled milk as soon as it takes the bottle. Vomiting of food or drink as soon as taken. After nursing, the bowels move. Stools watery, containing fecal lumps, or costive, the stools being white, dry, irregular or hard lumps of curd; marasmus.

Antim Tartaricum has nausea and retching, with vomiting, sweat on the forehead, afterwards langour, sleep. The stools are brown-yellow, fecal, watery, profuse, with sharp cutting colic. There are frequent jerks of the limbs during sleep.

In temperament the *Antimonies* display marked irritability; the child will be neither touched nor looked at.

Antim. Crud. is adapted to complaints arising from the heat of summer. While in *Sulphur* all bathing aggravates, in *Atim. Crud.* it is particularly cold bathing which cannot be borne.

The gastric symptoms and intolerance of summer-heat place *Antim. Crudum* with *Bryonia*. But the *Tartrate* favours more *Veratrum Album*. (See Bell on Diarrhœa).

Borax reserved from the nurses, who gave it no higher function than that of a wash for excoriated nipples or infant's sore-mouth, takes a useful place in our list of remedies.

The child grows pale, relaxed, flabby, cries, loathes the breast and falls into a heavy sleep. The head and palms of the hands are hot, the face is pale, clay-coloured. Impaired nutrition is shown by the hot mouth and aphthæ on the tongue and cheeks, bleeding when rubbed. When awake or not sound asleep, the child is nervous, startled by sudden noises, as thunder, distant cannon-firing, etc. When rocked or lowered into its bed, it screams as if affrighted. It can bear no downward motion. Every attempt to nurse causes screaming. The stools are light-yellow, slimy, green, consist of small pieces of yellow fæces, or are painless and if fermented, thin, brown, smelling like carrion.

Dr. Bell, in his oft-quoted monograph, refers to the danger of mistaking *Borax* for *Bellad*. Both have screaming out and starting from sleep, with tossing about, clinging to those near, etc., but only *Borax* has the fear of downward motion and the aphthous mouth.

Sepia bears some resemblance to Borax, as indeed it does to all soda compounds. The child wastes rapidly, eyes are sunken, palms and soles burning hot. During dentition the child cannot take any milk, especially if boiled. The stools are green and painless; the child awakens frequently, especially wakeful after 3 A.M. Possibly suitable to females. Moist scabs on the scalp; forehead rough.

Sarsaparilla is of service in those cases in which the child soon wastes away and looks withered like an old man and the skin hangs in folds. Eruptions are prone to appear in the spring, their bases are inflamed, the crusts detach readily out of doors, and the adjoining skin becomes chapped. On the forehead the crusta lactea is thick, becoming moist when scratched. Herpes and offensive sweat about the genitals, as in children of sycotic parents.

The child becomes very restless and uneasy, screams before passing water, afterwards the diaper is found covered with a white sand.

The stool is accompanied by much flatus, and is often followed by fainting.

Graphites is selected by its skin symptoms principally. Like in all carbons, the discharges are apt to be offensive. Thus breath, stools, urine, sweat, all are offensive. The diarrhœa is brown, thin, fetid, mixed, containing half-digested food, or watery and scalding, or composed of white mucus, which also coats what fecal matter passes.

The child is impertinent and laughs at reprimands. It has a harsh rough skin, disposed to chafing. Eczema capitis forms thick dirty crusts, which ooze a glutinous humour, matting the hair. The eyelids thicken, their tarsi thicken, crack and bleed; crusts form in the nose, with soreness and oozing; a gluey discharge oozes from a raw surface behind the ears. The groins become sore and the inguinal glands swollen. Best adapted to fair plump children who look like the typical *Calcarea* child but with well-marked skin symptoms.

Carbo Veg. is generally called for late in the disease, when the vital powers are failing and there is little or no reaction to well-chosen medicines. The skin is cold, pale, or blue, the face having a greenish hue. The feet and legs to the knees are as cold as death. The child may have an anxious look, but it is too lifeless to move or exhibit much restlessness. The breath may be cold and the pulse weak and rapid. The stools are dark, thin and cadaverous-smelling. Useful, too, in protracted sultry weather, when the days are hot and damp.

Arsenic steps in here as a worthy concordant of *Carbo. Veg.* The skin is dry, parchment-like; the face is sunken, pale, or earthy, and expressive of deep-seated distress. When eruptions are present the crusts are thick, on an angry, excoriated surface, or dry, forming branlike scales. As the child grows weaker the eruptions assume a darker hue, and intertrigo may look even purple. *Arsenic* develops a perfect picture of gastritis, acute and subacute. Food and drink cause instant vomiting and diarrhœa. The constant burning thirst demands iced drinks, ice, etc., but they invariably cause distress in the stomach, making the child writhe in agony until they are ejected.

The stools are green, slimy, bloody, dark, watery, undigested, excoriating and intolerably offensive. The urine may be suppressed, and the child lies in a stupor, hot and twitching. When aroused he is restless, demanding frequent change of position. On awaking he is cross and violent, his pinched features looking more hideous as he contracts the muscles and draws the lips more tightly over the gums. The tendency is surely deathward; but in some cases, when the symptoms appear more slowly emaciation follows, but dropsy and great debility set in. The child looks like a living skeleton, cannot be raised from his pillow, vomits his food and purges when given drink.

Arsenic is adapted to such mummified cases, to bottle-fed babies, and to rapid decline, suddenly appearing in chronic cases.

When the symptoms rather favor *Sulphur, Arsenicum Sulph. Flav.* may be substituted. Stools are green, slimy, watery and offensive, worse during the day, while it is well-known that the *Arsenicum Alb.* has diarrhœa worse at night, after 12 P.M. When the glands are engorged with the usual arsenic symptoms *Arsenicum Iodatum* may be substituted.

Argentum Nitricum is adapted to emaciated children who look old, yellow and wrinkled. The face is pale, sunken, the weakness is so great that every motion is attended with trembling. This exhaustion is the result of rapid loss of fluids, as in cholera infantum, or of long-protracted diarrhœa and defective nourishment. The gastro-enteric symptoms, which indicate it in marasmus, are somewhat akin to those of *Arsenic;* but the inflammation is less intense, while the paresis is more marked in the silver. Thus, with anæmia, weakness and emaciation, it is noticed that fluids taken seem to gurgle through at once. Also diarrhœa of green fetid mucus, with noisy emission of flatus at night. Child craves sweets, yet they aggravate the trouble.

Natrum Muriaticum is to be preferred when the child is emaciated, notwithstanding it has a good appetite. The tongue is mapped, and vesicles or herpes form about the mouth. The wasting is especially marked about the neck. (Campare *Verat. Alb.*)

In one case a child who, though old enough, could not talk, was cured with salt. The defect here was not paralysis, but arose from imperfect development of the muscles of the tongue and larynx. So, similarly, *Natrum Mur.* may be used internally and topically for weak ankles in children; they stumble, or their feet turn under them. Salt here compares with *Causticum, Sulphuric Acid,* etc., which, cæteris paribus, may relieve weak ankles.

Causticum is adapted to children who grow tardily, and who seem to suffer from a sort of paresis. The abdomen is swollen and hard, but the body is wasted and the feet are diminutive. They walk unsteadily and fall easily. This arises not only from weak ankles, but from weakness of brain also. Such children are timid, fear going to bed in the dark, and have a weak memory.

ANTIPSORICS IN THE ATROPHY OF INFANTS

They also have intertrigo during dentition, and eczema on the occiput.

Baryta C. is very similar to *Causticum* in mental weakness, timidity and slowness in learning to walk. Both, also, have an eruption chiefly on the occiput. But in *Bary. Carb* the brain may be actually undeveloped, as in the sclerosis of infants. The child is dwarfish; it does not want to play, but sits idly in a corner. It cannot be taught, for it cannot remember. The face is red, the abdomen bloated, the rest of the body being wasted; stools imperfectly digested, loose and pappy, or hard and dry. Glands are enlarged, especially the cervical and the tonsils. Child wants to eat all the time, but is averse to sweet things and fruits. A little food satiates.

Phosphoric Acid necessarily favors the *Phosphor.*, but the child is apt to be listless and indifferent rather than oversensitive. The abdomen is swollen, and, if diarrhœa is present, there is much fermentation in the bowels. The diarrhœa, though long-lasting, does not proportionately weaken.

Sulphuric Acid cures marasmus with restless, nervous, weakly children. They do everything hurriedly and yet without vim. The eruption, similar to *Sulphur,* is associated with bright yellow mucous stools, which are stringy or chopped. In addition, there is generally aphthous sore mouth, yellow and painful.

Natrum Sulphuricum is to be chosen when a sycotic constitution is inherited; when the abdomen is bloated, with much rumbling of wind, and when the stool is watery, yellow, gushing, coming on so soon as the child begins to move in the morning. (Resembling here *Bryonia.*)

Complaints from living in damp dwelling. Of the remaining soda preparation, *Natrum Phosphoricum,* we have sufficient knowledge to prescribe it in the marasmus of children who are bottle-fed. Abdomen swollen; liver large; colic after eating; stools containing undigested food.

Magnesia Salts, so abused in allopathy, are certainly neglected by Homœopathy. They correspond to forms of marasmus which seem to depend upon defective digestion. In *Magnesia Carb.* we find emaciation, swelling of the glands, abdomen bloated and heavy. The child suffers from gripping pains, colic, followed by green, watery, sour diarrhœa. At other times the stool, if it stands, forms a green scum resembling that on a frog-pond.

Magnesia Mur. Child suffers from ozœna; the discharge is acrid, and the nose obstructed at night; scurf in the nostrils, the alæ and point being red and swollen. The stomach is bloated, and the stools are in large hard lumps, or crumble as they pass the anus. Such a child is puny, rachitic, or has an enlarged liver. The glands are swollen, and, like in *Silicea,* sweat of head and feet accompany all the symptoms.

Magnesia Carb. most resembles *Colocynth* (colic), *Rheum* (sour diarrhœa and griping), and *Chamom.* (green, yellow stools, with colic).

Dr. Clifton confirmed many of the above symptoms of *Magnesia Mur.*

Conium has been of use when the abdomen is hard and distended; frequent sour stools, undigested. The effort at stool causes great weakness.

Gettysburg Water has proved efficacious in affections of the joints and bones. Hip-disease, Pott's disease, with ulceration, the discharge being thin, watery, and offensive. The child suffers from diarrhœa, worse at every change in the weather. (Introduced by Dr. Macfarlan.)

Lithium Carb. to which the *Gettysburg Water* chiefly owes its efficacy, may be successfully used when the child has a rough, harsh skin, milk crust and ringworm, itching violently. The skin is seldom moist, being generally harsh and dry. The nose is swollen, internally sore and dry, with shining crusts in the nostrils. The diarrhœa is light-yellow, fecal in the morning and offensive at night; worse after fruit.

Staphisagria is too often forgotten. It resembles *Coloc., Chamom.* and *Merc.* The child has a humid, fetid eruption; scratching changes the place of the itching, and increases the oozing. The face is sunken, the nose pointed, and blue rings encircle the eyes. The teeth, as they appear, soon turn dark or crumble. The mouth is aphthous, the gums appearing pale, spongy and bleeding when touched. Nostrils sore with the catarrh; eyelids and corners of mouth ulcerated. Fetid nightsweat. The abdomen is swollen. Colic after the least food or drink. Stools hot, smelling like rotten eggs, or dysenteric. The child is irritable, asks for things, and then indignantly pushes them away.

Viola Tricolor certainly leads the list when crusta lactea is the most prominent feature of the case. The incrustations are thick, and discharge copiously a thick yellow, purulent matter. The child cannot sleep because of the irritation. The urine is profuse, and has an odor like that of cats. During sleep the hands twitch, the thumbs are clenched, the face is red, and the whole body hot and dry.

Hydrastis, though not known to be an antipsoric, is introduced to show its value in excoriations in the groins, as confirmed by Anna E. Griffith, M.D.

In addition, it may probably suit when the following symptoms are present, though as yet clinical confirmation is absent. Eczema on the forehead at the border of the hair, oozing after washing. Thick mucous discharges (more excoriating than the botanically related *Pulsat.*). Marasmus; great debility, faintness at the stomach; aphthæ of weakly children; tongue swollen, shows marks of the teeth, or appears raw, dark-red, with raised papillæ.

Nitric Acid is called for in weakly children, after abuse of calomel, or who have inherited syphilis. The child is wasted, sallow, weak. The upper arms and thighs in particular are emaciated. There are aphthous ulcers in the mouth, with putrid breath. This acid attacks prominently mucus outlets; so we are apt to find ulcers or blisters about the mouth; soreness and rawness at the anus, etc. The diarrhœa consists of green mucus, sometimes fetid and undigested, and is worse in the morning. Stool followed by great exhaustion. Glands enlarged. Sometimes indicated for the *Calcarea* patient, when debility and wasting persist despite the use of *Lime*.

Muratic Acid stands between *Phosph. Acid* and *Nitric Acid*. Like the former there is present taciturnity; the child is too listless to move or take notice. Like the latter there are aphthæ in the mouth. The child has become exhausted from frequent vomiting and diarrhœa, and the stomach has become so weak it will no longer tolerate or digest food. This gastric atony is most marked about 10 to 11 A.M. The tongue is shrivelled and dry as leather, or covered with deep-bluish ulcers, having black bases; breath fetid; salivary glands tender, swollen. Stool involuntary when passing urine, followed by protrusion of purplish, extremely sensitive piles; prolapsus ani during urination. Also useful in muscular debility following abuse of opiates, soothing syrups, etc.

Theridion, recommended by Baruch for scrofulosis, has proved of great value in infantile atrophy, caries of the bones, rachitis, scrofulous enlargement of the glands, especially after the failure of *Sulphur, Calcarea* and *Lycopodium*.

Ozone. In some cases in which the symptoms clearly indicate *Sulphur,* but that remedy fails, ozonized water cures. The symptoms from provings are all but identical with *Sulphur.* In one case a hip-disease which defied the latter remedy was cured by ozone water, three tea-spoons daily.

Pinus Sylvestris has been recommended for rachitis, when children, from weakness in the knees, do not learn to walk.

Oleum Jecoris Aselli, according to the provings, corresponds to atrophy of infants. It resembles *Phosphor.* and *Iodium,* and especially *Calc. Phos.* The child is emaciated, with hot hands and head. Constant tendency to catarrhs. Bones affected; rachitis. Fever at night with sweat, mostly on the head, neck and hands. Cannot take milk. Vivid dreams; restless and feverish at night.

Hypophosphite of Lime, when the child from excessive and protracted loss of fluids, as from long-lasting diarrhœa, chronic suppuration, etc., is reduced almost to a skeleton. Face wan pale. Abdomen bloated. Limbs habitually cold. At times the pale face flushes, the head becomes hot, and the child nervous and excitable. Debility with copious exhausting sweats. (Compare: *Cinchon., Phos., Calc. C., Phos. Acid,* etc.)

Cistus Canadensis has hot, gray-yellow, spurting stools; worse after fruit, and from 12 P.M. until noon. The glands especially the cervical, are swollen or suppurating. All symptoms worse in wet weather. Tetter on and around the ears. Caries; indicated in thin scrawny children, of a well-described scrofulous diathesis.

Arum Triphyllum, though not well defined as a remedy in diarrhœa, becomes indispensable in some cases (especially after scarlatina), with boring in the nose, picking at one spot; restless tossing; irritability; mouth and nose sore, raw; alæ and corners of mouth cracked and bleeding; putrid odor from the mouth.

Mercurius has many similarities with atrophy of infants, but must be used with some reservation, as relapses often follow its administration. It is, however, admirably adapted as an intercurrent when *Sulphur* ceases to improve. Its distinctive symptoms are: Emaciation; skin dry, rough, dirty-yellow or clammy, especially that of the thighs; icy-cold sweat on the forehead, sour or oily sweat on the scalp; eruption like herpes, but soon becoming pustular or suppurating; glands swollen and suppurating; skin chaps easily, becomes raw and sore; thirst; frequent attacks of jaundice; skin yellow; abdomen and right hypochondrium swollen and sore to pressure; stool green, sour watery, with emaciation; diarrhœa bloody, slimy or green, with tenesmus often continuing after stool. In this latter symptom *Mercury* exhibits more constancy than in any other. It is often associated with colic, as from cold or indigestion. Prolapsus ani after stool, the tumor being dark-red and sometimes bloody. Genitals become sore and excoriated; urine causes pain; child pulls at the penis. The child is pale, weak and obtuse, or precocious and restless; face becomes hot and red; speech is hurried, all reminding one of *Belladonna*. The fontanelles are open, the head large and covered with an offensive sweat. The gums are soft and bleed easily. Ophthalmia is common, with suppuration, especially when the lids are involved—all worse from the heat of the fire. Sour nightsweats. It is rather inimical to *Silicea*, and must be carefully differentiated.

PART II.

REPERTORY OF PROMINENT SYMPTOMS

1. **Child Sad:**

    Hepar, Lycop., Sulph., Vio. Tricolor, Psorin, Graph.

CAUSTICUM	cries at the least thing.
NATRUM MUR.	cries if spoken to.
CALC. CARB.	cries persistently.
KALI C.	moans, 3 A.M.
BORAX	cries when nursed or rocked.

2. **Child Afraid, Full of Fear:**

CARB. VEG.	of ghosts.
CAUSTIC	of ghosts, of strangers.
BARYTA CARB.	of strangers, timid.
BORAX	of being rocked, of downward motion, of noises, clings to those near.
MURCURIUS	restless, full of fear in the evening.

3. **Child Apathetic, Indifferent:**

PHOS.	cares for nothing, is restless.
PHOS. AC.	wants nothing, listless.
LYCOP.	loses its wonted brightness and becomes quiet.
BARYTA CARB.	sits idly in a corner, cannot bear to read.
MURCURIUS	indifferent, stupid.

4. **Excitable, Anxious:**
   Phos., Petroleum, Silicea, Merc., Sulph., Sulph. Acid, Borax, Kali Carb., Magnes. Carb., Psorin.

5. **Child Irritable:**
   Sepia, Mercur.

SULPH	hasty, hard to manage.
CALC. PHOS	perverse, peevish.
ANTIM. CRUD.	will not be looked at.
ARSENIC	becomes unmanageably angry, will not be spoken to; more so on awakening.
CALC. CARB.	self-willed, cross before stool, also in afternoon; pupils enlarged.
CARB. VEG.	strikes, bites, kicks anxious.
LYCOP.	a mild child suddenly becomes refractory, cross, frightened, kicks on awaking, especially cross when trying to urinate; red sediment in the urine.
KALI CARB.	easily startled by noises, awakens cross, strikes, wants now this, now that.
PHOS.	restless at twilight, anger makes the child worse.
ANT. TART.	anger causes cough, will not be touched or looked at.
BORAX	startled by least noise.
STAPHIS.	cries for things, which received, he throws away.
IODIUM	especially with enlarged mesenteric glands.

ANTIPSORICS IN THE ATROPHY OF INFANTS

SILICA	nervous, timid.
PETROLEUM	easily angered.
PSORINUM	nervous, cries out at night.
SARSAPARILLA	restless, screams on urinating.
GRAPHITES	laughs at reprimands.
NATRUM MUR.	cries if spoken to.
SULPH. ACID	restless, hasty, nervous and weak.
ZINCUM	brain affected.
ARUM T.,	restless, irritable, caused by sore mouth, etc.

6. **Large Head, Sweating, Placid Expression, Mild Eyes, Want of Power to support itself (typical of rachitis):**
Silicea, Calc. Phos., Calc. Carb., Mercur.

7. **Child Precocious:**
Calc. C., Sulph., Phos., Mercur.

LYCOP.	mind active, body frail.

8. **Delirious, Restless:**

ARSENIC	tosses about, strikes its head with its fists.
ARGENT. NITRIC.	especially before and between convulsions.
LYCOP.	4-8 P.M., also awakens as if terrified, screams, knows no one.
PSORIN.	awakens terrified.
SULPH.	screams on awaking, becomes restless, cries at night start from sleep with screams.

Borax	starts from sleep with anxious screams, throws hands about.
Kali Carb.	awakens cross and screaming, anxious, reaches for things, startled at slight noises; worse after 12 p.m., generally about 3 a.m.
Calc. Carb.	restless, cries out at night, makes an anxious face when lifted from the cradle, face pale.
Calc. Phos.	restless, grasps with the hands, anxious face, difficult respiration when raised in the arms.
Oleum Jecoris	restless and feverish at night, hot hands.
Zinc.	on awaking screams, knows no one, brain affected.
Arum Tri.	bores the nose, etc.

9. **Stupor, Coma or Drowsiness:**

Apis, Sulph.	lies in a stupor.
Calc. Phos.	exhausted, limp, drowsy.
Calc. C.	drowsy, pale, scratches its head when aroused.
Phos.	comatose, wasted, pulse thready, cold.
Lycop.	sleeps profoundly, lower jaw dropped, rattling breathing, eyes dull.
Antim Crud.	drowsy all the forenoon.
Ant. Tart.	drowsy, sleepy, rattling breathing, cyanotic.

ANTIPSORICS IN THE ATROPHY OF INFANTS

BORAX	falls into a heavy sleep.
SEPIA	drowsy by day, sleepless after 3 A.M.
CARBO VEG.	lies as if dead, cold, blue pulseless.
ARSENIC	lies comatose, twitches, hot, restless, as if disturbed.
PHOS. ACID	listless, drowsy, but easily awakened.
MURIATIC ACID	in a restless, moaning sleep, slides down in bed during sleep, sudden red face with coma.
ZINC.	occiput hot, face pale, rolls head, hydrocephaloid.

10. Hydrocephaloid:
Sulph., Calc. C., Calc. Phos., Phos., Arsenic, Silicea, Lycopodium, Zincum, Apis, (Cinchon. prostration which precedes).

11. Fontanelles Remain Open:
Mercur, Puls.

SULPH., CALC. C.	sweat on the scalp.
CALC. PHOS.	especially posterior fontanelle.
CALC.I., SILICEA	head very large, whole head sweats.
SEPIA	jerks head backwards and forwards.

12. Face:

SULPH.	pale, cold sweat on forehead (hydrocephaloid); sunken with deep hollow eyes, red, old-looking, wrinkled, spotted red.

CALC. CARB.	pale, watery, chalklike, red at times, sunken, pale, pinched, veins show through the face and scalp (sweat).
CALC. PHOS.	sallow, sunken, blue around the eyes (hydrocephaloid).
SILICEA	earthy, waxen, sweaty.
PHOS.	hippocratic (hydrocephaloid), blue around the eyes, red cheeks, circumscribed, emaciated, with soft hair, delicate lashes, changing color.
IODIUM	yellow, brownish or sunken.
LYCOP.	earthy, blue around eyes, wrinkles, one cheek red, after eating sweet.
PSORINUM	sickly, pale, emaciated.
BORAX	pale flabby skin, sallow.
SEPIA	pale or sallow, sunken, yellow about mouth, yellow saddle across nose.
SARSAP.	yellow, wrinkled, old-looking.
CARB VEG.	anxious look, pale earthy hue, green, covered with cold sweat.
ARSENIC	hippocratic, waxen, sallow, skin drawn tightly over bones, green, cold sweat.
ARGENT. NITRIC.	old, wrinkled, yellow or brown.
NATRUM MUR.	pale, shining, greasy.

CAUSTICUM	yellow, especially about the temples, distorted.
BARYTA CARB.	stupid, silly look.
PHOS. ACID	pale, blue around eyes, hippocratic.
MAGNES. CARB.	red after meals.
MAGNES. MUR.	pale, yellow (from the liver).
CONIUM	pale, yellow.
STAPHIS.	pale, sunken, sickly, dark around the eyes.
NITRIC ACID	pale, eyes sunken, dark-yellow about the eyes, cheeks sometimes red, bloated around the eyes on awaking early.
MURIATIC ACID	suddenly red, pale, sunken with the exhaustion.
HYPOPHOSPHITE OF LIME	wan, pale.
ZINCUM	pale, now and then red.
MERCURIUS	pale, yellow, at times red.

13. Eyes, Ears, Nose, Tarsi Thickened:

Graph. (and raw and cracked), Staphis., Borax, Antim. C. (Canthi. raw.).

14. Styes:

Sulph., Lycop., Hepar, Silicea, Staphis. (hardened), Graph. (Pulsat.), Mercur.

15. Ophthalmia Scrofulosa:

Sulph., Calcarea C., Hepar, Nitric Acid, Silicea (Phosp.), Borax, Graph., Arsenic, Psorin, Mercur.

Arg. Nitric.	.	much pus, granular lids.
Natr. Mur.	.	pus, spasm of lids.
Conium	.	disproportionate photophobia.
Lycopod.	.	bland pus.

16. Otorrhœa:

Sulph., Calc. Carb., Calc. Iod., Cal. Phos., Graph., Lycopod. (Kali Carb., thin yellow cerumen), Arsenic, Ars.Iod., Cistus.C., Carbo. Veg., Psorin., Nitric Acid., Silicea, Borax, Hepar, Baryta C., Mercur.

17. Scrofulous Catarrh:

Sulph., Calc. C., Calc. Ph., Graphites, Phosp., Bary. C., Hydras., Psorin.

Arsenicum	.	every winter, thick yellow.
Arsenic Iod.	.	glands swollen.
Hepar	.	worse at every exposure.
Lycopod.	.	thick, purulent, nose stuffed up.
Nit. Ac., Silicea		ulcers bloody.
Muriatic Ac.	.	thin, excoriating, nosebleed.
Iodium	.	hot, watery, at every cold; glands swollen.
Kaolin	.	scabs in the nose, bleeding, nose sensitive.
Mercur.	.	recurs at every damp change of weather.
Stillingia	.	excoriating, syphilitic, similar to Kali Hyd.

18. Eruption like Milk Crust:

Calc. Ph., Carbo Veg., Caust., Bartya C., Phos., Sepia, Coni., Cistus C.

Viola Tri.	thick, pours out yellow pus, mats hair.
Sulph.	head and face bleeds easily; thick pus.
Calc. Carb.	spreads to face; thick mild pus; at times in isolated spots and white.
Hepar.	after salves; itches mornings.
Silicea	more back of head; pustules.
Lycop.	thick, offensive, angry, oozes pus, worse on occiput.
Sarsaparilla	worse out of doors; pus spreads the eruption.
Graph.	sticky.
Arsenicum	angry excoriating discharge; branlike on forehead.
Hydras.	forehead.
Argent. Nitric.	nape of neck.
Natrum Mur.	nape of neck, impetiginoid.
Sulph. Acid.	with stringy stools.
Lith. Carb.	skin dry, harsh, itching.
Staphis	humid, fetid, occiput and behind ears.
Psorinum	down over ears, temples and cheeks; moist, fetid, or scaly.
Petroleum	eczematous, purulent, cracking.

ANT. C.	. hard thick crusts.
ARUM TRI.	. corners of mouth sore, cracked, bleeding, alæ nasi bleeding.
MERCUR .	. herpes, becoming scaly; pustules; eruption worse in warmth of bed.
STILLINGIA	. moist, brown, excoriating, on the scalp.

19. Aphthæ, Stomacace:

BORAX .	. mouth hot, mucous surface of palate shrivelled; child cries when nursing; red blisters on tongue.
NITRIC ACID	. offensive ulcers, yellow ulcers, blisters on lips, salivation, gums sore, etc.
MURIATIC ACID	. very weak, deep blue ulcers, etc.
SULPHURIC ACID	whitish ulcers, ptyalism, easily bleeding gums, ecchymoses.
SULPHUR .	. sour fetid smell; gums bleed; blisters and vesicles; saliva mixed with blood; excoriated about the anus, etc.
CARBO VEG.	. gums recede and bleed easily, oozing of blood, mouth hot, bloody saliva, edges of gums yellow, indented.
NATRUM MUR.	. blisters in and around the mouth, scorbutic gums.

CALC CARB.	dry mouth alternating with salivation, constitution agreeing.
BRYONIA	beginning, mouth dry, so the child cannot nurse until it is moistened.
STAPHIS	gums ulcerated, spongy, white, receding, bleed easily; blisters; child weak, sickly; sunken eyes and surrounded by blue rings; cervical glands swollen, etc.
SEPIA, HYDRASTIS	tenacious mucus hangs in shreds from the mouth; tongue, red, raw, blistered; weak children; eczema on forehead at margin of hair, worse from being washed; bloody purulent mucus from the nose.
ARSENIC	ulcers or blisters turn livid or black, ptyalism, restlessness and great exhaustion.
KALI CHLOR.	with extreme fetor, follicular stomatitis.
CONIUM	grayish ashy hue to ulcers; gangrene.
ARUM TRI.	great swelling of lining membrane and tongue; will not or cannot open the mouth; mouth raw, burning, bleeding; putrid odor; lips as if scalded;

	lips and nose chapped and bleeding; picks the nose or lips.
Lachesis . .	ulcers bluish, fluids return through the nose can bear no clothing to touch the face or neck, etc.
Ranunc. Scel. .	tongue looks as if covered with "Islands".
Ammon. Carb. .	tonsils large, bluish; mouth raw; nose stopped up arousing the child at night.
Apis . . .	rosy-red mouth and fauces; mucus surface swollen; tongue swollen and studded with small blisters; also in clusters on the tongue or along its border; slight thirst.
Baptisia . .	gums ooze blood and look dark, purplish, fetid odor; tongue brown; great exhaustion; can swallow only fluids.
Capsicum . .	suitable to fat, but flabby, sluggish children; small burning blisters in the mouth, having a carrion-like odor.
Mercur. . .	scorbutic gums; saliva copious, offensive, bloody; ulcers with bases like lard; glands swollen; diarrhœa with tenesmus.
Hepar. . .	white aphthous pustules on the inside of lips and cheeks and on the tongue.

ANTIPSORICS IN THE ATROPHY OF INFANTS 209

SALICYLIC ACID . mouth dotted with white patches; burning, scalded feeling; ulcers on the tip of the tongue; many cases.

KALI BICHR. aphthous ulcers eating deeply; stringy mucus in mouth and throat; nasal catarrh.

IODIUM . aphthous eruption in the mouth; offensive odor; copious saliva; nasal catarrh, thin, excoriating.

MERCUR. CORROS.. mouth terribly swollen; lips swollen and everted; ptyalism; nose sore and stuffed up with a gluey secretion.

20. Tonsils Enlarged:

Baryta Carb., Calc. Iod., Iodium, Lycop., Arsen. Iod., Calc. Carb., Hepar, Nitric Acid, Sulph., Mercur., etc.

21. Goitre:

Iodium, Spongia, (Calc. Flour.), Calc. Iod., Calc. Carb., Hepar, Conium (Lapis Alba), (Kali Hyd.), Lycopod., Natrum Mur., Causticum (Apis), Sulph.

22. Appetite or Hunger:

Nat. Ph., Staph., Nat. M. (Zinc).

SULPH. . . weak and hungry 10 to 11 A.M., also at night, grasps at everything and thrusts it into the mouth.

CALC. CARB. . craves eggs.

CALC. PHOS.	craves bacon, etc.
SILICEA	no appetite, or voracious hunger, but on attempting to eat, loses all desire.
PHOSPH.	even at night craves cold food.
PETROLEUM	after stool.
IODIUM	very restless if hungry; appetite excessive; better while eating.
HEPAR.	child seems stronger just after eating.
LYCOPOD.	inordinate, but soon surfeited.
PSORIN	even at night.
GRAPH., BARY. C.	constant desire to eat, but averse to sweets.
ARGENT. NITRIC	wants sweets, but they disagree.

23. Thirst:

Carbo V., Nitric Acid, Natrum Mur., Silicea, Mercur., etc.

CALC. C.	especially P.M., and night.
SULPH.	much thirst, but no appetite.
ARSENIC	burning, unquenchable, or little and often.
PHOSPH.	for cold drinks.
PHOS. ACID.	for something refreshing.

24. Vomiting:

Silicea, Arsenic, Phosph. (Calcarea Acetica), Ant. Crud., Ant. T.

Sulph.	chronic.
Calc. Carb.	curdled, sour milk.
Æthusa	vomits, green curd, exhausted afterwards.
Kreos.	even hours after nursing; stomach so weak it will tolerate no kind of food.

25. Eating, cries as soon as he Eats:

Arsenic, Calcarea Phos., Sulphur, Staphisagria, Croton Tig., Staphis., Phosph., Phos. Acid, Sulph., Lycopod., Sulp. A., Carbo V. (Cinch, Fer.).

Arsenic, Argent. Nitric.	eating or nursing causes diarrhœa.

26. Fruit provokes Diarrhœa:

Arsenic, Lith. Carb., Magnesia Carb., Sulphur, Muriatic Acid, Kali Carb., Cistus Canadensis (Laches).

27. Milk Disagrees:

Arsenic, (Kali C.).

Sulph.	passed undigested, vomited, causes colic.
Calc. Carb.	vomitted in sour lumps, passed in white curds.
Magnes. Carb.	colic, indigestion, sour, white and green stools.
Antim Crud.	vomited or passed undigested.
Sepia	also if boiled.
Carbo. Veg.	abdomen swollen.

    Nitric. Acid. . will not digest.
    Silicea . . vomits mother's milk.
    Conium . . abdomen inflated.

28. Worse from Bottle-Food—From Artificial Foods:
Arsenic, Sulph., Lycopod., Calc. C., Calc. Phos., Magnes. Carb., Natrum Phos.

29. Worse from Fresh Meat:
Causticum.

30. Worse from Smoked Meat:
Calc. Carb.

31. Better from Ham, Bacon, etc.:
Calc. Phos.

32. Worse from Eating Potatoes:
Alumina, Sepia.

33. Worse from Cold Water:
Arsen., Lycop., Sulph., Carbo. Veg.

34. Worse from Sweets:
Argent. Nitric., Zinc., Calc. C.

35. Abdomen Swollen:
Sulph., Calc. C., Phosphorus, Lyco., Graphites, Caust., Arsenic, Baryta C., Staphis. Stillingia.

    Mag. Mur. . from enlarged liver.
    Natrum Sulph. . from flatus.
    Conium . . hard and distended.
    Phos. Acid . with gurgling, rumbling flatus.

MERC. . . swollen especially about liver with sensitiveness.

36. **Remedies known to have enlarged Mesenteric Glands:**

    Sulphur, Calc. Carb., Calc. Phos., Calc. Iodata, Iodium (Conium), (Silicea), (Baryta Carb.), (Arsenic). Probably we may include: Hepar, Phosph., Graphites, (Natrum Phos.), Staphis.

37. **Fatty Degeneration of the Liver (Common in Tuberculosis):**

    Phosph. (Aurum, with caries of bones or syphilis), Arsenic, Silicea.

38. **Enlarged Liver:**

    Sulph., Magnes. Carb., Magnes. Mur., Mercur., Lyco., (Nux Vom.), Sepia, Silicea, (Chelid.), (Teucr.), (Leptand.).

39. **Diarrhœa, Undigested:**

    Sulphur, Baryta Carb.

CALC. C. . .	contains curdled milk.
GRAPH. . .	thin, brown, half-digested and fetid.
CALC. PHOS. .	and hot.
PHOSPH. . .	with great exhaustion.
PHOS. ACID .	without much exhaustion.
HEPAR . .	and sour, white or green.
ANTIM. CRUD .	hard lumps of curdled milk.
ARSENIC . .	at once when eating.
ARGENT. NITRIC.	on eating at night, gurgling through.

Nat. Phos.	bottle-fed.
Conium	and sour.

40. Watery:
Calc. C.

Sulph.	sudden urging.
Calc. P.	hot.
Phosph.	white.
Psorin.	black, offensive, at night.
Antim Crud.	containing fecal lumps.
Ant. Tart.	profuse.
Graphites	half-digested.
Carbo Veg.	rather a dark thin, fecal diarrhœa, very offensive.
Arsenic	brown or black, with restlessness and anguish.
Phos. Acid	like Phos., but with much gurgling in abdomen.
Sulph. Acid	with irritability and weakness.
Magnes. Carb.	green, sour, frothy.
Natrum Sulph.	yellow.
Nitric Acid	yellow, white.
Merc.	green, watery, sour.

41. Smell.
Iodium, Graphites, Lycop., Sepia, Psorin., Lith. Carb., Sulph. Ac.

Sulph.	sour. fetid.
Calc. Carb.	like rotten eggs, pungent, sour.
Calc. Phos.	with offensive flatus.
Phosph.	sour.

Hepar	. .	sour, like rotten cheese.
Argent. Nitric.		fetid.
Arsenic	. .	like carrion.
Carbo. Veg.	.	putrid, offensive.
Silicea	. .	small, liquid, putrid.
Borax	. .	like carrion.
Staphis	. .	like rotten eggs.

42. Purulent:
Arsenic, Iodium, Calc. C., Kali C., Lycop., Sulph., Sepia, Silicea.

43. Mucous:
Nat. Sulph., Sulph.

Sulph.	. .	with fever.
Sulph. Acid	.	chopped, stringy, frothy.
Phosph.	. .	white, granular.
Borax	. .	yellow.
Silicea	. .	fæces.
Graphites	.	coated fæces.
Calc. Carb.	.	green.
Sepia	. .	green.
Calc. Phos.	.	green, slimy.
Magnes. Carb.	.	green, like scum in frog-pond.
Argnt. Nitric.	.	green at night, with much flatus.
Arsenic	. .	brown.
Iodium	. .	frothy.
Ars. Sulp. Flav.		green, slimy, offensive.
Nitric Acid	.	green, fetid.
Merc.	. .	green, with tenesmus.
Stillingia	.	white, pasty.

44. With Much Flatus:
  ARGENT. NITRIC. at night.
  CALC. PHOS. . fetid.
  CARBO VEG. . putrid.
  SARSAP. . . with much flatus; faint afterwards.

45. Bloody:
  Argent. Nitric., Arsenic, Phosph, Sepia, Silicea, Mercur.

46. Bilious:
  Arsenic, Sulph. (Ars. Sul. Rub.), Phosph. (golden), Mercur. (green).
  SULPHUR . . in streaks.

47. White:
  CALC. C., HYDRAS. chalklike.
  HEP., ANT. CRUD.,
  PHOSPH. . grains.
  MAGNES. CARB. . like tallow.
  KALI CARB. . gray, fecal.
  LYCOPOD. . pale, fecal.
  (STILLINGIA).

48. Diarrhœa with Excoriation or Redness of the Anus:
  Sulph., Arsenic., Phosph., Graphites, Antim. Crud., Staphis. (Natrum Mur.), Mercur.

49. Stools Costive:
  Sulph., Lycop.
  MAGNES. MUR. . crumbling as they pass.
  ANT. CRUD. . hard white lumps.
  GRAPH. . . mucus-coated.
  CALC. CARB. . claylike, gray, fecal.

Calc. Phos.	. hard, causing great depression.
Causticum	. urging causes red face
Hepar	. . hard, difficult, often with eruption in bends of joints.
Silicea	. , more than diarrhœic; rectum inactive, spine weak, stool slips back.

50. Alternately Costive and Diarrhœic (said to denote mesenteric disease):
Antim. C., Phosph., Lycopod., Sulph.

51. Urine Suppressed:
Sulph. (with hydrocephaloid), Lycopod., Silicea (hydroceph.), Carbo Veg., Arsenic (Zinc), (Apis), (Camph.).

52. Wetting the Bed:
Sulph., Calc. C., Graph., Silicea, Ars., Nat. Mur., etc.

Sepia	. . first sleep.
Caustic	. . worse in winter or when coughing.

53. Stool passes with Urine:
Muriatic Acid.

54. Urine.

Calc. Carb.	. strong, fetid, but clear.
Nitric Acid	. strong, like that of the horse.
Benzoic Acid	. strong, turbid.
Iodium	. . ammoniacal.
Phos. Acid	. milk-colored.
Ars., Phos. Acid., Carbo. Veg.	. fetid.

VIOLA TRICOLOR	smelling like that of the cat.
SARSAPARILLA	depositing a sandy sediment.
LYCOP.	red sediment with crying before passing.
GRAPH.	becomes sour or turbid with reddish sediment.
CALC. CARB.	sediment like flour.
ANT. CRUD., NAT. MUR., SEPIA	all have reddish sediment.
BORAX	acrid, fetid urine; aphthæ.

55. Hydrocele:

Silicea, Graph., Arsenic, Conium (Apis).

56. Bronchial Catarrh (often a symptom of atrophy; frequently, also, tuberculosis):

Calc. Ph.

SULPH.	dry cough, flushes of heat, rattling of mucus; sputum yellow, purulent.
CALC. CARB.	rattling of mucus; loose cough.
PHOSP.	violent cough, quick breathing, oppression of the chest; cough with diarrhœa, hoarseness, etc.
HEPAR	croupy, harsh even if loose.
IODIUM	croupy, hoarse, worse in warm wet weather.
CONIUM	dry teasing cough, worse when lying.
LYCOP.	loose rattling cough, moist rales; sputum yellow, purulent.

Sepia	dry cough, causing bilious vomiting.
Arsenic	dry cough, or with frothy sputum and emphysematous dyspnœa.
Baryta Carb.	glands of neck enlarged, also those of the bronchi.
Ant. Tart.	cyanotic symptoms: dyspnœa, child cannot nurse, cries with cough, also cough when angry.
Hypophosphite of Lime, Silicea	rachitic children: pain under sternum; loose cough, with purulent sputum, nightsweats.
Sulph. Acid.	belches when coughs.
Oleum Jecoris, Kali Hyd.	lungs hepatized; sputum frothy, green, looking like soap-suds.
Kali Carb.	predominant stitches; shortness of breath; sputum contains pus globules.

57. Jerks the Legs on dropping off to Sleep:
Sulphur, Arsenic, Borax, Ant. Tart., Lycopod. (Zinc.).

58. Hands Twitch, Thumbs Clenched:
Viola Tric.

Arsenic	twitching, hot; stupor.

59. Ankles Weak:
Causticum (Natrum Carb.), Natrum Mur. (also topically) Sulph. Acid, Sulphur, Calc. Carb., Calc. Phos.

60. Will not stand: Spine Weak:
   Sulphur, Calc. Carb., Calc. Phos. (head drops), Silicea.

61. Every Wound or Abrasion Festers:
   Sulphur, Calc. Carb., Hepar, Silicea, Petroleum, Carbo Veg., Graph., Lycopod., Mercur.

62. Ulcers on the Fingers:
   Sepia, Borax.

63. Appearance of Health, Plumpness:
   Sulphur, Calc. Carb., Calc. Iodata, Antim. Crud. (Arsenic), Graphites, Hepar.

64. Skin clear, thin, veins shine through (often in tuberculosis):
   Phosph., Calc. Phos., Calc. Carb., Lycopod.

65. Induration of Soft Parts:
   Silicea, Sulph., Conium, Hepar, Iodium, Baryta Carb., Phos., Magnes. Mur., Graph., Lycopod. (Carbo Anim.), Carbo Veg., Staphis., Sepia.

66. To Soften Cicatrices:
   Graph. (Phytolac.)

67. Emaciation:

SULPH., CALC. C., IOD., SARS., ARG. NIT., ARSENIC .	child looks like an old man.
SULPH., IOD., CALC. C., CALC. PH., NATR. M., STAPHIS., (SELEN).	emaciated, yet appetite good
NAT. MUR., CALC. PHOS. . .	emaciation of the neck.
SELEN., PHOSPH. .	of the face and hands.

ANTIPSORICS IN THE ATROPHY OF INFANTS 221

SULPH., CALC. C., CALCAREA PHOS., LYCO., SILICEA, PHOSPH., PHOS. ACID, PETRO., BORAX, SEPIA, SARSAP., MERC., GRAPH., CARBO VEG., ARSENIC., ARG. NITRICUM, BARYTA CARB., CAUSTI., SULP. ACID, MURIAT. ACID, NIT. AC., HYDRAS., STAP., OLEUM JECORIS, PSORINUM . of whole body.

NITRIC ACID . of arms and thighs.

LYCOPOD. . . of upper part of body:

68. Glands Enlarged:

Sulph., Calc. C., Calc. Phos., Calc. Iod., Phosph., Phos. Acid, Silicea, Oleum Jecoris, Natrum Mur., Graph., Carb. Veg., Arsenic Ars. Iod., Cistus, Mercur., Therid., Petrol., Baryta Carb., Nitric Acid, Staphis., Sepia, Caustic., Psorin., Conium, Magnes. C., Magnes. M., Sulph. Acid, Hepar.

69. Bones: Imperfectly Developed:

Sulph., Phosph., Hypop. of Lime, Sili., Calc. P., Calc. Iod., Therid., Hepar., Iodium, Phosph. Acid, Oleum Jecoris.

CALC. C. . . and soft joints large.

MERCUR. . . pains worse at night.

70. Bones: Brittle:

CALC. PHOS. . skull.

71. Caries, Necrosis:

Phos. Acid, Therid., Calc. Carb., Lycopodium, Chlor. of Gold, Chlor. of Platinum, Iodium, (Stillingia).

PHOSPH. . .	especially lower jaw.
SULPH., SILICEA .	fistulous openings, thin pus.
GETTYSBURG WATER .	. of vertebræ or at joints.
NITRIC ACID .	mastoid, skull.
STAPH. . .	necrosis of fingers.
AURUM .	. syphilitico-mercurial cases, of mastoid, nasal bones, skull.
ASAFŒTIDA	. skin around bluish, adherent, sensitive even to light dressing.
STRONTI. .	. necrosis of femur, diarrhœa.
FLUORIC ACID	. like Silicea, but symptoms relieved by cold.
MEZER. .	. with intolerable pains at night after mercury.
OLEUM JECORIS .	fistulous openings; pus flocculent, nauseous.
CISTUS CAN.	. submaxillary or maxillary bone.

72. Bony Tumors:

Silicea, (Calc. Flour.), Sepia, Carlcarea. Carb., Cal. Iod., Cal. Phos., Sulph., (Hecla lava), (Aurum), Lycopod., Asafœt., Merc.

PHOS. . . of skull, or clavicles.

73. Spinal Curvature: Bones Curved:

Sulph., Calc. Carb., Calc. Phos., Lycopod., Silicea, Gettysburg water, Nitric Acid, Phosph., Phos. Acid, Oleum Jecoris, Iodium, Hepar, Sepia, Mercur.

74. Complicated with Syphilis:

(Kali Hyd.), Nitric Acid, Hepar, (Mezereum, mercurialized), (Aurum), (Fluoric Acid), (Phyto.), (Stillingia), (Asafœtida), Mercur.

75. Joints:

SULPH., CALC. C.	white swelling, pains intermit at night.
CALC. PHOS.	suppuration, pus contains spicule of bone, tendency to articular pains at every damp change of weather.
SILICEA	fistula, caries.
GETTYSBURG WATER	caries, thin, ichorous discharge.
LYCOP.	awakes screaming, cross, violent; beginning of hip-disease.
IODIUM	swollen, doughy; fistulous openings, with watery pus.
OLEUM JECORIS	fistulæ, with flocculent pus.
APIS	synovitis, with copious exudation.
ARSENIC	fetid pus, œdema, great exhaustion.

Carbo Veg.	similar to Arsenic, but with less irritability of fibre, restlessness, etc.
Baryta C.	white swelling, pains intolerable at night.
Ozone	hip, see Part I.
Caustic	burning pains, caries.

76. Tuberculosis (Remedies known to have been useful):

Phosph.	brain or lungs.
Sulph.	in the beginning, but must be selected strictly.
Calcar. Carb.	follows the former well.
Spongia	of lungs, with dry, harsh cough.
Hepar	after the former, cough harsh, but at the same time much phlegm.
Calc. Ph., Hypo. of Lime, Caust.	of the spine.
Baryta Carb.	of the spine; also with indurated glands.
Lycop.	lungs; also of the liver.
Silicea	with purulent breaking down, abscesses, lungs, liver.
Magnes. Carb.	of liver.
Argent. Nitric., Helleb., Apis.	of brain.
Kali Carb., Phos. Acid.	of lungs.

Nitric Acid .	of lungs; follows Calc.; morning diarrhœa; sputum purulent; great emaciation.
Mangan., Dros., Argent.Met. .	of the larynx.
Ozone . .	of the larynx.
Glanderin .	is said to have caused it in lungs.
Laches. . .	one of the best after pneumonia when tubercles are present.
Iodium, Oleum Jecoris, Hydr.	of lungs, with weakness at the stomach and diarrhœa.

77. Serous Membranes (commonly attacked in tuberculosis):

Sulph., Arsenic (Bryonia), Hepar, Phosph. (Kali Carb.), Ant. Tart. (Apis, Synovitis).

78. Feels bruised all over, worse from any motion (often anticipates rachitis):

Calc. Phos. (Ruta), Hepar, Silicea, Phosph., Oleum Jecoris.

79. Skin has an offensive odor, despite frequent washing:

Sulph., Psorin.

80. Skin Dry, Hot:

Sulphur, Calc. Carb., Lycop., Arsenic, Oleum Jecoris, Viola Tric.,

81. Skin Cold:

Arsenic, Carbo Veg., Sulph. (Camph.), (Verat. Album), Cal. Carb., Calcarea Phos., Mercur. (Clammy).

82. Kicks the clothes off (said to be a symptom of rachitis): Sulph.

83. Aggravations:

Natrum Sulph. .	worse living in damp dwellings.
Sulph., Psorin., Gettysb., Calc. Phos., Calc. C., Mercur. .	worse when the weather changes.
Sarsap. . .	worse in the spring.
Antim. Crudum, Natrum Mur., Sepia, Carbo.V., Silicea . .	worse in summer, in hot weather.
Sulph. . .	eyes, worse in hot weather.
Conium . .	photophobia, worse in summer.
Phosph., Silicea, Petrol(Rhod.)	worse in electric changes.
Sulph., Calc. C., Antim. Crud., Sepia, Hydras., Nit.Ac., Sarsa. etc.	worse when washed.

84. Relations of the Remedies in the symptoms given:

Sulph., followed by:

Calc. C. . .	child nervous, pupils large, etc.
Lycop., Psorin., Sepia, Silicea, Ozone, Phos.	in general.
Mercurius .	is an appropriate intercurrent remedy when Sulph. fails or only aggravates.

ANTIPSORICS IN THE ATROPHY OF INFANTS

CARBO VEG.	similar to Arsenic, Camph. (collapse).
CALCAR. CARB., followed by:	
LYCOP., IODIUM PHOS., THERID.	
SILICEA	bones ulcerate.
NITRIC ACID.	debility continues, child thin.
BELLAD.	intercurrent.
CALC. PHOS.	similar to Sulph., Phosph.
SILICEA similar to:	
PHOSPH.	abscesses of glands, nervousness, etc.
FLUORIC ACID	bone diseases.
NITRIC ACID	bones, ozæna, etc.
GETTYSB.	spine.
MERCUR.	said to be inimical to Silicea.
PHOSPH.	similar to Arsenic., Silicea, Carbo V., Hypophos. of Lime, Petroleum.
CAUSTICUM	inimical to Phos.
ARSENIC	similar to Argent. Nitric., Cinchon, VeratumAlb., Ferrum, Graph., Phosph., Ars.Iod., Ars.Sulph.Rub., Ars.Sulph.Flav., Secale,
BARYTA C.	similar to Causticum.
CALC. I., CONIUM	similar to Baryta C. (glands).
LYCOPOD.	similar to Arsenic (cross on waking).
GRAPH., ARSENIC, SARSA., THERID, IODIUM, LACH.	similar to Lycopodium.
ANTIM. CRUD.	similar to Bryon., Sulph.

ANTIM. TART.	similar to Verat. Album. (diarrhœa).
ARGENT. NITRIC.	similar to Natrum Mur.
SEPIA	similar to Natrum Mur., Nat. Phos., Borax, Sulph.
PHOS ACID	similar to Arsenic, Cinchona: both suit in anæmia (brain exhaustion from protracted diarrhœa.)
MAGNESIA CARB.	similar to Calc. C., Coloc., Chamom, Rheum.
MAGNESIA MUR.	similar to Silicea.
STAPHIS	similar to Merc., Chamom., Carbo V., Graph., Coloc.
HYDRASTIS	similar to Silicea, Sulph.
LYCOPODIUM	similar to Hydrastis (intertrigo).
CLEMATIS	similar to Hydrastis in eruption, worse from washing.
MURIATIC ACID	similar to Carbo Veg., Ars., Phos. Acid., Nitric Acid.
RHUS TOX.	similar to Muriatic Acid (irritable weakness, etc.).
SULPH. ACID.	similar to Sulph., Pulsat.
NATRUM SULPH.	similar to:
THUJA, SARSAP., STAPHIS.	sycosis.
BRYONIA	diarrhœa.
SARSAPAR.	similar to Lycopod., Sepia, Calcar. Carb., Mercur., Viola Tric.

Mercurius similar to *Bellad., Hepar, Carbo Veg., Nitric Acid, Staphis., Hydrastis, Sulph.* It symptomatically resembles *Calc. Carb.* and *Silicea* so closely as to require great caution in its choice. The latter remedy is said to be inimical to *Mercury.* When *Sulph.* ceases to improve, or acts too energetically, *Mercury* may be interposed. *Arum Tri.* similar to *Nitric Acid, Lycopod., Silicea, Ailanthus, Arsenic* and *Phosphorus.*

PROGNOSIS OF PANCREATIC DISEASES

SO few cases of disease of the pancreas have been recorded that but little can be said in regard to the prognosis of the various forms of affection to which this gland is liable, but from the known favorable action of remedies, when applied under the *law of similars,* in the treatment of diseases of kindred glands, we would be led to believe that a favourable prognosis might be given in many cases of *Acute Pancreatitis,* also in the early stages of *Chronic Pancreatitis.* As regards morbid growths, cysts, concretions, etc., we are at present unable to speak favorably, as most of such cases, thus far recorded, have been unrecognised prior to the autopsy. In general, owing to the uncertainty surrounding the diagnosis of pancreatic disease as well as the fact that many cases of supposed gastric, hapatic, or intestinal origin, have in reality been dependent upon disease of the pancreas, it is but fair to infer that many unrecognized cases have recovered.

PANCREATIC THERAPEUTICS

The therapeutics of diseases of the pancreas are very deficient. Works on poisions, as those of Wormley, Taylor, Reese and Ziemssen, seem to make no mention of the action of poisons on this viscus; nor do they include its pathological changes in their description of autopsies. Equally unsatisfactory is the medical literature of all schools.

In our own text-books and works on therapeutics, *Iris Versicolor* is mentioned as a leading remedy in acute inflammation of the pancreas; and *Phosphorus* and *Arsenic,* in fatty degeneration.

Since a prominent function of the pancreas is the contribution of a juice, which behaves like saliva, we may, perhaps be allowed to examine drugs which act upon the salivary glands and determine if they have any of the symptoms supposed to indicate pancreatic disease.

We add, then, in tabular form, the symptoms of *Bellad., Mercur., Conium, Carbo Animal., Carbo Veg., Rhus Tox., Hepar Sul., Kali Carb., Dulcam., Baryta C., Lycopod., Silicea, Sulph., Thuja, Calc. Ostr., Iodium, Podoph., Nitric Acid* and *Colchic.,* with a few others, whose symptoms are suggestive.

Soapy taste: *Iris Vers., Iod., Dulcam., Rhus Tox.*

Raises a watery fluid: *Bellad., Carbo Veg., Dulcam., Mercur., Hepar Sulph., Uranium Nitrate, Iris Vers.*

Icterus: *Mercur., Iris Vers., Podophyl., Lycopod., Dulcam., Sulph., Digital., Aurum.*

Pains in the region of the cœliac axis: *Iris Vers., Colchic., Phosph., Arsenic, Plumb., Rhus Tox, Stann., Plat., Kali Bich.*

Pains deep in between the pit of the stomach and navel: in addition to the above: *Zinc, Carbo Animal., Carbo Veg., Conium, Thuja.*

Ulceration of the duodenum: *Arsenic, Kali Bich., Uran. Nitrate.*

THERAPEUTICS OF PANCREATIC DISEASES

Stools contain fat: *Iris Vers., Iod., Phosph., Arsenic, Asclepias Tub., Thuja, Polyp. Offici., Sulphur, Cauc. F., Fagop., Fer Met, Pic. Acid.*

Stools undigested: *Arsenic, Phosph., Calc. Ostr., Iris Vers., Graph., Sulph., Nitric Ac.*

Stools with emaciation: *Arsenic, Phosph.*

Fatty degeneration of the pancreas: *Phosphorus, Silicea, Arsenic.*

Diabetes mellitus: *Phosph., Arsenic (Uranium Nitrate).*

Dr. Buchner recommends the following:

Catarrh of the salivary ducts: *Belladonna,* follow with *Mercurius.*

In chlorotic girls: *Pulsat., Calc. Ost.*

For hypertrophy of the pancreas: *Salts of Lime.*

Inflammation: *Bellad., Con., Hepar, Merc.*

Inflammation with suppuration: *Calcarea, Hepar, Silicea.*

Erythematous patients, or skin affections: *Calc. Acet.*

Cardiac or renal diseases: *Calc. Ars.*

Tuberculosis: *Calc. Phos.*

Melanosis: *Calc. Oxal.*

Gangrene or softening: *Kreos., Secale C.*

Pancreatic stones: *Bell., Salts of Lime, Potash* and *Soda.*

Cancer: *Phos., Silicea, Calc. Ars.* (latter with burning).

Icterus: *Bell., Merc., Digit., Aurum.*

Atrophy: *Phosph.*

Diabetes: *Phosph.*

In epidemic diseases: *Rhus Tox.,* then *Calc. Ars.*

Iris Versicolor : Burning distress in the region of the pancreas; vomiting of a sweetish water; saliva has a greasy taste; green watery diarrhœa, worse from 2 to 3 A.M., offensive flatus, smelling like copper. Diarrhœa contains undigested fat; bilious vomiting; sick headaches return periodically every week; dull, throbbing or shooting over one eye, usually over the right, with dim vision, nausea and vomiting.

Congestion and rupture of minute vessels in the pancreas of a cat poisoned with *Iris.*

Iodine : Great emaciation: hungry, anxious if he cannot get food at the appointed times; eats enormously, yet grows thin; soapy taste; fat in the stools; glands enlarged, or atrophied; lungs affected.

Phosphorus : May prove valuable in tuberculous patients; or when there are evidences of fatty degeneration of various organs; especially of the heart, liver or kidneys; distressing burning pains in the cœliac axis; stools undigested, containing particles of fat; face pale yellow; anæmia; atrophy of the pancreas with diabetes mellitus. One of the best remedies in neuralgia of the cœliac plexus.

The **Phosphorus** diarrhœa containing small particles like sago, or, as expressed by some, like tallow, is not the fatty diarrhœa which suggests the drug in pancreatic diseases.

Arsenicum : Organic changes similar to those mentioned under *Phosphorus;* but distinguished by greater restlessness and anxiety, as if the pains would drive him to despair. Ulceration of the duodenum, which, by extension, involves the pancreatic duct. This ulceration may be a result of burns, of malignant disease, etc. Neuralgia of the cœliac plexus. Stools undigested, containing fat.

THERAPEUTICS OF PANCREATIC DISEASES

Uranium Nitrate: Causes ulceration of the duodenum and also of the pyloric end of the stomach. It should, therefore, be remembered as a possible remedy, when the pancreas is secondarily involved. The stomach symptoms are: vomitting of a white fluid; putrid eructations; pains worse from fasting. The kidneys are usually affected; the urine deposits a mucopurulent looking sediment, and contains albumen, Phosphates, Lithic Acid, in excess. *Glycosuria.*

Lycopodium: According to Dunham, causes a chronic duodenitis; pressure on the hypochondrium produces tender pains in the epigastrium and *vice versa*. If, then, the pancreatic duct is involved, and we have the well-attested dyspeptic symptoms of *Lycopodium* and jaundice, it may prove curative. It should also be remembered in pancreatic stones.

If a pancreatic tumor is diagnosed, we may study the *Calcareous* preparations, as advised by Buchner, and also: *Conium,* deep-seated lancinating pains; tumor feels hard, nodulated: *Zinc* Carboan., Carbo Veg., Iodine, Phosph., Silicea* and *Arsenic.*

---

* Zinc has a hard tumefaction over and below the stomach. It has relieved enlargement and induration of the left lobe of the liver. We introduce it here merely as suggestive of its employment when the tumor is pancreatic, instead of hepatic.

MANGANESE FOR WOMEN

WE possess in some of the minerals, medicines of inestimable value in the treatment of organic lesions. Thus, for instance, fatty degenerations, cirrhoses, albuminuria and paralysis have been cured by *Aurum, Argentum, Manganum, Cuprum* and *Plumbum,* and, cœteris paribus, will be benefited by one or other of these same metals.

The minerals may also be advantageously employed as nutritive remedies. I know that I am treading upon debatable ground in advocating the use of the term nutritive. Still, I claim that there are some medicines which, when employed according to the *law of similars,* favour bodily growth and repair more than other drugs do. And it is with this fact in mind that I prefer regarding certain substances as nutritive remedies; *Cal. Phos.,* for example, symptoms indicating it, favors the deposit of lime at points of union of fractured bones. So, in reference to the metals under consideration, Dr. Burnett, an excellent Homœopathist, has found that gold will hasten the manly growth of the puny boy; Grauvogl has proved that *Platina* will aid in the resuscitation of the child whose health has been broken by pre-pubic masturbation. And, similarly we know that lead is needed often in paralysis with atrophy, *Argentum Nitricum* in ill-nourished nerves, *Copper* when mental and bodily over-exertion have impaired the strength and led to emaciation; and finally, I think that *Manganese* may, under certain circumstances, be regarded as a nutritive remedy for women.

A few months ago, Dr. Ringer published his experiments with the Permanganate of Potash, claiming that it was the *Manganese* in the compound that effected almost invariably a restoration of suppressed menses.

If, now, we turn to the provings of *Manganese* as collated in Allen's Encyclopædia, we find such symptoms as these: Pressure in the female genitals (Hahnemann); gripping, pinching above the pubes, eructations, weakness of the feet—all characteristic symptoms—followed by heaviness in the head, and a menstrual flow that is thick and black. (Nenning).

These effects show plainly that, if given in the large and crude dose employed by Dr. Ringer, *Manganese* can assuredly force the menses. To us, however, this fact is invaluable, not because it teaches us a rough and unnatural means of establishing a tardy or inoperative function, but because it becomes a symptom worthy of consideration in the application of the only law of cure to one of the ailments of women.

Last of all I had occasion to treat a young lady who, ever since puberty, a period of eleven years, had suffered from scanty and delayed menses. *Pulsatilla, Caulophyllum,* etc., failed. Finally, taking a new *"totality of symptoms",* I found in addition to the menstrual tardiness, general emaciation, weak pulse, pale sunken face, and great weakness of the back and limbs after the least exertion. These symptoms are all to be found in the provings of *Manganese,* and remembering, too, the symptoms of Nenning and the experiments of Ringer, calling to mind, also, the fact that workers in *Manganese* emaciate and develop symptoms of nervous weakness even to paralysis, I saw in this drug a *similimum* for my patient. To make my choice even more certain, and to test the power of the drug to cure amenorrhœa with ineffectual urging pains, I enquired particularly concerning the symptoms incident to the menstrual epochs. The reply was that there was always at these times much pressure and pain, but the system seemed too weak to secure the establishment of the flow. *Manganum Acet* 3 was given twice daily for two weeks before each menstrual period.

The effect was all that could be desired. For the first time in her life the menses came in proper time, and, what was more pleasing to the patient, with but little inconvenience. The lady has slowly but steadily improved in strength, and now menstruates quite naturally.

Lest I be misunderstood in my support of the term 'nutritive', I wish, even at the risk of repetition, to say that I mean simply the expression of the fact that drugs which can cause lesions characterized by mal-nutrition are often, of necessity, homœopathically adapted to the restoration to a normal state of bodily nourishment. Such medicines will act more profoundly and more lastingly than drugs which bear only a superficial resemblance to the disease to be treated. But in all cases the selection of the remedy must be made by the rules of the Organon, by the similarity of the symptoms. There is no other known way of finding a curative drug. And there is no law of cure—not 'rule' or 'method' as some teach—known to the scientific world but the *law of similars*.

SPASMUS GLOTTIDIS

SPASMUS glottidis, whether considered as a symptom, or as an indiopathic disease, possesses considerable interest, since it occasions much alarm and distress.

As a symptom, it causes the croupy cough and dyspnœic paroxysms incident to laryngitis. It also constitutes the main symptom in the non-inflammatory or the spasmodic croup. It is produced, too, during hysterical attacks, and as a reflex effect of tumors which press upon the par vaga or their branches, especially upon the recurrent or superior laryngeal. In the convulsive stage of tubercular meningitis it forms a frightful complication.

As a distinct disease, as a neurosis, it appears independently in inflammation, tumor or any organic affection, although it may be complicated thereby. It appears almost always in infants between the fourth and eleventh month. Very few cases of indisputable diagnosis have been noticed after the fifth year, and scarcely any among adults, except in cases of hysterical origin.

Of exciting causes the principal are: dentition; rachitis; over-feeding, or improper food; intestinal irritation; emotions, especially in children of nervous and excitable temperament. Enlargement of the glands, especially of the thymus, has been considered as an exciting cause, but of this pathologists are uncertain. It would seem that goitre might act as a provoking cause, since its pressure on the larynx is often sufficient to produce dyspnœa, and might create an irritation of the recurrent laryngeal nerve. Tumors, enlarged bronchial glands, atelectasis, in fact any abnormality which can embarrass the pneumo-gastric nerves, may give rise to the spasm.

The disease is unattended by fever, cough or catarrh, and the intervals between spasms, except in far-advanced cases, are free from all symptoms. The general health, however, is always below par.

Its essential phenomenon is difficult breathing, caused by a spasmodic closure of the rima glottidis. According to the intensity and persistency of the spasm are the accompanying symptoms. In mild cases the child is observed to suddenly stop breathing as if holding its breath. In a moment the paroxysm ceases and with it the mingled expression of astonishment and fear on its face. In rather severer cases the child is affected with the so-called 'crowing breathing', especially when excited or on awaking. When the disease is well-developed, the child is suddenly seized with dyspnœa; inspiration is crowing and prolonged, expiration all but impossible. The frequent inspiratory efforts, not followed by successful expirations, distend the lungs enormously. The child kicks, throws back its head, clenches its jaw and exhibits a very characteristic flexion of both fingers and toes. The face, at first red, becomes livid, the eyes project, and general convulsions may follow. In some instances the diaphragm becomes convulsed, thus adding to the distress. In others, the spasm continues so long that the child presents a complete picture of asphyxia. The general convulsions rather mark a second stage of the affection.

Complicating affections are rachitis, which exhibits the symptom so often that it might be considered as a part of the rachitic disease; scrofulosis, with its enlarged glands and delayed dentition, marasmus, favouring the spasm by impairing growth and weakening resistance to disease; too rapid growth, as in the children of tuberculous parents, etc.

SPASMUS GLOTTIDIS

The neurosis may end in recovery. which, however, is generally tardy, or the paroxysms may become so frequent and so severe as to result in death, either during an attack from asphyxia, from convulsions brought on by cerebral congestion, or between attacks from secondary affections.

The disease may be easily diagnosed. From Croup: It differs in the absence of cough, and fever, etc.

From ŒDEMA GLOTTIDIS: It is distinguished by the absence of serous infiltration about the rima and by the breathing, which is worse during inspiration in the œdema, expiration readily pushing up the dropsical sacs above the rima of the glottidis.

From ASTHMA: It is distinguished by the seat of the dyspnœa, the noisy respiratory murmur heard over the chest and the free glottis belonging to that complaint.

SPASMS of the respiratory muscles may indeed complicate spasmus glottidis, but as an independent symptom it is plainly separable.

If TONIC, the thorax is retained in a position of inspiration, so that breathing is disphragmatic.

If CLONIC, inspiration and expiration are rapid and noisy.

Synonyms of spasmus glottidis, most of which are inaccurate, are: asthma millari, asthma wigandi, asthma spasmodicum, asthma thymicum, laryngismus, stridulus, "crowing" spasm, etc.

Treatment may be divided into preventive, palliative and curative. As preventive, avoid all excitement, as violent emotions, fright, anger, etc., provoke a paroxysm. See that the child is not overfed, and that its food is properly selected. If the mother's milk does not seem to agree, substitute cow's milk mixed with sweetened barley water, or milk with Ridge's food. If the stomach is excessively irritable, a preparation of barley, milk and a small addition of Glycerin may be needed. All so-called table-food should be prescribed if the child has not yet cut the majority of its teeth. Even oatmeal, though strained carefully, is often injurious to children under six months' old. If dentition is difficult or tardy, see if the diet is nutritious enough, and select a remedy principally from those useful in teething. If worms excite the disease, administer honey twice daily. If constipation acts as a provoking cause, make frequent use of enemata; or, in every young children, stimulate rectal contractions by inserting a plug of castile soap or a suppository of cocoa-butter. If the child is old enough, say eight to ten months or more, prepare the food with oatmeal, strained but cooked only ten to fifteen minutes, and, if its stomach is not weak, sweetened with brown sugar.

As palliative, instruct the mother or nurse to warm the hands or the feet when they become cold. During the incipiency of an attack, pat the child on the back or on the nates; plunge the child's hands into hot water, or into hot and cold water alternately, press down the tongue, tickle the fauces with the finger or, in extreme cases, employ artificial respiration, as in drowning or in asphyxia neonatorum.

Remedies calculated to cure the disease must always be selected in accordance with the rules of our Organon. ·Nevertheless our labour may be lightened, and our memory refreshed for an emergency, by a review of those drugs most likely to be called into service.

Remedies causing more or less spasm of the glottis: *Aconite, Arsenic, Asafoetida, Atropin, Belladonna, Bromine, Calc. Phos., Chamom., Chelidon.,*

SPASMUS GLOTTIDIS

Chlorine, Coral. Rub., Cuprum, Fluorine, Gelsemium, Hepar, Hyoscyam., Ignatia, Iodine, Ipecac (Kaolin), Laurocerasus, Lachesis, Lobelia Inflata, Lycopodium, Mephitis, Moschus, Naja, Nux Vom., Oleum Animale, Opium, Phospor., Phytolacca (Physostigma), Plumb., Sambucus, Silicea, Spongia, Stramon., Strychnine, Sulphur, Verat. Alb.

These may conveniently be divided into three classes, only two of which strictly belong to the subject under consideration. 1st. For the acute paroxysm, *Chlorine, Cuprum, Belladonna, Lachesis, Sambucus, Stramonium, Chamomilla, Arsenicum, Hyoscyamus, Oleum Animale, Phytolacca, Veratrum Album, Fluorine, Mephitis.*

2nd. Chronic cases, constitutional accompaniments: *Plumbum., Calc. Phos., Phosphor., Silicea, Lycopod., Sulph., Baryta C., Iodine, Hepar.*

3rd. Remedies adapted to diseases in which the spasm is a symptom, as croup: *Spongia, Bromine, Iodine (Kaoline), Lachesis.*

Hysteria and various nervous affections: *Ignatia, Asafoetida, Moschus, Strychnine, Zinc, Cicuta, Physostigma, Gelsem.*

Asthma: *Ipecac., Lobelia Inflata, Camphor, Sambucus.*

Brain affections: *Bellad., Hyosc., Stramon., Cicuta, Agaricus, Cuprum, Opium, Atropin.*

Spinal affections (causing the spasm by reflection): *Nux Vom., Zinc, Physostigma, Strychnine, Bellad.*

Affections of the par vaga, or of their origins: *Lobelia, Gelseminum, Laurocerasus, Naja, Arsenic.*

Suppressed hives: *Arsenic.*

It is not necessary to enumerate the especial symptoms of any of the above, excepting those which indisputably apply to the acute and chronic symptoms of the neurotic spasmus glottidis.

Chlorine, as proved and confirmed by Dr. Dunham, corresponds thoroughly to the paroxysm; inspiration unimpeded and natural, expiration absolutely impossible from a closure of the rima glottidis; inspiration again made was found easy enough, but attended with a slight crowing sound, expirations again impossible. Face livid, lungs fearfully distended from frequent inspiration without any corresponding exit of air; partial coma followed, the spasm relaxed and respiration become free. Although all the Halogens and even *Spongia* cause this spasm of the larynx, none so completely typifies the spasmus glottidis as *Chlorine*. Similar to *Mephitis*.

Lachesis is of service when the spasms occur during sleep; the child, as it were, sleeps into an attack, and is aroused, gasping for breath. At other times the paroxysms recur after each nap. The external neck, about the larynx, is very sensitive to the slightest touch.

Belladonna. The smallest quantity of fluid drunk, excites a spasm; larynx painfully dry, yet the child refuses all drink. Larynx feels suddenly constricted. Breathing during sleep is intermittent or irregular. On falling asleep the child awakes and starts as if frightened. Sleep restless, tossing about the bed, talking or crying out. Kicks about, quarrels in sleep. Brain excited; face red; eyes injected; strabismus, or dilated pupils; opisthotonic convulsions; clenched teeth; skin hot and dry or bathed in hot sweat, or fearful convulsions

NOTE.—General convulsions may possibly be palliated by firmly grasping the child's thumbs, or by forcibly flexing the thumbs and toes.

of flexor muscles. Over-susceptible to impressions, and hence made worse by strong light, noises, the least contradiction or cross word, by the irritation or dentition or the presence of irritating or indigestible substances in the abdomen. Urine stains a deep yellow or is scanty even suppressed. Larynx sensensitive to pressure.

Sambucus, employed by Hahnemann. Suffocative paroxysm after 12 P.M.,; aroused with anxiety, trembling, shortness of breath to suffocation; wheezing in the chest, difficult inspirations; face blue, eyes and mouth half open, profuse hot sweat. Its symptoms do not seem to point distinctively to a spasm of the glottis, however.

Moschus causes a spasm of throat, larynx, and lungs. Sudden sensation as if the larynx closed on the breath, as from inhaling sulphur-vapor. It is more applicable during the course of diseases which exhibit impending paralysis of the pneumogastrics.

Stramonium. Child arouses from sleep frightened and clings to those around. Becomes blue in the face; muscles of the chest also spasmodically affected. Violent convulsions.

Chamomilla. Sensation of oppression and slight constriction in the region of the larynx. Dyspnœa as from suffocative catarrh (the larynx feels constricted), constant irritation to cough. Hot swea on face and head, especially during sleep. Child becomes stiff and bends backwards, kicks with his feet when carried, screams and throws everything off. Staring eyes, child reaches and grasps for something, draws the mouth back and forth. Peevish, irritable; cries for things and pushes them away when given to him. Worse from anger or other violent emotions; worse from exposure to cold winds. Worse during dentition, accompanied by "wind asthma"; "liver-grown" or green, watery, hot, offensive stools.

Opium, especially after a fright.

Chelidonium Majus causes a sensation as if the larynx was pressed from without on the œsophagus, but swallowing, not breathing, is made difficult. Constrictive sensation in the trachea mounting towards the larynx. Constrictive spasm in the gullet, forcing him to swallow. Choking sensation in the throat, worse by breathing. It has no similarity to the disease under consideration.

Oleum Animale. Larynx feels as if it would be closed by outward pressure when lying on the back with the head bent forwards.

Gelsemium. Long croupy inspiration and sudden forcible expiration.

Phytolacca. Frequent spasmodic closure of the larynx; drawing of the thumbs into the palms; flexion of the toes; face distorted; muscles of the eyes so affected that the motions of one eye are independent of the other.

Plumbum causes closure of rima with sudden difficulty of breathing and asphyxia. Convulsions, during which expiration is suddenly arrested as if a valve closed the glottis. Emaciation. Stool, with much urging; hard balls.

Cuprum is well adapted to cases which have advanced to the convulsive stage. On attempting to take a deep breath, dyspnœa, stridulous inspiration. Face blue and sometimes covered with cold sweat. Body stiff, spasmodic twitchings; thumbs clenched. Gurgling down the œsophagus.

Mephitis. When drinking or talking, is liable to get foreign substances into the larynx. Inspiration difficult, expiration all but impossible; convulsions. Similar to *Chlorine.*

Iodine. Tightness and constriction about the larynx, with soreness, hoarse voice, etc. (See *Record,* 1873, p. 89). Glands, cervical and mesenteric, enlarged and indurated. The child has a tendency to marasmus. Excellent appetite, yet grows thin; or is indifferent to food; stools clayey; urine high-colored, scanty. Skin yellow; heart's action feeble, and increased by every motion. Child unbearably irritable. Well-marked, painless goitre.

Bromine. Gasping for breath, with wheezing and rattling in the larynx; child awakens gasping, hoarse, cries for water, which relieves. The face is hot and red and the eyes often injected and inflamed. Suitable rather to light-complexioned and blue-eyed children.

Spongia. Starts from sleep with contraction of the larynx; whistling inspiration; breathes as through a sponge; breathes with head bent backwards.

Veratrum Album. Spasmus glottidis, with protruded eyes; weakness and cold sweat on the forehead.

Arsenicum. Sudden dyspnœa at night, threatening suffocation. The child breathes freely between spells, but appears weak and is restless. Caused by suppressed hives. Pale waxen face. Convulsions; body hot, sweaty, and pale.

Phosphorus. Select by constitutional symptoms. The child is unusually tall, but not fat. The skin is clear and transparent. Easily catches cold on the chest and becomes hoarse. Parents tuberculous. Stridulous inspiration in the evening on falling asleep.

Laurocerasus. Cases in which the heart is affected. The child becomes blue, gasps for breath, face even livid, pulse thready.

Silicea. Not from local symptoms, but from constitutional. The child is rachitic; the head is disproportionately large; but the body emaciated. The head and feet sweat; in the latter locality there is offensive sweat. Is nervous and excitable; hence external impressions readily awaken convulsions. Dentition retarted.

Calc. Phos. Delayed dentition; the child sweats easily, especially during sleep; becomes emaciated, but the abdomen remain flabby. The skin looks yellow. The child gets suffocative attack when lifted from the crib. Is subject to rachitis. There is diarrhœa with green, hot and watery stools. Craves salt meats, bacon, etc. Compare *Calc. Ost.*

Sulphur. Attacks come on when dropping off to sleep. Sudden jerks of the limbs in sleep. Slow dentition. Disposed to fever, etc.

Baryta Carb. The child grows slowly and becomes dwarfish and timid. Cannot learn rapidly. Glands, especially the tonsils become swollen and indurated. Tonsilitis after every exposure to cold and damp air.

THE MOUTH SYMPTOMS OF THE MINERAL ACIDS

THE mineral acids, by their caustic action, cause a violent inflammation of the parts which they touch, leading, as when the buccal mucous membrance is the part attacked, to destruction of epithelium, coagulation of tissues, ulcers, and even gangrene.

Symptoms vary, therefore, from slight increased redness and raw appearence of cheeks and tongue to the production of blisters and the formation of ulcers and sloughs. Agreeably to such disturbances the neighbouring glands are affected, notably those which empty into the mouth; and there is also decided systemic prostration.

But the several acids vary in their intensity of action and in their respective characteristic effects. *Muriatic* and *Sulphuric Acids* cause deep ulcers; *Nitric Acid,* ulcers with hard, everted edges, paining as from splinters sticking.

All these cause inflammatory swelling of the tongue; but *Muriatic Acid* seems, more than the others, to cause a hardening of the tongue, with or without deep bluish ulcers. Hence Hahnemann employed it in cancer.

All increase and alter the saliva; *Nitric Acid* most intensely developing a ropy, fetid ptyalism; *Sulphuric Acid* a saltish saliva, with much frothy mucus in the mouth; *Phosphoric Acid,* a frothy, sour saliva.

The mineral acids, however, have another, and, to the homœopathician, a very important effect. I refer to the debility which they induce. In small doses they are termed tonic. They stimulate digestion, except, perhaps *Sulphuric Acid,* which precipitates albumen in an insoluble form (Ringer). But soon they induce true characteristic debility. This debility is not simply that of functional weakness, it is more like that which arises from impoverished blood, from severe and malignant disease, from mal-nutrition. And it is here we find the grandest use of the acids.

So far as mouth symptoms are concerned, this debility is manifested in one of two ways,—either the tongue is red, raw-looking, dry and smooth; or it is pale, flabby, and denuded of epithelium. In either form aphthæ may be present, though they are more common with the first form. Let us see if we can discriminate between the acids in these classes of symptoms.

Phosphoric Acid offers a tongue with a central red streak, widening as it approaches the tip. But in this acid anæmia is more pronounced than inflammation; pale smooth tongue, coated with a sticky mucus. If, as is claimed by Galloway, lemon juice contains *Phosphoric Acid,* we can expect the latter to do good in scurvy. In addition to symptoms named, it has swelling of the gums; they bleed when touched, etc.

Nitric Acid has an especial affinity for the junctions of mucous membrane and skin; it attacks margins or borders. Hence we find as valuable accompaniments of stomacace, aphthæ, etc., sores in the corners of the mouth, and vesicles and sores on the margin of the mouth.

Its buccal symptoms are very closely allied to those of mercury, and therefore it excels the other acids as an antidote to mercurialization, and as a remedy in secondary and tertiary syphilis.

Muriatic Acid is of inestimable value in debility, traceable to atony of the stomach, with prolonged refusal of food, or with persistent vomiting of what is taken. There seems to be no reaction. The muscles are utterly exhausted, and the vitality is so low that the sphincters relax, permitting defecation with each attempt at urination. The mouth is full of fetid, bluish-white aphthæ, with here and there deep, dark ulcers.

Sulphuric Acid is scarcely second in what we may term this "gastric debility." All substance is at once vomited, though brandy diluted is retained for a time. The patient, if old enough and conscious, complains of a general tremor. This may be purely subjective, or it may be also objective.

The aphthæ are whitish and also yellowish. This last color is, I think, worthy of especial note, since we know how charecetristic are yellow, slimy stools in this remedy; and since, moreover, Dr. R. M. Smith has confirmed the use of the drug in diphtheria, when the membrane is of a marked lemon-yellow color, hanging in strings from the posterior nares.

This remedy, resembles *Kali Bichromicum,* but is distinguished by the tough fibrinous quality of the secretions of the latter.

While these several acids agree in the kind of diseased effects produced, we see that they differ so essentially as to render their indiscriminate use unscientific.

NOTES ON THE TREATMENT OF PERITONITIS

IN no disease is it more important to observe strictly every homœopathic rule of prescribing; for the vital forces are quickly and profoundly depressed, and a mistake in the choice of the remedy may precipitate a fatal termination. Local symptoms must be carefully compared with the general condition, especially with the state of the circulation, the bodily temperature and what is of equal importance, the mental state.

Mucilaginous drinks acidulated with tamarinds or lemon-juice are often grateful and soothing to the irritated stomach. If the lemonade be made hot and then allowed to cool it is less likely to cause intestinal gripping. Effervescing drinks may increase the tympany, and should usually be avoided. During the early stages, when the fever run high, farinaceous foods may be given; but if the liver is so diseased as to interfere with biliary secretion, starch and oily foods will not be readily digested, and must be mainly substituted by mutton, beef, or chicken broth. In such a contingency the broth should be allowed to cool first, that all the fat may be skimmed off. In large cities poultry is brought to market so poorly and improperly fed, that great care is needed in its purchase.

Alcoholic drinks should be interdicted except in advanced cases, in which vitality is very low, or where blood-poisoning demands them.

Aconite. Burning-cutting pains, worse from the slightest motion and from lying on the right side; hard, frequent pulse; skin hot and dry. Abdomen hot and sensitive to touch. Face anxious; restlessness; fear of death. Caused by checked sweat, exposure to dry, cold winds, drinking ice-water while fatigued and hot. Puerperal cases especially in full-blooded women, when violent emotions seem to have caused a checking of the lochia. Hahnemann's advice here is imperative, not to give *Aconite* simply because there is fever or because there is synochal fever, but to be guided by the infallible accompaniments of restlessness and mental agony.

Verat. Viride has come into fashion as a rival of *Aconite*. It is selected in the beginning of inflammations by the pulse, which is said to express great arterial excitement. But the two remedies are really not at all similar. The *Veratrum* rather pictures asthenic fever of a low type. Congestions and inflammations are accompanied by delirum, great prostration, and, what is very characteristic, a red streak down the centre of the tongue. It has no action on serous membranes, like *Aconite*.

Belladonna. Abdomen distended, hot, and exquisitely sensitive to touch or to the least jar of the bed; pains in sudden attacks, which come and go suddenly: or less frequently, gradually increase and gradually decrease (see *Allen* Vol. II, p. 102). Sometimes enteritis co-exists, with clutching as from nails at the navel; bloody, slimy diarrhœa. Bodily temperature very high. On raising the bed-clothes a hot steam rises. Head very hot and dry; or hot and yet bathed in sweat. Feet cold, head hot. This is not the coldness indicative of collapse, but of upward congestion. Urine scanty and sometimes golden yellow. Delirium, varying from simple starts in sleep to furor, with red, congested face and throbbing carotids. The face instead of being red, may appear pale, hot, and expressive of deep-seated distress. There are drowsiness and stupor but is easily aroused.

Belladonna especially attacks the uterus and ileocœcal region, and should be studied in metritis with peritonitis, and also in typhlitis. In the former case the lochia will be checked or hot, and occasionally in offensively smelling clots. There is also backache; she feels as if her back was broken.

Cantharis. That portion of the peritoneum which covers the bladder is particularly affected; frequent and painful urination; the urine passes in drops and may be bloody; tenesmus vesicæ and burning, cutting continue after micturition. Cutting, griping, burning, and wandering pains, worse in the lower abdomen. Face indicates extreme suffering; eyes sunken. Also indicated when effusion has taken place; and still more when collapse results from internal suppuration; surface cool; he lies unconscious with outstretched arms, which occasionally jerk; convulsions; suppressed urine.

Bryonia, Cantharis, Merc. Corros., Apis and *Sulphur* are useful especially when exudation has taken place. It would be an egregious mistake to select one of these, or of any other group, merely because they have been known to produce seroplastic effusions. The individual symptoms must always determine the choice.

Bryonia acts well, especially in rheumatic patients and when the diaphragm is attacked as shown by stitches with each breath or motion of the body. Tongue dry, and possibly white down the centre. There is none of the restlessness and agony of *Aconite*. He desires to lie perfectly still and be quiet. Still, his face is a perfect picture of anguish; he breathes in quick, short inspirations, which oppress him, and in some instances he is impelled by his distress to move, but desists, for the pains become thereby aggravated. The fever runs higher than with *Cantharis,* and the urine is scanty, dark, red, and clear.

Merc. Cor. has produced in toxic does peritoneal effusion. The exudate is purulent, and is accompanied with creeping chills, sweat without relief, and cutting, stabbing, griping pains. There is less of the well-defined stitch which characterizes *Bryonia*. Both *Merc. Corros.* and *Cantharis* have strangury with intense burning and if enteritis complicates, both may have slimy, bloody stools. The latter, however, is relieved by perspiration.

Apis Mel. is recognized by a distressing aching soreness of the abdomen, which will tolerate no pressure; burning stinging pains, or sudden knife-like thrusts through the abdomen. Urine scanty, dark and often albuminous. Absence of thirst, or drinks little and often. Œdematous puffiness of the face. In bad cases, with enteritis combined, he passes thin yellow stools with every motion of the body, as though the anus and rectum were paralyzed. Infants and those predisposed to tuberculosis scream out in their sleep a sudden shrill cry from cerebral irritation. Face looks distressed, he feels as if he would die; but he is not so full of fear as to indicate *Aconite*. Sleepy but cannot sleep. This differs from *Belladonna;* the *Apis* patient can't sleep because he feels so nervous and fidgety.

When typhoid symptoms develop, *Rhus. Tox., Lachesis, Lycopodium, Arsenic* and *Baptisia* stand foremost.

Rhus Tox. is most frequently indicated. Tongue red, dry; red at the tip; tympany; restless change of place; change of position relieves his pains, though it increases his weakness and compels him to desist. Muttering, not violent, delirium. His dreams are full of laborious effort; he thinks he is swimming, climbing hills, etc. If enteritis is present the stools are bloody, and each movement is accompanied with tearing down the thighs.

Baptisia deserves the preference when he is confused as to his personal unity,—thinks himself double, scattered in pieces, etc. Tongue is brown, especially down the centre. Stools dark, bloody, painless. Fever and temperature show decided evening exacerbation.

Lachesis inflames the cœcum. Even if unconscious, he will resist the slightest touch to the abdomen; parts most distant from the heart are cool; pulse rapid, feeble, or intermittent; arouses from sleep smothering. This smothering may also suggest *Baptisia,* but the conditions are different. The tongue trembles and catches behind the lower teeth.

Lycopodium. Rumbling in the splenic flexure. Diaphragmitis, with feeling of a cord marking the costal attachments of the diaphragm; tympany. Especially useful when the brain shows signs of giving out; he becomes more and more drowsy; eyes half open, expressionless, and covered with a film; the lower jaw tends to drop; one foot cold and the other warm; no urine in the bladder, or it passes involuntarily and stains the sheets with a red sand.

Arsenic is invaluable when the patient is pale and hot, eyes half-open, with absence of winking; "gum" on the eyes; restlessness or great anguish after 12 P.M. These symptoms are not uncommon in infants.

Hyoscyamus must be remembered when there are spasmodic jerking delirium; she suddenly sits up, looks around and lies down again; uncovers herself; lascivious talk; or, stupor, stool and urine involuntary; the urine leaves a streaks of red sand on the clothing.

Terebinthina. Burning in the uterus; tympany; tongue dry and smooth; urine scanty, dark, smoky, with strangury.

Kali-Carb. Stitching pains all over the abdomen; tympany; urine scanty, dark, nervous; easily startled if touched, especially if the feet are touched; unconsciousness in puerperal peritonitis; or, stupid, cares for nothing; when questioned is at a loss what to reply; pulse rapid, weak, or intermittent.

In peritonitis of infants, generally tuberculous, compare with the above, *Sulph., Silica, Calc. Ostr., Calc. Phos., Phosph., Iodine, Ars. Iod., Baryta C., Psorin.,* etc.

Calc. Ostr., general symptoms agreeing, must be remembered when, in child or adult, the abdominal pains are relieved by cold applications. This exceptional symptom of lime is recorded in Raue's Pathology, and may be inferred from the provings. In Allen, Vol. II, p. 365, we read: "Frequent attacks of colic after the disappearance of a severe coryza that had lasted two days, with great weariness and sickly look of the face, lasting several days, and then suddenly and completely relieved by bathing in cold water."

For typhlitis, which frequently leads to peritonitis: *Bellad., Lachesis, Mercur., Merc. Corros., Rhus Tox., Nux Vom., Ginseng, Hepar, Opium, Plumbum, Rhamn. Frangula,* etc.

The tympany which so annoys the patient is a very dangerous symptom when occurring late in the disease. For this compare: *Opium, Lycop., Kali C., Terebinth., Rhus Tox., Colchic., Carbo Veg., Phosph., Cinchona, Verat. Alb.* and *Cocculus.*

Raphanus produces distended abdomen; no emission of flatus either upwards or downwards. Dr. Bell's case confirming this symptom is suggestive, and should lead us to a careful study of the drug.

INDICATIONS FOR SOME OF THE METALS IN NEURALGIA

AURUM is useful in neuralgia after abuse of mercury. The pains are of a stinging and tearing character, and are almost always associated with anxious and hasty movements. The circulation is certain to be involved, and you have that anxiety and dread and haste that belong to heart affections.

In **Metallic Silver, (Argent. Met.)** the pains gradually increase and suddenly cease. They occur usually in very nervous people who are subject to vertigo. The neuralgia is especially apt to occur in the joints.

The pains of **Nitrate of Silver (Argent. Nitr.)** have this character: They gradually increase until they reach their acme, and drive the patients almost mad. Then they radiate in all directions.

Platina has for its characteristic gradually increasing and gradually decreasing pains. We will see presently that *Stannum* also has gradually increasing and gradually decreasing pains. The distinction between the two remedies lies in the concomitant symptoms. With *Platina,* these pains are followed by numbness or cramp in the affected part. With *Stannum,* there is more pure nervousness, the muscles jerk, and the patient is low-spirited and sad.

Plumbum has neuralgic pains, and they are relieved by hard, firm pressure, and they are associated with emaciation of the affected part. You will find it indicated in neuralgia of the abdomen, with pains that almost drive the patient crazy. If these are relieved

INDICATIONS FOR SOME OF THE METALS, ETC. 257

by pressure, *Plumbum* is usually the remedy, whether there is retraction of the abdomen or not.

Cuprum Metallicum is indicated in suddenly appearing pains in the involuntary muscles, and usually associated with a great deal of congestion and cramps.

The **Arsenite of Copper (Cup. Ars.)** is a very superior remedy in neuralgia of the abdominal viscera. I do not mean neuralgia of the abdominal walls, but of the viscera themselves. The pains are periodical in their recurrence.

The **Ferrum** pains are usually relieved from slow motion: in fact, they compel the patient to get up and move about for relief. They are worse at night and are usually accompanied by false plethora.

Manganum is chemically similar to *Ferrum,* and suits similar cases. Like the latter remedy, it produces chlorosis and anæmia. But this chlorosis and anæmia are not so erethistic as in *Ferrum*. There is not so much ebullition of blood. In addition, *Manganese* seems to produce a sort of periostitis, or if not periostitis, periosteal pains which are worse at night and worse from touch.

Kobaltum acts upon the spine and its nerves, particularly upon the lumbar spine, causing intense backache, which is worse sitting than it is walking. Such back-ache usually follows sexual excesses and is associated with weakness of the legs. The legs tremble and the knees give out.

Niccolum I do not know much about. It promises very well, however. It is particularly indicated in tearing pains in the head, worse in the left eye and recurring every two weeks. This is a periodical remedy. It has hoarseness occurring every spring. It also has a cough which, I would like to have you remember, is a dry, teasing cough compelling the patient to sit up, it jars the head so.

Mercurius is useful for neuralgia of the face, extremities and back, especially when the pains are rendered intolerable by the warmth of the bed and are worse at night. It is especially indicated in facial neuralgia, starting from decayed teeth.

GOUT

GOUT is a disease as obstinate as it is painful. It owes its origin usually to high living, although heredity has much to do with its development. Murchison, in his able lectures on funtional diseases of the liver, traces gout to lithæmia; that is, to imperfect oxidation in the liver with the consequent production of excreta less oxidized than normally—lithic acid and lithates, instead of urea. Now, Dr. Garrod determined that the gouty joint contained a concretion of lithate of soda. This salt accumulates in the blood by reason of its excessive production, which excess is favoured by over-indulgence in rich foods and by a functionally imperfect liver. The surcharged blood seeks to rid itself of the offender through the kidneys, and also by depositing it in various tissues removed from the central organs. This deposit would seem to be made first in the smaller joints, later in larger joints, and finally it encroaches on several of the viscera. If the kidneys are able to eliminate the lithates, the patient maintains comfortable health; but when these organs fail in their work or are overburdened, or, again, if perchance, exposure start an articular inflammation, the joints become involved. As the disease progresses, the kidneys may become affected with morbus Brightii, the heart may suffer from inflammation, the stomach becomes deranged, and arthritic headache and ophthalmia complicate the case, rendering the torture intolerable. The Frenchman's diagnosis between rheumatism and gout is trite and painfully true: "Put ze finger in ze vice and screw him tight: zat is ze rheumatism; now give him one under screw—zat is ze gout."

But why is it that all who indulge to excess in the pleasure of the table are not affected with gout? And, too, why is it that this lithic deposit so frequently selects the great toe for its punctum saliens?

The answer is involved in that great unanswered problem of constitution,—the soil in which disease is to grow, and by which disease is so materially modified. Hahnemann and Grauvogl gave us each three constitutions, but there must be many more. The physician who daily cauterizes the chancre or checks gonorrhœa with injections, is forming a "constitution" for his patient which will last him through life and seriously impress his offspring. No disease is ever cured except it be removed to the periphery. When we begin to treat our patients according to their several tendencies to disease, rather than according to the acute symptoms only, we will attain an amount of success never yet even dreamed of. Until then let each physician endeavour to make his prescription as accurately as his materia medica will permit, always valuing symptoms from the centre to the circumference; from mind to body; from more to less vital parts; from function to organ.

The treatment of gout may be divided into that of the acute paroxysm and that of the general symptoms.

In an acute attack the following have been most successfully used:—

Colchicum: In the evening fretful, cannot tolerate any annoyances; any external impression, noise, odor, touch or bright light makes him irritable. Toe joint becomes inflamed, dark red, hot and intensely painful; he is beside himself with agony. The foot becomes œdematous. Urine scanty and dark red. The smell of food makes him sick at the stomach. Greatly prostrated.

Ledum Palustre: After abuse of alcoholic drinks; pimples on the forehead; face bloated awakened with a hot, tensive swelling of the toe and foot, with tearing, shooting, grinding pains; cannot bear the least covering or the warmth of the bed; foot becomes œdematous, and yet the urine is copious and frequently passed. Old nodes, the sequelæ of former attacks, become excessively painful.

Arnica: Inflamed joint is shinning, red and hard. He dreads the proximity of any one, having a constant fear that they will touch him. Pains unbearable during the night; the bed feels too hard.

Sulphur: Especially for drunkards or those who indulge in too rich food and take but little exercise; face blotched red; nose red habitually; as soon as he drops into a sleep the affected limb jerks and arouses him with excruciating pains. Pains are erratic and leave a sensation of numbness. Often indicated.

Eupatorium Perf.: In some cases, when the big toe is swollen, the foot œdematous, the urine profuse and the body aches all over as if the "bones were broken."

Sabina: Probably more for women; great toe hot, swollen, paining at night, worse from warmth in bed; high fever.

Antimonium Crudum: Especially when the stomach is involved; tongue white, bowels costive; vomiting and retching.

Bryonia: Joint swollen, tense, not very red; if he raised his head he feels deathly sick; tongue white down the centre; patient unbearably cross.

Nux Vom.: The patient is irritable, overbearing; leads a sedentary life, and yet eats to excess; habitually costive; face sallow, but often also a flushing of the cheeks; aroused at 3 A.M. with pains in the great toe. Useful for drunkards.

Rhus Tox.: After exposure to wet; must move, though it intensifies the pains.

Benzoic Acid: Usually his urine has an offensive odor and deposits a reddish, clouded sediment, but now it is nearly clear and he complains of tearing in the joints; old nodes become painful. As these pains abate, palpitation of the heart sets in, ceasing only when they increase.

Berberis Vulgaris: Tearing, burning, stinging pains; patient subject to the formation of biliary calculi; darting, sharp pains radiate from the kidneys, usually downward and along the ureters; urine cloudy, grayish, depositing a sediment; fistula in ano.

Manganum: Toe or other joint dark red in spots; tendo Achillis shortened; pains shift, seem to be in the periosteum, and are worse at night.

Cinchona: Painful; oversensitive to pain; great weakness; pains worse at night.

For subacute and chronic cases, choose from the following:—

Causticum, nodes on the joints; joints stiff, toes or fingers contracted; pains relieved by the warmth of the bed.

Guaiacum, similar to the above and following it well. Limbs drawn up and curved; worse from motion.

Collocynth, stiffness of the joints, with boring pains.

Lycopodium, nodes; fingers and toes pain more at night; swelling of the dorsa of the feet; numbness; flatulence; rumbling in the splenic flexure; full feeling after a mouthful or two of food; lithic acid deposit in the urine. Must rise often at night to pass water.

Calc. Carb., especially when the well-known "lime-constitution" exists. Useful for drunkards, who feel worse at every change of weather. Also, when standing or working in water aggravates the disease.

Graphites, tearing in the toes; awakens at night and springs out of bed suffocating; eating relieves; gastralgia. Fleshy, bloated; nose red; skin rough, herpetic.

Rhododendron, always worse at the approach of a storm, especially of a thunderstorm.

Staphisagria, pain from the eyes to the teeth; eyes burn and feel dry despite the profuse lachrymation; patient weak, exhausted by dissipation; face sallow; eyes sunken.

Kali Hyd., periosteum affected; distressing pains at night, preventing sleep; limbs contracted; morbus Brightii. Abuse of mercury.

Kali Bich., pains in the fingers alternate with gastric ailments.

Natrum Phos. caused pains about the heart, which ceased when pains returned in the toe.

Lith. Carb., heart affected; worse stooping; tearing down the limbs; urination relieves the heart. Deposits on the valves of the heart; pain from heart to head; burning in the great toe.

Iodium, inveterate noctrnal pains, but not much swelling of the joints.

Amon. Phos., to remove deposit in the joints.

Aurum Mur., gnawing deep in the joints, which were recently inflamed.

Gout affecting the Head or Eyes.

Bryonia, sharp pains, worse on motion, neck stiff, eyes sore when moved, sclerotica red; glaucoma.

Coloc., boring pains in head or eyes, better from firm pressure.

Ipecac., pains from head into tongue, with nausea.

Nux Vom., headache with persistent retching.

Kali Hyd., lumps on the cranium; chemosis of the conjunctiva.

Colchic., Spigelia, severe pains in and around the eyes.

Sulphur, persistent headache; eyes inflamed, feel as if sticks or splinters were piercing the eyes.

Lycopod., Rhus Tox., tearing about the head; iritis, glaucoma, piercing, tearing pains through the eye to the occiput, worse at night; lids spasmodically closed, scalding tears.

Staphis., eyes feel dry, yet there is lachrymation; pains from eye to teeth.

Sepia, pains shooting upwards, with nausea and sour vomiting.

Stomach or Abdomen.

Antimonium Crudum, white tongue, vomiting and retching.

Bryonia, tongue feels dry, is coated, especially down its centre; deathly sick on sitting up; pains worse from any motion of the body.

Nux Vom., Nux Moschata, Sulph., Lyco., Arsenic, Coloc.

Heart.

Benzoic Acid, Lith. Carb., Kalmia. Lati., Colchic., Phosp., Arsenic.

Kidneys.

Benzoic Acid., Berberis, Lycopod., Sarsap., Sulph., Kali Hyd., contracted kidney.

Arsenic, Colchic., Phosph., Phos. Acid., Zinc., (can pass water only while bending backwards; the urine deposits yellow sediment).

Terebinth., urine dark, cloudy, depositing a dirty pink sediment.

Plumbum, Aurum, contracted kidney.

CUPRUM IN DEFECTIVE REACTION

THERE is an interesting side to *Cuprum* which deserves a more thorough study than has as yet been bestowed upon it.

If we examine the symptoms of copper, we shall see that despite their stormy, convulsive character, they express a tendency towards torpidity, prostration or lack of reaction.

Looking over the symptoms of spasms, we find them bearing a superficial resemblance to *Bellad.* and *Stramon.,* when resulting from repercussed eruptions, with consequent meningitis. But the cases calling preferably for *Cuprum,* are more serious. There is not the impetuous haste and quick motion of *Bellad.*, and though there may be fear on awakening, clinging to those about the patient, the deathly pale face, and paralytic weakness afterwards, are too severe for *Stramon.* to cure.

The uræmic eclampsia of copper, as in cholera, is characterized by loquacious delirium and asthma; but very soon apathy sets in, with cold tongue and breath, and death-like prostration.

Again, in gonorrhœa there is slow recovery: discharge changeable, now more, now less; urethral orifice glued.

Copper develops a fever, which is slow to yield, tending towards typhoid or becoming of an irregular, relapsing type.

To cap the climax, Haynel, with his wonted astuteness, used *Cuprum* in all diseases traceable to exhaustion from a combination of overwork with mental worry. Long lasting weariness; slow recovery.

How often is the busy practitioner, fretted with an accumulation of petty annoyances, deprived of needed sleep, and hurried in his day's work, so exhausted that he is reduced to the verge of typhoid. Medicines fail to relieve him. In such a case *Cuprum* should be thought of as a probable *similimum,* second to none, not even to *Sulphur.*

The analogues of *Cuprum* in imperfect reaction, may readily be distinguished. Hahnemann placed *Camphor* and *Copper* side by side in Cholera-collapse. Both are characterized by coldness, blue surface, deathly nausea, suffocation, epigastric distress and cramps. The former, however, suits more with significant absence of vomiting and purging; the latter, with predominant spasms and cramps, vomiting relieved by sips of cold water.

Arsenicum holds a supplemental relation to *Cuprum,* following it in Cholera, and relieving the protracted exhaustion from its misuse.

With *Sulphur,* its relation is very intimate, as shown in the defective reaction. In fevers, *Sulphur* has been found essential when, despite the most careful choice of a remedy, the heat continues unabated, or, at most, remits slightly, with total absence of critical perspiration. The patient becomes more and more drowsy, thought is sluggish and a typhoid condition develops. *Cuprum* is not greatly dissimilar in persistency, but causes more an irregular but oft-repeated renewal of the fever, with dry, withered skin, pale or grayish face. If the lungs are involved, paralysis may exhibit itself by sudden difficulty in breathing, followed by great prostration.

MALARIAL CACHEXIA; REMOTE EFFECTS OF MALARIA; TREATMENT

WHEN the malarial poison, instead of being eliminated from the system, remains to pursue its ravages, a series of constitutional effects follow, which are called the Malarial Cachexia.

The symptoms of this cachexia vary from those which mark merely chronic disease to those which indicate remote changes in functions and tissues.

When a patient is continually exposed to the miasm which gives rise to chills and fever, he no longer displays the typical, recurrent symptoms of an intermitting fever; except, perhaps, in the height of the "season", when a fresh supply of the poison arouses the system from its condition of non-resistance. But he is constantly suffering from a series of symptoms which indicate that depraved state of the body we call cachexia. As this state becomes more and more fixed, nutritive changes develop and increase, and finally a condition is reached which constitutes what we may term the remote effects of Malaria.

We are to consider, then, two conditions differing only in degree—the one the ultimate effect of the other.

In the early manifestations of the Malarial Cachexia, the patient suffers from general *Malaise*. Clear, crisp days are enjoyable, but every damp day, especially every warm and wet change, makes him gloomy, weary and cold.

One suffers from biliousness; another from diarrhœa; a third is tormented with neuralgia. Still another feels tolerably well, but the onset of any disease is the occasion for an arousing of the malarial poison, greatly to his discomfort as it complicates his case and renders recovery tardy and uncertain. As the cachexia becomes more permanent, the victim displays more constant symptoms, indicative of organic lesions. He is pale or sallow, jaundiced when the liver is diseased or its ducts obstructed, but yellow whether icteric or not. The mouth is dry, there is bitter taste and the tongue is furred. He is melancholic, suffers from tinnitus aurium, and complains of spinal irritation and even of paretic symptoms. He is always dizzy, even when not bilious.

Soon he becomes anæmic; and liver and spleen are enlarged forming what are termed "ague-cakes"—a term most frequently applied to an enlarged spleen, though no less applicable to the swollen liver, too.

Still later there develops a sort of cirrhosis of liver, spleen and kidneys. "Ague-cakes" are now replaced by contracted organs, congestion and hæmorrhage giving place to softened pulp, fatty degeneration, amyloid changes and hypertrophy of the connective tissues. The basement membrane of the kidneys is thickened and uriniferous tubules are filled with cast off epithelium.

The heart, like muscular tissue elsewhere, becomes softened and flaccid; finally it is dilated.

Anæmia is an early and progressive symptom. Dependent at first upon defective manufacture of blood, arising from diseased spleen, etc., it soon finds other causes in the advance stage of the Malarial Cachexia; especially in imperfect digestion and in defective assimilation from intestinal catarrh and alterations in the intestinal glands.

Disintegration of red corpuscles leads to two sets of accidents; one hæmorrhage, which most commonly appears as epistaxis; the other, the effects of emboli.

These emboli, if they may be so-called, arise from a clogging of small vessels with pigment granules, derived from the broken down blood-cells in the spleen.

A common symptom is dropsy. This may appear as œdema of the ankles, as ascites, or as anasarca, according as it arises simply from anæmia or from lesions of liver, spleen, heart or kidneys.

Finally, as still more remote effects of Malaria, we may refer to the wrinkled and half-imbecile state referred to by Watson, as resulting from a protracted residence in miasmatic districts. Children reared in such places are dwarfed and idiotic; adults are shrievelled, stoop-shouldered, and also mentally impaired.

So similar are the effects of Malaria to those of Quinine that when *Cinchona* has been misapplied or extravagantly employed, it seems to intensify the perniciousness of the former, and thus to aid in the permanency of a cachexia.

TREATMENT.

To give in detail the treatment of the Malarial Cachexia would be to reproduce the Materia Medica. Still, there are several drugs, the pathogenesis of which so closely resemble the chronic effects of Malaria, that we may confine our studies to them.

These drugs are: *Arsenicum, Carbo Veg., China, Chinin Sulph., Sulphur, Aranea Diadema* and *Natrum Mur.*

When practicable, the patient should be removed to another and more healthy district. If he is taken to a mountainous country, it must be dry and free from stagnant pools and dense woods. Remaining out of doors after sunset and leaving the house at or before sunrise should be be strictly interdicted. Such invalids are very susceptible to exhalations from the ground and also to the dampness of nightfall. If the patient is taken to the sea-side, care must be used to see that the locality is well-drained. Sandy soil soaked with either the offal of the kitchen or that of water-closets is particularly objectionable to malarial patients, and will hinder their recovery if it does not increase their maladies.

When acute paroxysms now and then develop, select one of the following: *Lachesis, Sulphur, Carbo Veg.*

If the spleen is affected, *Arsenic, Carbo Veg., Aranea, Sulphuric Acid, Sulphur, Ceanothus,* (the last one if its pain is present).

If the liver is diseased, with or without duodenal catarrh, *China, Arsenic* (duodenitis), *Lachesis, Sepia, Polyporous Officinal, Sulphur, Calc. Carb.*

Dropsy calls for *Arsenic, China, Ferrum, Sulphur, Apis., Apoc. Cann., Helleborus* (when Arsenic fails), *Digitalis* (circulation weak, pulse thready with every little exertion).

Chronic neuralgia: *Chinin. Mur., Arsen., Cedron* (left supra-orbital), *Chinin. Ars., China, Chinin. Sulph* (spinal irritation).

For protracted debility, sallow complexion but no dropsy: *Sulphur, Arsenicum, Chinin. Ars., Carbo Veg., Ferrum, Chelone, Alstonia.*

Hysterical symptoms require, probably, Tarantula (Jousset). As several of the mineral acids cause a sort of liver-cachexia, they should be considered in severe cases.

To remove the cachexia, it may be necessary to institute a careful and exhaustive analysis of the case under consideration, from the initial chill on. In this manner we sometimes find a meaning for existing symptoms, otherwise apparently—insignificant.

A skilful physician may often trace indications for a remedy, which, though originally indicated, was awkwardly applied or utterly forgotten, but which still suits the main features of the case. And again, it may be that the early paroxysms were suppressed by crude drugs and no remedy can be found for the disconnected malady of existing symptoms. Under such circumstance, *Ipecacuanha* 30 should be prescribed to prepare the way for a more profoundly acting medicine. Quite frequently, too, heredity and various acquired dyscrasiæ step in to complicate and perplex, and must be considered in prescribing.

When the patient suffers in damp places or in wet weather, *Aranea, Nat. Sulph.* and *Rhus* may be studied. When the spleen is the seat of sharp pains, we can thank Dr. Burnett for an efficient remedy in *Ceanothus*. When the liver is affected and the patient is annoyed with sick headaches, yellow tongues, nausea, dull dragging pains in the liver through to the back, etc., *Polyporous Officinalis* is required. If, however, the patient is a child, or a well marked "lime-subject," *Calc. Carb.* acts rapidly for enlarged liver with a feeling of fullness to bursting in the right hypochondrium, worse from stretching, or, which is equivalent, from bending over to the left.

PERSONAL OBSERVATIONS.

A case of *Morbus Brightii* of malarial origin was cured chiefly with *Sulphur* 30 and 2c. The urine was albuminous and contained casts; the patient was sallow, emaciated and dropsical. *Sulphur* was chosen because of hunger in the forenoon, burning of the feet, restless sleep and a tendency to relapse after apparently well indicated drugs. The urine was examined every two weeks, at first by Dr. Tyson and later by Dr. E. Seguin.

A young lady who contracted chills and fever in St. Louis in 1880, was not cured despite homœopathic and allopathic treatment. In the fall of 1882, after conducting a kindergarten for three months, she was so prostrated that she was obliged to take to her bed. Chills came regularly accompanied by jerking of the head backwards, opisthotonos and general tremors. *Cicuta* 2c was the only remedy that helped. For the remaining spinal exhaustion and general muscular weakness, remedies were wholly ineffective. Galvanism and massage were relieving. After the disease assumed the nervous form, a persistent vomiting (which, by the way, nothing but grain doses of Quinine would stop, showing their origin), ceased. It has not yet returned.

An elderly lady, living in a marshy region in Maryland was so prostrated by Malaria and Quininism that she became bed-ridden. Her extreme weakness, together with such symptoms as flatulency, inability to take the simplest food without turning in the stomach or vomiting, cold feet and legs, led to the selection of *Carbo Veg*. In four or five months, she was able to go about the house, and is now well.

LACERATION OF THE CERVIX UTERI
(PREVENTIVE TREATMENT)

THE prevention of cervical laceration includes every hygienic and therapeutic measure which can possibly be needed during the entire period of gestation; hence, the whole Materia Medica is tributary to the obstetrician. Still it may not be amiss here to refer to several points most likely to present themselves in the usual run of cases.

I am, however, treading upon new ground. Clinical experience in this direction is, as yet, so meagre that it offers no guide to therapeutic study. And added to this, is the lamentable truth that our Materia Medica is deficient in clear and well-characterized symptoms of the cervix uteri. Gynæcologists, instead of following Dunham's advice to institute provings on females, have too frequently discarded homœopathy, and has resorted to local devices suggested in allopathic works.

What I shall offer, then, will be chiefly suggestive, to be accepted and tried, or to be rejected, according to the judgment of the reader.

My predecessor has presented a graphic description of the causes of cervical laceration, some of which may be met with therapy or mechanical device.

The professional care of the enceinte woman usually dates from her distressing morning sickness. It is now recognized that this symptoms is often, if not always, an evidence of disease of the cervix, disturbed uterine vascularity, etc. It constitutes an early evidence of disease which may lead to the accident we desire to prevent. We should, therefore, pay careful attention to this symptom, and combat it with medicines, or, in the event of their failure, with mechanical means. One of the most promising medicines for morning sickness, reflex from a hard tumfied cervix, is *Sepia*.

The physiological softening of the lower uterine segment, which suddenly develops about the seventh month and progresses thence until full term, may be interfered with in various ways:

If by undue congestion: SEPIA, NUX VOM., *Sulph.*, Aloes, etc.

If by weak heart, which favors venous stasis, the cervix appears patulous, congested, even livid, or œdematous: *Digitalis, Lachesis,* Lycopus, *Arsenic, Apis,* Lilium Tig., Puls., Gels., Naja, Elaps.

It has been determined that heart-diseases are regularly and progressively aggravated by successive pregnancies. Since, therefore, weak heart may permit uterine engorgement, why should we not treat the heart when diseased, both with a view to stay its tendency to grow worse during gestation and labor, and also with the view of counteracting its baneful effects upon uterine nutrition?

If softening is interfered with by swelling or induration of the cervix: Con., CARBO ANIMALIS, SEPIA, *Phytolac., Iod., Kali Iod., Thuja, Ars. Iod., Ferr. Iod., Calc. Carb., Natr. Carb., Aur., Aur. Mur., Aur. Mur. Natronat., Hydrastis, Alumen, Canth., Mitchella, Plat., Arg. Met., Hydrocotyle, Kreosote, Nux Vom.*

Years ago Dr. Lippe stated that on being engaged to take charge of a lady in labor, she remarked that he must certainly bring instruments, for they were always necessary, and, according to her former physician, always *would* be necessary, because she had an indurated cervix. Dr. Lippe gave the patient *Sepia*, and she was delivered in due time *without* instruments.

In many cases *Carbo An.* will doubtless suffice.

Conium is suggested when there are stinging pains.

Phytolacca deserves a trial when the hardened neck is dark red.

Kali Iod. claims attention in syphilitic or in scrofulous cases with swollen and contracted neck.

Aurum (preparations of gold) particularly the *Aurum Mur. Natronat.*, may be needed especially when there is much vascular engorgement, with melancholy, weariness of life.

Platina is preferable when there are shooting pains.

Alumen is required when the cervix is swollen, painful and narrowed.

Mitchella answers for a dark-red, sore and swollen cervix.

Hydrocotyle should not be neglected when there is unnatural redness of the cervix, hot and red vagina with pricking and itching at the vulva; scaly eruptions on the skin.

Hydrastis will undoubtedly assist if the cervix is red, shining, or engorged and ulcerated, with gluey or ropy mucous leucorrhœa.

The *Salts of Iron,* since they notably disturb the circulation, and include the uterus in their sphere of action, may serve a purpose here too. *Ferr. Iod.* has been proved to affect the uterus, inducing prolapsus, bloating of the abdomen, deepseated intra-pelvic soreness, and a confirmed symptom,—on sitting she feels as if she was pushing something up into the vagina.

Argentum Met. may possibly come into service if the cervix is corroded and spongy.

Kreosote if it is tender, as if ulcerated.

Natum Carb. if ill-shaped.

Ustilago if patulous, oozing blood when touched, etc.

Copaiva if there are stitches, with dragging in uterus and bladder; burning spots in the vulva, itching; acrid leucorrhœa.

If the softening process is excessive, we may study with advantage: *Ustilago, Secale,* and also remedies and hygienic measures looking to general uterine as well as systemic nutrition. For, if the body is illy-nourished, the new-tissue will be weak and readily susceptible of retrogressive changes. It would be folly to attempt a summarizing of such a vast subject as this.

The whole range of therapeutics must be consulted. Attention may be drawn, however, to two or three drugs which seem especially adapted to uterine debility. These are *Aletris Farinosa, Abies Canadensis, Cyclamen, Pulsatilla, Helonias, Caulophyllum, Secale, Ustilago, Sepia,* etc.

Aletris suits when there is persistent morning sickness, debility, constipation, slow digestion.

Abies Can. should be thought of when there is abnormal hunger, with faint feeling, swimming tipsy sensation; she feels as if the womb was soft and feeble; craves pickles. Compare *Sepia*.

Cyclamen causes weak digestion, even the plainest food cannot be digested; nocturnal flatulency, from atonic bowels, causing distension, relieved only by getting up and walking about. Nausea referred to the throat.

Helonias, as is well known, causes a quantitative loss of blood-corpuscles. There are, consequently, lan-

LACERATION OF THE CERVIX UTERI 277

guor, tiredness, as after long exertion, aching of all the muscles, etc. If it fails, *Picric Acid* has proved a successful substitute.

If cicatricial tissue retards the necessary cervical changes, compare *Graph., Phytolac., Thuja.*

Flexions, cervical contractions, and uterine deviations must be corrected by mechanical means. Tampons of cotton, so placed as to hold up the uterus, and so to straighten the flexed neck and permit free circulation, will be needed. If the uterus is retroverted or retroflexed, we have found Cutter's pessary necessary until the uterus shall be large enough to rise out of the pelvis.

Rigidity of the various parts needed in labor, as well as inharmonious action of these parts, may also lead to lacerated cervix. It becomes the accoucheur's duty, then, to see to it, that his patient be free from any of these conditions. False labor pains, which, as it were, mark the preparatory drilling of the uterus, should be controlled if they become excessive and spasmodic. The best remedies here are *Caulophyllum, Ignatia, Nux Vom., Viburnum Op., Actea Racemosa, Cuprum* and *Coffea.* The first is usually all-sufficient.

If the labor is too rapid, not permitting time for normal dilatation, we may select such drugs as BELL., *Cham., Coffea, Actea Rac.,* CAULO, SECALE C., *Apis.*

Belladonna is suggested by the suddenness of the pains, coupled with their too quick bearing down, as if everything in the pelvis would be ejected.

Caulo and Secale are indicated by a prolonged bearing down without any intermission. The woman may talk or otherwise make inspiratory and expiratory motions, and yet the pain continues.

Apis has bearing down in the early stage of labor, and so may be needed to retard the too rapidly progressing second stage.

If, however, these fail, or if rapidity is due to a large roomy pelvis, we may press steadily, but not too strongly, upon the advancing head during the pains.

If the danger arises from too early escape of the amniotic fluid, from dry labor, or from protracted labor, frequent and thorough lubrication of the cervix and vagina will materially aid. Medicines, too, are of service. For dry labor, the parts feeling hot, give *Aconite, Coffea,* or *Belladonna,* especially the last, though mental symptoms will decide.

Delay at the pubic arch is very common. The anterior lip of the cervix is felt swollen, hot, and dry, between the advancing head and the pubic bones. By continued compression it loses its tone and readily yields latterly, when the head finally, and often suddenly, descends upon the perineum.

The tumefied lip, if there is not too much stretching of the tissues by the advancing head, may be held above the bones during two or three pains. The woman may be directed to lie upon the abdomen, or the accoucheur can press with the hand upon the hypogastrium.

Neuralgia and rheumatism of the uterus, by leading to protracted labor, favor the accident under consideration. Prominent remedies are, for the former: *Actea Rac., Xanthoxylum, Lilium, Sepia, Puls., Ignatia, Helonias, Viburnum Op.*, according to their respective indications. And for the latter, *Actaea Rac., Rhus Tox.,* and *Pulsat.*

Still another source of causation is a want of consentaneous action between fundus and cervix. The pains are intensely *painful,* but either lack expulsive force, or produce irregular contractions, the uterine surface being felt as if full of lumps.

The most effective drugs here, are: CAULOPHYL., SECALE C., PULSATILLA, *Gelsem., Causticum,* COFFEA, BELLADONNA, *Cuprum,* and lastly Brandy.

Some years ago Dr. Burdick published it as his opinion that Brandy acted on the fundus uteri. Since then several opportunities have been afforded to test the value of this observation.

On one occasion I treated a lady whose labor pains ceased to do any good, the fundus remaining uncontracted. Despite the utmost care in selecting my remedies, the patient steadily grew worse until her distressing moaning, her rapid but weak pulse, upturned eyes, and wandering speech, warned me of her imminent danger.

The os was rigid and but slightly dilated, rendering instrumental interference very difficult if not impossible. A few drops of cognac in a half wine-glass of water, a teaspoonful every three or four minutes, quickly restored strength, and, likewise, brought on vigorous and effective labor pains.

More directly concerned in cervical laceration is a rigid or spasmodic state of the neck. For the first condition the best remedy is undoubtedly GELSEMIUM. Pains are cutting from before backwards and upwards, the uterus seems to go upwards. Pains leave the womb and fly all over the body—(Allen). (Compare *Causticum* and *Caulophyllum.*)

We may also consult *Conium* when there are stinging stitches in the rigid neck; *Calc. Carb.,* stinging and cutting; the uterus seems to ascend, *Actea Rac.*

For spasmodic rigidity, the most reliable remedy is BELLAD.; though we may need *Actea Rac.* and other remedies. If nausea is a prominent reflex symptom, relaxation will follow the use of *Ipecac, Lobelia Inflata, Ant. Tart.,* or *Morphinum.* Too much credit, however, may here be misplaced, for the oncoming of nausea frequently indicates the commencement of the wished for relaxation. I do not advocate any of these drugs in emetic doses as has been advised. I refer solely to their homœopathicity, according to their respective symptoms. Partiality to allopathy is never becoming in a homœopathician; but an emetic here is especially objectionable, for, by causing laxness, it might precipitate the very accident we are anxious to prevent.

Finally, since Dr. Burnett and several others have shown, indisputably, that the growing fœtus may be influenced through the mother, why should we not avail ourselves of this fact?

DISCUSSION ON THE TREATMENT OF INTERMITTENT FEVER

By Dr. E. A. Farrington, M.D., and others.

AT the December (1881) meeting of the Philadelphia County Homœopathic Medical Society, the following discussion was held upon the treatment of intermittent fevers, the subject having been reported upon by the Bureau of Clinical Medicine and Zymoses:

Dr. McClatchey, having been invited by the President to open the discussion, did so as follows: "The society will bear me out on the statement that my voice is not often heard in these discussions, and that I rarely refer to my cases,—least of all, to my cures. But I feel that I must not be silent, being called upon to speak, and must even do a little bragging too. On comparing my success in treating cases of intermittent fever, with that of others that I hear or read about, I feel that I have been very successful. I attribute my success entirely to this,—that I treat my cases homœopathically, rigidly adhering to the principle, *similia similibus curantur* in all cases. I follow the precepts of Hahnemann, and prescribe for the totality of symptoms. I individualize each case, and get all the symptoms together, those that are most prominent and those that are least so, the modalities, etc., and having done this, I choose that which is the *homoeopathic* remedy for the case, and I find that this is, in most cases, or at least, in a very large percentage of them, QUININE, and I believe that all my success in treating such cases is due to my close adherence to homœopathy.

Is not QUININE the *similimum* to intermittent fever, *par excellence?* By QUININE, here, I mean *Sulphate of Quinia, Peruvian Bark., China, Cinchonidia,* and others of that ilk. These are nearly identical so far as their pathogenetic or curative effects are concerned. I have heard quite a good many lectures on homœopathy, and one of the most frequently repeated statements, made on such occasions, was to the effect that Hahnemann, while engaged in translating Cullen's Materia Medica into German, was dissatisfied with the explanation given by Mr. Cullen as to the action of *Peruvian Bark* in the cure of ague, and that he set himself to experiment with that drug, and, very greatly to his surprise, found that the drug, when taken by a person in good health, produced symptoms very similar to those produced in an attack of ague. This, together with other experiments, led to Hahnemann finding that drugs would cure symptoms similar to those that they were capable of producing, or *similia similibus curantur*. Thus homœopathy may be said to have had its foundations laid on bark. Now was Hahnemann mistaken in all this? And if he was, is it not possible that he was mistaken in other things just as well, and might not homœopathy be an error altogether? But my experience proves to me that it is not, for just as Hahnemann found that bark would produce symptoms analogous to those of intermittent fever, I have found that bark, or its alkaloid, or alkaloids, will cure genuine and true malarial intermittent fever.

There are other remedies for intermittents besides QUININE, as every physician knows, and it is not always necessary to give QUININE or *China* to cure intermittent, as is also known to every physician. But there is not one, in my experience, so frequently indicated as QUININE, nor so often the *similimum* for a case of ague. In that magnificent treatise, which we should all read daily, Allen's *Encyclopaedia of Materia Medica,* you will find a complete record of the pathogenetic effects of QUININE and *China,* and in these records you will find nearly every symptom of a very large majority of intermittent fever cases. If I were to ask this assembly to give me the keynote or notes for *Natrum Muriaticum* in intermittent, the reply must be: "Chill commences at eleven o'clock in the morning," and "Herpes labialis." The QUININE chill may commence at eleven o'clock, and there may be herpes labialis also. In regard to *Capsicum,* I would be told that the chill "commences in the back, thence spreading," and so on. The *China* chill also begins in the back. The indications for the concentrated essence of bed-bugs (I confess I do not know what the indication for this delicious medicine is), a voice behind me says, "always worse at night." If that be true, the chills of QUININE may be worse at night or at many other times.

In using QUININE it is not necessary to give it in the large doses of the old school, for if you do the effect of the drug will be superadded to those of the disease, the curative effect will be crowded out by the toxical effect, and the patient is apt to be made worse. I have never been quite able to understand why our school objected so to the use of QUININE, and seemed almost afraid of it. That the old school uses it is surely no good reason why we should not. It is homœopathic to ague, no matter who uses it. The old school are almost daily making use of our remedies, and shall we abandon them so soon as Ringer, or Harley, or Phillips introduces them and their methods to their old-school brethren? They are constantly making such experiments. There is a man almost within the sound of my voice, and his name is Horatio C. Wood, who is constantly making such experiments—rediscovering homœopathic screws. If we are to abandon our remedies so soon as the allopaths take them for their use, our whole Materia Medica is in great danger.

The physician who fails to use QUININE for ague because of its allopathic history, and with knowledge of its action, casts dirt on the graves of his ancestors, and is also belittling homœopathy.

DR. C. E. TOOTHAKER: In what doses does Dr. McClatchey give QUININE?

DR. MCCLATCHEY: In whatever doses I please or think will be best in the given case. "Let no pent-up Utica contract our powers. The whole boundless continent is ours."

DR. TOOTHAKER: I cured a child of chills with *China* 30, after it had been extravagantly dosed with QUININE.

DR. FARRINGTON: I have been waiting for some other member to get up and reply to the remarks of the gentleman on my left. The insinuations which he has thrown out concerning Hahnemann are so outrageous that I wonder that so many did not rise, eager to defend, that the chair would find it difficult to decide as to who should be the first to reply. Is it possible that the gentleman's eloquence has wrought this wonderful effect? If so I had better sit down, as I cannot compete with him. The assertions that he has made tonight in all truth (of course he does not mean them for a farce) show that Hahnemann claimed *Peruvian Bark* to be the remedy for intermittent fever. That is a "reading between the lines" which is rather too broad for me to comprehend. Hahnemann thought when he was translating Cullen's *Materia Medica,* that certain of the symptoms attributed to *Purivian Bark.* were rather peculiar. So he determined he would test them. He was astonished to find that he produced the same symptoms which he had when he suffered from chills and fever. Now my good friend asserts that Hahnemann considered that, with few exceptions, *Peruvian Bark.* was the remedy for intermittent fever. Hahnemann distinctly says that *China* is the remedy when the chill comes so and so, the fever so and so, and the thirst so and so, and this is a flat contradiction to the assertion that QUININE is *the* remedy for intermittent fever. I deny, too, that those symptoms which he found under QUININE are as characteristic of QUININE as they are of the others referred to. In my experience *China* is frequently indicated. If his remarks had ended here, I should have applauded. I find that the potency must not enter into the question at all. I do not believe in any "pent-up Utica." I have given the drug high, low and crude. But the worst cases that I have ever had to handle were those in which QUININE had been abused. The results of the administration of QUININE are two, either a cure, which often results, I confess, or a spoiling of the case, which oftener results. If the case has been one of malarial poisoning, and is taken in the beginning, if there is no systemic taint, psoric, sycotic, or syphilitic, QUININE will often, by its power of destroying germs, prevent the manifestations of the disease. If there is anything in addition to the malarial poison, QUININE will ruin the case. The question is a broad one and is one which seriously involves homœopathy. It is a question which calls up the power of homœopathy to cure any disease in which there is a substantial poison, rheumatism, scarlatina, diphtheria, and the puerperal fevers. I never saw a clearly indicated remedy given which was not followed by relief. I have had many failures in the treatment of intermittent fever. I agree with the gentleman that it is more important to mention our failures than our successes. I do not pretend to say that I have cured every case. But when my remedy has been properly selected, it has never failed, and that remedy has not always been *China*. I will not be confined to *Cinchona*, but I will take the whole of nature's gifts, and use them according to law, and not according to empiricism.

DR. MCCLATCHEY: I rise to correct an error on the part of Dr. Farrington. I said that Hahnemann claimed that while taking bark he produced in himself symptoms very similar to those of an intermittent fever. This he surely did say, and if he misstated these circumstances, then might he not have misstated all other things from which he and we have deduced homœopathy? I did not accuse Hahnemann of stating that bark is the chief remedy for ague. It was I who stated that on my own behalf. I find the symptoms of ague well and prominently marked in the provings of *China* and *Quinine*, much more so than any other drug in the Materia Medica, and I have abundantly proved, and seen it proved by others, by countless homœopaths and allopaths, that Hahnemann's provings and those of others are true and correct, and that *Cinchona*, as QUININE, is the remedy for ague, and that *similia simi-*

libus curantur is here proven to be true. I am not responsible for the mischief which allopaths do by giving those large doses of *Quinia,* and producing the pathogenetic effects of the drug to be added to those of the disease. I only wish to get curative effects.

Dr. Farrington: Dr. McClatchey said that if the father is not right in saying that Quinine is the *similimum* for chills and fever, is he not wrong in everything else? Hahnemann never said it; and, besides, what he said or did in the beginning of his work should not be charged against him; for later he said that *China* is the remedy when certain definite symptoms present. In one place he states that *China* is not the remedy for intermittent fever, because it is not even an intermittent remedy at all.

Dr. McClatchey: I don't care whether Hahnemann said that *Cinchona* is an intermittent remedy or not. I know that it is a remedy for intermittent fever, and does cure it, in contradistinction to the suppression or palliation it is charged with. Indeed, it acts as a true cure, and not by the suppression or palliation of symptoms.

Dr. Dudley: I expected that something would be said about Quinine to-night, and as I have a weakness for Quinine, I prepared my speech in advance. If I could get along without Quinine, as some claim to do, I could get along without homœopathy altogether. Dr. McClatchey stated that the symptoms of a majority of our cases of intermittents can be found under the symptoms of *China* or *Quinia*. I believe that this is strictly true, and, consequently, physician who prescribes *China* or one of its preparations for ague, is not far from homœopathy, whether he gives it in large or small doses. Why, therefore, should men be afraid to use Quinine? Is it simply because allopaths use it? Dr. Dudley then read a collation of symptoms of *China* and *Quinia*, taken from Allen's *Pure Materia Medica*, showing the prevalence of ague symptoms of all kinds in the pathogeneses of these drugs, as follows:

Chill.—In the morning; in the forenoon; before dinner; in the afternoon; the whole afternoon; in the evening; the whole day.

Chilliness.—Slight; violent; transient; persistent; constant; periodic; with cold hands; with cold feet; with external coldness; without external coldness; with internal coldness; without internal coldness; with nausea; without nausea; with vomiting; without vomiting; with thirst; without thirst; alternating with thirst; followed by thirst; preceded by heat; with heat; followed by heat; alternating with heat; over the back; over the stomach; in the stomach; over the arms; over the legs; over the thighs; over the forehead; above the elbows; above the knees; on the chest; all over; external; internal; when walking; when sitting; when lying; when standing; in open air; in a warm room; in bed; after eating; after every swallow of drink; with heat; without heat; alternating with heat; before the heat; during the heat; after the heat; with red face; with yellowness of the face; with pallor; with gooseflesh; with chattering of the teeth; with weakness; with headache; followed by heat, then thirst; without subsequent heat, and without thirst.

Coldness.—Of hands; of feet; of nose; of left hand or of both hands; of left leg or of both legs; of stomach; internal; external; periodic; preceded by heat; followed by heat; with shivering; followed by heat, then thirst; followed by heat, then sweat.

Heat.—Preceded by coldness; followed by coldness; transient; in flushes; internally; externally; with sweat; without sweat; with nausea; without nausea; with slight thirst; with intense thirst; without thirst; of face; of abdominal region; of head; of trunk; of thighs; of cheeks; of extremities; of whole body.

Sweat.—At night; in the morning; after 3 A.M.; during sleep; after waking; incessant; profuse; cold; with feverish heat; oily; exhausting; after fever; on face; on forehead; on neck; on back; on trunk; all over; with thirst; without thirst; in warm room; in open air.

Thirst.—In the morning; in the evening; before the chill; during the chill; after the chill; before the heat; during the heat; after the heat; without heat; for water; for beer; for wine.

Nausea.—With hot risings; in pit of throat; with vomiting; without vomiting; during the chill; during the heat.

Headache.—Confusion of the head; with vertigo; with dizziness; tensive pain in forehead and orbits; heaviness and heat in the head, worse on turning the eyes; jerking pain in the temples; headache now in one part and now in another; dull, stupefying headache, as though the skull would burst; as though the brain were pressed together from both sides; as though the brain were pressed out at forehead; like a congestion in the head (this symptom ought to be italicized); violent pressive headache deep in the brain, with sense of constriction in forehead and occiput; jerking-tearing headache, worse on motion; headache, as if the brain were sore; headache, which changes its location on moving the head.

Urine.—Dark-colored, scanty, with brickdust sediment.

Pain.—Across lower portion of chest and the stomach, with anxiety and shortness of breath, and oppression; in or between the shoulder-blades; tensive

DISCUSSION ON TREATMENT OF INTER. FEVER

and intolerable in small of back, as if crushed or bruised; jerking tearing in bones of upper or of the lower extremities, in almost every part of their length, with numbness or paralyzed sensation.

Besides these we have the jaundice, prostration, œdema, and a host of other symptoms which I have not undertaken to include. Now about the cases which have suffered relapses while taking *China*. I have had cases come back at the end of a week and tell me that they have had a relapse. I have had the same thing happen under *Eupatorium, Belladonna, Capsicum, Arsenicum* and other remedies. The trouble is that we have not learned *how* to administer our drugs in all cases. There is a difference of opinion as to when and how to administer QUININE. I learned how to administer it from Professor Dickson. He said that the proper time was shortly before the onset of the rigor in typical cases. I have nearly always found that I obtained the best effect by administering it three, two, and one, hours before the chill. The same is true of all other homœopathic remedies. I caution the patient not to take it after the chill comes on. I am satisfied that QUININE, *Eupatorium,* or any other *homoeopathic* remedy, if administered during the chill, will make the case worse and cause trouble afterwards. *China Tincture* I have given in from one to five drop doses. When I am sure of QUININE as my remedy I give from one to three grains. All my cases are well with one exception, and that is the case of a lady from Washington, who caught Potomac flat chills and took immense quantities of QUININE before I saw her. I have not cured her and I doubt if I ever will. Hypertrophy of the spleen complicates the case.

DR. MOHR: Dr. Dudley appears to make out a very good case, and I only wish that I had thought to take my Materia Medica and write down the chill and fever symptoms of *Arsenicum, Baptisia,* and *Eupatorium.* I could have done the same thing, and the symptoms would have appeared as characteristic. Until this fall I have never given QUININE in substance, although I have used *Cinchona.* When I have given *Cinchona* it has usually been for what I esteemed to be characteristic symptoms. I have always given *Sulphate of Quinine* in potency when I found the chill anticipating. Dr. Dudley asks us why we look to allopathy in administering QUININE for chill and fever patients. Yet he says that he learned how to administer the drug from Professor Dickson, who was an allopath. I do not believe in looking to allopaths, so far as the administration of QUININE is concerned, as I have made up my mind that they do not know how to administer it. While they can prevent chills and fever, they cannot prevent relapses. Dr. Dudley refers to the fact that *Eupatorium* is much like *China* in regard to the bone pains. My interpretation of the symptom is somewhat different; while *Cinchona* has jerking-tearing pains, *Eupatorium* has more of a broken, aching feeling in the bones. If I had jerking-tearing pains I would give *Cinchona;* if it was a bruised, sore feeling I would give *Eupatorium.* My own preference has been for giving the remedy before the chill, and stopping it when the chill begins. I would not hesitate at all to give QUININE when it is indicated. I must confess, that in the case in which I resorted to QUININE, it did not help me out. Dr. McClatchey, in his remarks, refers to the fact that he will find *Natrum Mur.* and *Capsicum* symptoms under *Cinchona.* It is a mistaken idea to give any remedy on any one symptom. I never prescribe *Natrum Mur.* because a man has a chill at 11 A.M., because I have cured cases having that symptom with *Cinchona* and *Eupatorium.* I do not give *Capsicum* because the chill commences in the back; I must have other symptoms.

Dr. Farrington: I have willingly admitted that some preparation of Quinine is frequently indicated in chills and fever. Dr. Dudley's quotations from the provings, giving all sorts of symptoms of chill, and fever, and sweat, do but confirm my statement.

A German homœopathic physician, quoted by Dr. Dunham, gives *China* when no other remedy seems to be called for. I have no objection to this method. It is a sort of reduction by exclusion. But the main issue between us, as I understand it, is whether or not Quinine is so often the remedy, so precisely similar to all, or nearly all cases, as to deserve the specific use which Dr. McClatchey gives to it.

Now a misinterpretation may be taken from Dr. Dudley's paper. Let me illustrate by two examples. Dr. Bœnninghausen made the remarkable assertion that the anti-psoric symptoms may be found under any anti-psoric remedy. Dr. Hering was astonished at the remark, and he inferred that Bœnninghausen said that any anti-psoric would do when psora was present. But Bonninghausen meant that these remedies were so well selected by Hahnemann that each one seemed to grasp the whole constitution, yet there are individual distinctions in each anti-psoric which render its selection certain. I say this in order to counteract the effect of the remark that all these symptoms being under *Cinchona,* therefore *Cinchona* is the remedy *par excellence* for chills and fever. *Arsenicum* is a remedy that covers 90 per cent. of the symptoms of cholera Asiatica, and yet I would not say that it is to be given as *the* remedy for cholera Asiatica. The rules of the *Organon* for the selection of a drug are true or they are not true. Let the discussion turn on that. If they are true, then we must be careful how we draw inferences from the remarks of Dr. Dudley.

DR. MOHR: I believe that the question of hygienic treatment is one of great importance. I make the patient avoid the use of stimulants. If I had to depend, in the treatment of intermittent fever, on either the remedy or hygiene, I most certainly would prefer to depend on the hygiene.

DR. R. C. ALLEN: About three months ago, I had a young lady patient suffering from intermittent fever. I gave her QUININE, *Rhus Tox., Nux Vomica, Dextro-Quinine,* without avail. One day I went to see her, I found cold, pale face, anxious-looking, thin lips, and sweat on the face. I thought of *Camphor,* and gave it, and cured her. Since then I have given *Camphor* to every case with uniform success.

DR. TRITES: I have collated a number of sure cures for chills, such as tying a tarred rope around the waist, walking across running water, going down stairs backwards, etc. Yet when you come down to the real treatment I know of nothing upon which I have more confused ideas. I was unfortunate enough to be brought up in the midst of malaria. Just after I graduated at this college I succeeded in contracting malarial fever. I was treated by the best methods, but I shook for three months. QUININE will suppress the disease but will not cure it; yet in my practice I resort to QUININE. I cannot find cases that will go to bed, or patients that will shake three or four weeks. They say I must give relief right away. When I give it, I give it as an allopath would. I give it in two-grain doses until ten grains have been taken, generally on the day between the chills. Probably they will have no chill. After that the patient is comparatively well. I always tell such patients that they are not cured. It seems to me that by and by Pasteur will have something to tell us about this disease. There is some poison in the system which QUININE has the ability to smother, but will not wipe out. The assertion that after using QUININE the homœopathic remedy will not act, is not according to my experience. The difference in our experience is because you do not see the disease as I see it. I have a very severe case. It is the wife of a lock-tender, who has had chills and fever since September. She sent for me a week ago disgusted with QUININE. I gave her *Ipecac.* and she has improved somewhat. There is a case that shows that after long dosing with QUININE the homœopathic remedy will act. I agree with Dr. Martin, that people who have once contracted malaria are never free from it. It is so in my own case. Every spring I have a periodical trouble which usually yields to QUININE, but it will return. I was in hopes that I would learn how to treat these cases. I live where we have chills and fever to perfection. I have not succeeded in curing any case excepting with QUININE or the *Tincture of China.*

DR. DUDLEY: Neither Dr. McClatchey nor I said that there was *constant* curative relation between Cinchona and intermittent fever. We both insisted on the remedy when indicated, and we both asserted that there are cases when it is not indicated. The point that I wish to make is this, a homœopath should no more be ashamed to administer QUININE than he should be to administer *Natrum Mur.* Suppose you are treating a case of dyspepsia, and the patient apparently gets well; you stop medication and back comes the trouble, in the same way as do chills and fever. In this case, has the disease been suppressed? No; you have not given your remedy long enough to do its work. I I believe that cases are suppressed by QUININE, and I as fully believe that cases have been cured. I heard of one case that had been suppressed by QUININE for thirty-eight years, and reported as such by a homœopathist in New York State. The disease may come back after that sort of "suppression" by any other remedy. Let us follow the law of cure, whether it leads us to QUININE or *Natrum Mur.*, and let us use it in the preparation which we know will cure.

DR. MCCLATCHEY: I made no claim for QUININE in intermittent fevers except that which is founded on its homœopathic relations to the disease. I said that I believe my success in curing chills to be due to the fact that I always prescribe homœopathically. I do not give QUININE or *China* in chills, except when it is indicated homœopathically, which is pretty nearly always. I wish to tender my congratulations to the society on the very remarkable degree of unanimity exhibited in this discussion. We all seem to be of one mind on the subject, our differences being all minor and unimportant ones. If there is one physician present who has not used QUININE, it is not because QUININE is not homœopathic to ague, but it is because certain medical popes or boses have said he must not use it, and that it is not homœopathic to ague at all. Now, I take no stock in medical popes or bosses, and I do not even believe in the blind worship of Hahnemann and his opinions simply because they are his. I do believe in the truth, and always try to find it. If there is anything true in homœopathy, it is that Quinine is homœopathic to fever and ague,—it presents the periodicity, the alternation of states, and all the symptoms ordinarily presented by an attack of intermittent fever, more so than any other remedy. It has the symptoms that have made other medicines famous in intermittents, such symptoms as have passed as the keynotes to these remedies. I referred to a number of these from memory, but Dr. Dudley has taken the time and trouble to collate the symptoms from Allen. Dr. Mohr says he could do the same with other remedies, such as *Arsenic, Pulsatilla* and *Eupatorium*. I think not. *Arsenic* would fill a good many such symptoms, but not so many as QUININE. If I had *suppressed an ague*, or a diarrhœa, for thirty-eight years, I should feel that I had done a good thing. I think QUININE *cures* ague, and not merely suppresses it. If my patients have a relapse after a given time, I give more QUININE; if they relapse again, I give still more. I find that they return again and again, in spite of QUININE, I try something else, whatever I think is best indicated homœopathically, and having done this I feel that I have done all I can. Some cases won't get well, and some patients must die. Such frequent relapses are rare; I don't know that I ever saw even one. I give QUININE in the 1st and 2nd decimal trituration up to five grains of the pure drug. My favourite dose is pills of two grains each, once a day, for a week or two, and then wait future developments. Lately I have been using two-grain pills of *Cinchonidia* with very good effect. I prescribe homœopathically, but how the medicine acts when in the system I don't pretend to know. I don't know that any one does. *Similia similibus curantur* is the only guide for the selection of the medicine.

I do not wish to be held responsible for the heavy drugging of the old school. They have the right remedy, but, as is often the case with homœopaths, the wrong dose.

It is rather late in the day to deny the curative powers of *Cinchona* in ague. I have read somewhere, that in the seven years preceding the introduction of Peruvian bark into England, there were 15,000 deaths from ague, while in the seven years after its introduction there were but 13 deaths. Now, Sidney Smith has said that there is nothing more fallacious than facts, except figures; but surely such a table means and proves something, especially when Quinine has carried the banner to this day despite all the abuse heaped upon it.

DISCUSSION ON DR. WILLIAM SHARP'S PAPER ON "THE FOUNDATIONS AND BOUNDARIES OF MODERN THERAPEUTICS".

R. FARRINGTON: In reviewing Dr. Sharp's paper, I cannot but think that he was founded his arguments upon fallacious premises. "Among the precious fruits which Hahnemann gathered," writes the doctor, is "The use of much smaller doses than had before been given." And yet in a subsequent paragraph, because Hahnemann began to employ infinitesimal doses, the doctor deprecates the practice as one which has been "an almost insurmountable barrier against the progress of his system." Hahnemann, as we well know, was not the first to discover the law of similars, no more than he was the first to make experiments on the healthy. Yet no predecessor ever investigated the subject so thoroughly or systematically as he, because no one had so clear a conception of the great fact. What was original with him was this disputed potentization of medicaments, "this precious fruit," which Dr. Sharp acknowledges, but refuses to profit by its cultivation. When Hahnemann began to dilute his remedies to avoid aggravations, he did not find, as he expected, that their action ceased. Indeed, they multiplied, though their nature was considerably altered.

At this stage, in his mental growth a new world opened to view. He saw, in the unexplored panorama before him, means for the relief of the sick hitherto unnoticed, or silently rejected. He was enabled to penetrate the secret recesses of the body, holding, as it were, communication with the soul within, working thence to coarse and less vital parts. He began to appreciate the delicate qualities of symptoms, their relative value, and their adjectiva. Thus the effect of emotions, of temperature, of weather, time, position, etc., became of practical value. And is not science to-day elucidating these very points? Does not physiology teach us that certain hours in the daily cycle mark positive changes in the human economy, such as maximum electric tension at 10 A.M. (*Natrum Mur.*), minimum, 4 to 8 P.M. (*Lycopod.*)? And who will deny the opposite physical changes by north and south, or north-west and north-east winds?

So, too, in the domain of psychology none but the potencies will develop the many mental symptoms which Hahnemann and experience make the most important in practice. It is no wonder, then, that he made every remedy have a general action upon all parts. Each drug has its prominent points of attack; but the system is a unit, and suffers as such. Centrally are those symptoms which distinctly characterize the drug: while concentrically distributed are those of less import, receding like the centrifugal ripples following the splash of a stone into water. The highest potencies will produce and demonstrably have cured symptoms, primary and secondary, subjective and objective. In this one indisputable fact lies the answer to all arbitrary attempts to limit the range of potencies.

That large and small doses have a contrary action is only an apparent truth; or, at least, is of no importance to us.

Years ago, the question was asked, "What is the peculiar, the characteristic, which cures?" The answer came simultaneously from both sides of the water, "Those symptoms of a drug which have distinct opposites, all the rest being only accessory." Then came the experiments with *Glonoin.* and the sphygmograph, proving incontestably that those opposites are but variations in the waves of motion. The smallest doses will cause them just as certainly as will the largest.

From my standpoint the doctor's charge against Hahnemann, that he was an iconoclast, "breaking the old, but worshipping new images of his own make," seems as unjust as it is unmerited. Until it can be proved that potentized medicines do not act, do not cure, all attempts to bound therapeutics to their exclusion must fail, because fallacious.

Again, we are asked to exchange Hahnemann's scheme for Sharp's organopathy. Call the former, if you choose, a kaleidoscope; you do but express its immensity, not its uselessness. The kaleidoscope is constructed on scientific principles, as is homœopathy. The kaleidoscope obeys fixed laws, as does homœopathy. "The kaleidoscope," says one authority, "is of great use to pattern-makers, to whom it supplies endless varieties of figures;" so with Hahnemann's homœopathy. It supplies the student with an endless variety of *similima* from which he may choose that corresponding to his case. As the pattern-maker thus increases his usefulness, so does the homœopathician increase his opportunities to heal the sick.

The time will come when this new science of homœopathy will become definitely systematized, but *never through organopathy;* In the words of our good friend, Dr. Lilienthal,—"only a master, but not the apprentice, dares override fixed rules." We are all apprentices. Let us gather up material until time shall develop the master who is to lighten the burden, but not lead us astray."

DISCUSSION ON DR. RICHARD HUGHES' PAPER ON "THE VALUE OF HYDROCYANIC ACID" IN EPILEPSY

R. FARRINGTON: I would like to say a few words regarding Dr. Hughes's paper. Dr. Hughes has very clearly revealed the similarity between epilepsy and Prussic Acid (Hydrocyanic Acid) poisoning, especially in that form which has been termed *la grand mal.*
Hydrocyanic Acid has already been used by homœopathicians in spasms from various causes. Thus Buchner recommends it in uræmic convulsions, placing it with its relative, *Tabacum,* or *Nicotine.* H. N. Guernsey characterizes it thus: "Gasping for breath; bluish tint of the skin; muscles of back, face, and jaws principally affected." So there is an agreement between these two authorities,—Dr. Buchner terming the condition asphyxia, from its known power to suspend blood-oxygenation; Dr. Guernsey picturing the cyanotic surface resulting thereform.

It would appear, then, that the *acid* corresponds to those forms of epilepsy which present this marked dyspnœa and cyanosis. Hence it is not applicable to *la petit mal,* with its mild paroxysm, and which progresses insidiously towards irreparable imbecility.

We must, however, remember that the remedy simulating the paroxysm only is, at best, merely a palliative. In our therapeutics there are so many contingencies to be noted that we are safe only in a recognised study of *all* the symptoms of the patient. A remedy may cure a case even though it possess a very imperfect resemblance to the symptoms of the paroxysm. For instance, *Sulphur,* after suppressed itch; *Calcarea C.* in fleshy, scrofulous women with profuse menses, after suppression of chronic eruptions. *Bufo,* after internal suppurations; *Nux Vom.* when the aura starts from the solar plexus; *Silicea,* scrofulo-rachitic persons, etc. Each of these remedies may possibly produce a picture of an epileptic convulsion, but its distinctive characteristic lies outside this similarity. While, then, we welcome this addition to our armamentarium, let us not treat it as a specific; but, in the language of Dr. Hughes, let it aid us in the task of curing this formidable disease, epilepsy.

HAHNEMANN AND MISAPPLIED HOMŒOPATHY*

play the part of instructor, demands that the teacher shall have carefully ascertained the truth of what he would impart.

One's judgment is always based on the store of ideas already incorporated in his mind. If, by meditation, he would create new ideas, they must be limited and qualified by the extent and importance of the parental ideas, already accumulated; hence, how easy, with the beginner, whose ideal stock is necessarily meagre and whose eager spirit seizes on every new thought, to impart fallacies which, received and appropriated, make a fearful basis upon which to erect his future temple of knowledge!

I can recall a medical acquaintance, whose early days had monopolized the study of *Ammonia.* This was the superstructure. Mention to him, a perplexing case of pneumonia or croup, cholera or dysentery, and

---

* Being a reply by Dr. Farrington to an article of Dr. P. Dudley, published in the *Hahnemannian Monthly* of February 1872 under the above caption.

after long and deep thought his invariable answer would be "Have you tried *Carbonate of Ammonia?*"

This is the basis of hobbyism. No true scientist ever rides a hobby. Each new truth shines with a fresh lustre which delights but never dazzles him. He has a long-prepared niche for it; his orderly system missed a something which he knew must be forthcoming, and which once seen was recognized as the missing link.

There are some in the ranks of homœopathy whose names at once recall their favourite medicine, so inseparably united have they become. Scarcely a work of the "Great Translator" but makes us feverish with a multitude of *Aconite* notes! Never teach hobbyism.

But this one-ideaism is not the worst result of a false education. It is rather the result of a paucity of knowledge. But let the student of medicine be invited to listen to medical discussions, such as monthly engross our various societies, and if truth be not there taught, will he not suffer a worse fate than hobbyism? What is the grand cause of the reckless, meaningless theorizing of the day if it be not a false basal education? Begin wrong and the gap between right and wrong widens with each onward step. Let us say with Hahnemann, "TOLLE CAUSAM".

Quite recently, a society meeting of physicians and students was called upon to listen to an article on "Homœopathy Misapplied." Its tenets seemed to me too unscientific to disturb even a student's mind; and yet, on leaving the hall, one of them remarked: "I liked that lecture very much." The author, a gentleman of education and integrity, was thoroughly in earnest, and no doubt thought he was promulgating the truth. So did the student think; the latter, because he knew no better; the former, because his collegiate impression of homœopathy was incorrect.

His tenets are, however, in the light of modern science, false. He seems to know nothing of molecular action, direct and indirect action, and disease itself. He asks, speaking of post-parturient hæmorrhage: "Will *Ipecac* or *China* coagulate healthy liquid blood? .... Will *Bell.* or *Sabina,* or *Crocus* contract and retract a broken vessel which has already contracted and retracted so much as is consistent with the laws of its own health?" Now, how can such a sentence be answered unless the interrogator first study the manner of nature's cure of hæmorrhage and still more, how medicines act?

But errors of one's own invention may be nursed *ad libitum* if they remain respectfully at home, but when one's aspirations make him a critic of Hahnemann, whose pure teachings, not comprehended, are misjudged, patience ceases to be a virtue.

MISAPPLIED HOMŒOPATHY BY HAHNEMANN is a phrase as shocking as it is false, and its author deserves unmitigated censure. Poor Hahnemann, how could he so misunderstand his own discovery as not to see, with our learned author, that his cures of frost-bite and burns were not homœopathic! Strange, too, "that so many of his followers in our day should have made the same mistaken application!"

Now, "in the name of reason, in the name of science" we call upon all to renounce *Aconite* in "foreign substances in the eye;" *Silicea* in the "removal of splinters;" *Cicuta* for "fish-bone in the throat;" *China, Bell., Croc.* and *Ipecac* for post-partum hæmorrhage; *Berb., Nux Vom.,* and *Merc.,* in the renal colic; else all are, with Hahnemann, guilty of Misapplied Homœopathy.

CORRESPONDENCE

To

The Editor, Hahnemannian Monthly.

Dear Editor,

Our mutual friend, author of "Misapplied Homœopathy" and "Criticism Misapplied," has so complicated our discussion by new issues, which I did not criticise and which are hence foreign to the point, that I must needs bring the matter to a timely close, that you may be no longer annoyed, and your space be better filled. In doing so I shall endeavour to take no advantage which my "last say" might give opportunity to exercise.

First I am sorry that Professors Lee, Gause and Brooks are dragged into the contest; for the fact that one of their students acquired an incorrect impression of homœopathy does not prove that they mistaught him.

Secondly, if I have misjudged my offended colleague by calling him a gentleman of education and integrity, and at the same time asserting that his impression of homœopathy is false (cannot an educated man be wrong in anything?), I can retract thus much: I surely deemed him honest in his remarks: and that he is educated, witness his acquaintance with Socrates and Galileo, the fables, and his euphonious quotation from Shakespeare.

But serious discussions invariably bring forth the bitterest sarcasm, and never do either party any good. I forbear noticing any slurs applied to me personally, whether quoted from Marcy, or exhibited, school-master fashion, in a review of my style. But you must allow me to reassert, that *Aconite* is homœopathic to foreign substances in the eye (but it won't pull them out); that *Silicea* will hasten the superficial appearance of needles lost in deep tissues; that medicines are homœopathic to renal colic (of course not as solvents to the calculi); that *Sabina,* "a shred of Cinchona bark," if prepared rightly, will check post-partum hæmorrhage. All these can be explained by molecular motions.

I was animated by no personal feelings; hence I censured him professionally, and must still be allowed the privilege of considering his remarks as not correct (even if my "pot" is seven years junior to his "kettle"), and as contrary to the teachings of Hahnemann, and I find that I am far from being alone in my judgment.

Very truly yours,
ERNEST A. FARRINGTON.

CONFIRMATION OF SYMPTOMS

Among the agreeable duties of the active practitioner is that of confirming symptoms; for thereby he materially aids in contributing to the construction of a reliable and stable Materia Medica.

Every symptom of a proving or series of provings may be genuine, and yet all genuine symptoms are not equally valuable. Some are vague, indefinite, or commonplace, while others are peculiar, distinctive, characteristic. It is the latter we desire to see confirmed. And yet, before clinical experience lends its aid, we are often at a loss to premise which effects of a drug are probably characteristic. Many of the prominent features are so plain that they are easy of recognition; but

CONFIRMATION OF SYMPTOMS

in nice prescribing we need fine qualities and it is the recognition of these latter that is so difficult. Who, before testing it, could expect such a simple symptom as pain at the costal cartilage of the third right rib to indicate a remedy in hæmoptysis and in enlarged liver? Who, until he has tried it would believe that tuberculosis could be retarded by a drug, the characteristic of which is merely pain in the apex of the left lung? It is clinical confirmation, then, confirmation made in accordance with the rules of homœopathic institutes, that we most need for the firm establishment of our system of proving and prescribing.

1. Several months ago I had the pleasure of reporting to the club of which I am a member, a confirmation of the *Carduus Marianus* in jaundice. The patient was suffering from chills and fever, tertian type. Several remedies failed when finally, guided by a painful liver, full feeling, stool void of bile, and urine surcharged with bile,—all symptoms in the provings of *Carduus,—* I prescribed it. To my gratification, not only did the icterus disappear, but also the chills and fever; so, if in the future I shall be called upon to treat ague with jaundice, I shall think of *Carduus,* along with the other more tried remedies. The drug was given in the tincture, three or four drops in a glass half full of water, two teaspoonful every two to three hours.

2. Recently, a consumptive was attacked by hæmoptysis—no rarity, you will say. True; but its stubbornness was very unwelcome, if not uncommon, and I failed with such oft-used remedies, as *Hamamelis, Erigeron,* and *Pulsatilla.* After repeated careful inquiries, I finally elicited from my patient this peculiarity, that the bleeding was always worse while she was lying down. Several remedies have this symptom, but of the list only *Sepia* has harsh night cough and suppressed menses,—additional symptoms in the case under con-

sideration. The 30th potency was sufficient to cure the hæmoptysis, and to give my patient so much strength, that she is now able to go out and take comfortable walks.

In Gregg's useful illustrated Repertory—I wish he would give us a second and enlarged edition—will be found the following symptom, an exact counterpart of which I cured with *Arnica*: "Stitch at every inspiration in the right side of the back, extending from the last rib up to the axilla."

Would not many of us, in the hurry of business, hastily give *Bryonia* for such a symptom? In my case, the patient had unsuccessfully tried the latter drug, and so I was saved the humiliation of a failure.

3. We are accustomed to regard nausea as a sort of *sine qua non* of *Ipecacuanha*—and almost, if not quite correctly.

The other day, I had an opportunity of seeing it work promptly in a case without nausea. The lady had miscarried or rather was in the midst of her expulsive efforts, and there was much bright red hæmorrhage. An annoying attendant was a violent cutting pain across the abdomen above the umbilicus, a cutting going from left to right; no nausea. *Ipecac.* was given, and effected a speedy relief of both pain and hæmorrhage; the embryo, however, did not come away for several hours.

Cutting at or near the navel is very characteristic of *Ipecac;* and especially it is indicative of this drug, if worse to the left of the centre, or going from left to right. *Lycopodium* has cutting to the right, or, as Dr. Guernsey has confirmed it, going from right to left.

4. And now, having mentioned several instances, embracing potencies from the tincture—if I may call

CONFIRMATION OF SYMPTOMS

this a potency—to the 30th, I purpose relating a confirmation with a very high potency.

A boy who had suffered for five years with stomacace, never well, though occasionally much better than he was when his disease was fully developed, came to me for treatment. He had been prescribed for by allopathists and homœopathists, but always with unsatisfactory results. His symptoms were plainly those of *Sulphur*, and I doubt not, had received that medicine, though probably not in so high a potency as the one I purpose using, namely, the 100,000th.

Under this preparation the patient is improving, and has enjoyed more complete immunity from soremouth than for years.

I do not refer to this experience as an isolated one, but as confirmatory of the emphatic assertion, which a few make and many deny, that high potencies can and do cure.

But talking about attenuated drugs, one has reason to look with distrust upon the provings of *Thuja*, made by Wolf with one single globule of the 1000th potency, and extending over a period of two years! Think of the vicissitudes in twenty-four months, of the diversities of season, of weather, of modes of living, and then expect it to be possible to record the pure effects of a single, tiny pellet of the one-thousandth attenuation of the *Arbor Vitae!*

And yet, what am I to do? Wolf says *Thuja* caused diarrhœa daily, in the morning, after breakfast; foul diarrhœa; and others, as well as myself, have cured it with *Thuja* 6th.

That watery stools are caused by this drug is confirmed by the heroic provings of Watzke with 900 drops of the tincture. Is it all a coincidence?

Some of Wolf's symptoms are, as Hughes truly declares, "quite beyond the range of the drug's action," and so we must conclude with the author last cited, that Wolf's symptoms must be regarded as dubious, until otherwise confirmed. I hope that the diarrhœa symptom is now "otherwise confirmed,"—but time and rigid tests are needed.

DYNAMIZATION OF DRUGS.*

(Dr. Dudley's Platform.)

Editor Hahnemannian Monthly: Dr. Dudley's "Open Letter" in your August issue is the most remarkable paper against high potencies that has yet appeared. He charges the advocates of these potencies with being illogical and, yet, he lays down six "principles" which are supremely absurd, and altogether opposed to the plainest forms of logic. Surely, Dr. Potter, whom hearsay reports as astute and shrewd, will not "go on record" with Dudley upon such an insecure platform.

---

* Dr. Dudley's Open Letter to Samuel Potter.

I have read the paper on "The Logical Basis of the High Potency Question". Not having the pleasure of your personal acquainance, I must ask you to pardon my familiarity, in saying that you are a man after my own heart; not because you are evidently a low 'potency' man, but rather because you bring your medical principles to the bar of reason and logic, a custom all too rare among medical men, homœopathist especially. Your temerity, however, is amazing. Have you no conception of the nature of the dangerous elements you have invoked? Hail, dunder and blitzen, cyclones, volcanoes, earthquakes, tidal waves,

DYNAMIZATION OF DRUGS

His first plank is, that dynamization "is not sustained or even encouraged by a single fact yet discovered in the whole range of physical science". Now, this is not true; but if it were, what is its application? Is it the fault of the doctrine, or of science? Hahnemann established the doctrine of dynamization, just as he did homœopathy itself, by experimentation. He cared not whether science said yea or nay. His was an inductive philosophy. Will the doctor assert that the doctrine under consideration is at all affected because physical science does not sustain it? Who made physical science, as now formulated by man, a supreme judge? And who

---

profanity, scurrility, "open letters," and nitroglycerin; yet one thing you need not fear, and that is logic. Your opponents are too sharp to take the field in strange armour or to fight with unknown weapons.

Your article ought to be widely read. It is high time that the origin and the basis (?) of some of the so-called "doctrines of homœopathy", which have done, and are doing, so much to retard the progress of our system, should be thoroughly and universally known. There are hundreds of homœopathic physicians who have all along been decided with the idea that these "principles" were constructed on a foundation of preliminary observation and experiment, nor dream that they had their origin, some, in the purest and most baseless speculation, some in a desire for cheap notoriety, and some in a lofty ambition to defy the adverse criticism of allopathy and allopathists to the last extreme degree. Until these facts are made plain to all our colleagues, and homœopathy subjects her doctrines, one and all, to the test of rational experiment, and verifies them by positive demonstration in the presence of hostile critics, we cannot expect or ask that our system should receive a general public, much less a scientific recognition. When that is done, the very natural prejudice with which we now have to contend will rapidly disappear, and the final result of the rivalry between the two schools will be no longer doubtful.

The writer has never been foolhardy enough to declare that, the use of high potencies cannot be instrumental in curing disease,

dare claim that this science has yet grasped the full extent of the physical universe? The plank, then, is wholly inapplicable to the subject; so, Dr. Potter don't trust it.

As to the remaining planks, did I not know Dr. Dudley so well and so favorably, I should think that they were intended as a travesty on the whole question.

If the high potencies contain neither the material presence, nor the dynamic properties of the drug, they are mere nothings, yet we may resort to them "after a

---

any more than he would make a similar assertion respecting clairvoyance, mesmerism, triturated moonshine, or any other unlikely thing. But I am ready to go on record with you upon the following:—

PLATFORM OF PRINCIPLES RESPECTING HIGH "POTENCIES."

1. That the doctrine of "dynamization", as understood by high-potency homœopathists, is not sustained or even encouraged by a single fact yet discovered in the whole range of physical science.

2. That the latest investigation in physics render it probable that matter cannot be diluted beyond the tenth or twelfth centesimal.

3. That (consequently it is probable that no dilution above the tenth or twelfth centesimal contains either the material presence, or the dyanmic property of the drug employed in its preparation.

4. That in view of the probability that dilutions above the tenth or twelfth contain neither the material nor the properties of the original drug, their regular use is not warranted, until they shall have been subjected to the most thorough and exhaustive crucial tests that human ingenuity can devise.

5. That until high dilutions are shown to be capable of curing as regularly, as certainly, and as quickly as do appreciable

DYNAMIZATION OF DRUGS 311

lower dilution has been tried without success". And, again, as if to complete the fiasco, "No cure effected with any potency above the twelfth can claim to be homœopathic, because there is no evidence that the remedy administered contained any portion or property of the Similimum. Such cures must, for the present, stand beside those occurring under the influence of clairvoyance, mesmerism, spiritualism, and other occult agencies." So, then failing with the low, we may use the high even though they are not material, not dynamic, not homœopathic, not the similima! And if they stand beside occult agencies, by parity of reasoning, if one's

---

quantities of medicine, their use is not justifiable in any case until after a lower dilution has been tried without success.

6. That no cure effected with any potentcy above the twelfth can claim to be homœopathic, because there is no evidence that the remedy administered contained any portion or property of the similimum. Such cures for the present must stand beside those occurring under the influence of clairvoyance, mesmerism, spiritualism, and other occult agencies.

Your paper is exactly in the line of a good deal of modern homœopathic thought, and is, therefore, timely. It will accomplish much in directing our young men into the only correct methods of therapeutic investigation. It ought also to do good by showing our high-potency friends that, if they are actuated by the true spirit of reform, they will avail themselves of every possible chance to demonstrate the truth of their opinions so conclusively that all of us will be forced to accept them. No considerations of pride, no false idea of personal dignity can exempt the true reformer from the duty of promulgating his new doctrines at every opportunity. He must be "instant, in season, out of season." The Milwaukee test furnishes an occasion, which ought to be made the most of.

Besides the "high potency" question, my dear doctor, there are others looming up for our examination in the near future. One is: "Can a drug be persuaded to hasten its curative action

religion fail him, let him seek consolation in spiritualism; if the detectives fail to recover his stolen property, let him consult a clairvoyant; if *Coffea Cruda* fail to cure sleeplessness, let him use the *cm.*, and, if this fail, send for a mesmerist. Don't trust these planks either, Dr. Potter.

I, for one, welcome this "Milwaukee Test," because it will, if persistently and honestly conducted, add more evidence of the validity of Hahnemann's priceless boon, *"The Dynamization of Drugs."*

Experimenting with high potencies, having ample opportunity every winter I have proved satisfactorily that they produce symptoms severe enough to seriously incommode the prover, and even to compel him to keep his bed. I have proved the *20m* made on the Hahnemannian Plan of 1 to 99, and I have produced symptoms in many incredulous students annually.

---

simply because the case is urgent or desperate?" Another is: "Where, oh, where is the line between the broad realm, where the law of similars wields the sceptre of its beneficent empire, and that other contracted field of disease and of accident, over which it has no control?" I tried to answer this latter question in 1872, and whew! what a tornado I aroused! An ill wind that blew nobody any good. That's what makes me tremble for you.

You have shown our "High potentates" that the evidence they furnish in favour of their methods of practice is deficient, not in quantity but in quality. You might also have pointed out to them that any single "potency" of the different drugs would require for its proper testing and experimentation, at least one year of the undivided attention of the whole profession; that, if the eighty years of the existence of homœopathy had all been devoted to this work, we should still be below the one hundredth dilution, and that, therefore, the indiscriminate use of the high dilutions, with our present limited knowledge of their potency, is rash beyond measure.

I look forward then with no other concern than a fear lest the test fail for want of support. I am eager to place its confirmations along with the invaluable papers furnished by Watzke, Eidherr, and lately by T. F. Allen, in his able criticism of Houat in the N. A. J., Aug. 1879.

I have cured patients with high potencies, and so has Dr. Dudley. I can assure you he is vastly better as a partctitioner than he is as a theorist.

Genial, candid, able as a lecturer, and instructive in the Hahnemann Club meetings, I am all the more astonished that he should permit his pen to play such wild freaks with his better judgment. And I am still more surprised that he should accuse, among others one-half of his club of being a set of illogical fellows, who dare not rationally defend high potencies, because such an armour would be strange to them, such weapon unknown to them.

E. A. Farrington, M.D.

IS IT JUSTFIABLE?

CRIME, encouraged by defective and unexecuted laws, fostered by political partiality, and sheltered in the güise of wealth, spreads it baneful influence everywhere, threatening church and state, social security and family growth.

The murderer's knife or subtle poison adds its horrors to police news. But there is a crime as far spread as society itself. It is dead, finds no funeral pomp, no mourning friends, no christian burial. No monumental slabs inscribe their names; no solemn cemetery shelters their remains. Out of the homes of luxury, as well as from the hovel, they are taken unnamed, unknown, unloved. The cesspool or the dissecting knife hushes all suspicion. We may count the white sepulchres, and approximate to the dead which the sea has claimed; but could the unnumbered host, ushered into the world before their tender forms were fully moulded, speak to us, what a fearful tale of parental degradation would be theirs!

Rightly does the medical profession, denounce, as murder, the production of abortion, unless justified by the impossibility of live birth. But is it ever justified on any other grounds? We had thought not until we learned that the "offspring has no right to life without the consent expressed or implied in the sexual relation of both parties." (See Amer. J. H. M. M., Vol. V, No. 3, p. 122). The writer here, of course, refers to a particular class of cases presenting itself, "though rarely for our consideration and action." He states that a guiltless woman is violated and pregnancy follows. The discovery of her situation entails a life of disgrace for her and her family, and he comes to the above astounding conclusion!

He adds, "she has a right to relief, and her physician is right in granting it." "The relief of the injured woman from the burden of a pregnancy which is hateful to her, which has been forced upon her, and which she has a right to throw off. . . . as soon as it shall please her," and "to save her from the disgrace of the publicity of her misfortune," are his reasons for terming this justifiable fœticide. He believes it "right in the sight of God and in the judgment of men of good conscience and sound mind." And the "Society" accepted his article.

Is life the gift of man, and can he take it for social or any other reasons? Who shall foretell the destiny of the forthcoming child? Even though the distressing ban of illegitimacy be upon him, may it not be his cross, which bearing, he may rise above the sneer of society which our author so fears, and grace the noblest office of humanity? Or if he but walk humbly through life, true in his lowly condition, shall we deny him a hereafter, where, having been faithfull over a few things, he becomes ruler over many? Where both he and his unfortunate mother no longer bow beneath the curse of exposure and illegitimacy, but having borne their crushing burden faithfully, "enter into the glory of their Lord"? Is the woman any the less wronged if she destroys her "hateful" charge? Society is shocked, but the still small voice of a religious conscience tells her to live on, trusting to Him who alone gives life and who alone may take it, living above reproach, and teaching her illicit child the same faith that strengthens herself.

We can point to one case as touching on the one hand as it was fiendish on the other. But, to-day, the child her woman's heart must love, supports her in her old age, and is an ornament to society and the favourite of his employers. Until it can be proved that this man must die because of his unbidden birth, we must call it murder to destroy the fœtus under similar circumstances of conception, for they differ only in time, and time is nothing in eternity.

DETECTION OF INSANITY.

A DIAGNOSIS of a marked case of mental aberration, is comparatively easy, but in the court as in the camp, when life or liberty is threatened, the deceptions practised are often so ingenious as to defy detection.

No one cause is more perplexing to jury or more insidiously applied by the lawyers than this:—an attempt to prove the accused of temporary or permanent mental disease. An alibi, if it is to be successful, must be so conclusive that few ever dare to bring it into court and when circumstantial evidence points with bloody finger and seems to say, "That is the man," the law must hold him, unless his witty lawyer can prove him to have been insane at the time. To prevent deception on the one hand and to shield irresponsible parties on the other, is the high duty of the physician in court. His honor is, or should be above the bribe, above the law, above all, with no motive but the conscientious decision, "Is the prisoner sane or insane?"

Quite recently it became my painful duty to decide whether or not a certain individual, receiving aid from a beneficiary society, was insane or merely deceiving. Two prominent surgeons had pronounced him an imposter. I found him pacing his floor with an aimless tread, and as I entered, he greeted me with an insidious smile, which seemed to say, "I know what you are after." He was cross-questioned for an hour, his answers frequently contradictory, and yet a sane man might deceive thus much. A second visit was made, when finding him in a melancholy humor, I sought to work on his feelings. "Mr..... I am exceedingly sorry to see you suffer so. Isn't there some medicine that I could give you to help you? Your society is kind enough to help you pecuniarily, and I will volunteer my medical aid. Your pulse beats so regularly that I think your mental trouble might yield to proper treatment, if you" he stopped short in his walk and eyed me with a glance so searching, that my blood chilled within me, but I never changed my assumed compassionate look, but continued "if you will give me a history of your case, I'll try what I can do for you, and I'm sure my report to the society will satisfy them and you." Two great tears stood in his eyes and seizing my hand, he exclaimed "My family shun me, the world too, have I found a friend in you?" The last words were fairly hissed out and I felt very uncomfortable "Sit down, Mr.....," I ventured, "I'am anxious to hear your case." "Well, my friend" (emphasis on friend) "my wife's sick—at least so they say, she won't see me, won't sleep with me—hasn't for—for—I don't know—certainly a long time. If I'd gone with some woman—ha—ha— that would have been wicked, but———." "But what," I said: "Oh, there's an end to everything, I've said enough." I was puzzled, was he a Hamlet or not? An idea struck me, as he paced the floor, a hand on either hip. "Does your back pain you as much as it did the other day?" "Incessantly, yes, ever since I lost my nature."* "I suppose," I continued "in your solitary life you found some handy way of allaying your sexual

---

* Nature is a common phrase for sexual power.

appetite?" (The insane are often quick to appreciate a pun). He laughed and said, "Yes, once a week or so." Backache, trembling gait, stupid face, except when brightened by the fire of his passion, and an acknowledged onanist! "Wouldn't shutting your eyes make your walking better, you'd see fewer of those vision . ...." "I stagger like one drunk, in the dark!" he interrupted. I was satisfied, Tabes Dorsalis and softening of the brain from Onanism. Six months afterwards, he was admitted to Kirkbride's and placed in the ward of incurables.

Hahnemann, with incomparable astuteness, touched the very keynote, when he bid us treat the insane as though they were not insane. By assuming a state harmonizing with that of my patient, opposing him in nothing, I gained what else might have been impossible.

SUGGESTION FOR "A MODEL MATERIA MEDICA."

TO deserve the title "model" a materia medica must be more than an abridgment restricted to a maximum of five pages to a drug. The limitation of a drug must be measured by its own capacity, not arbitrarily.

To meet all the requirements of a "model" each drug should be arranged with due regard to the following points:

1. Its officinal name, its place in natural history and its composition.

2. A concise statement of such characteristic features as are nearly or quite universal in its symptomatology.

3. A clear compact but complete arrangement of its symptoms, subjective and objective.

> (*a*) These symptoms should comprise not only the effects of provings, but also such developments of provings and such merely clinical symptoms as are indisputably characteristics.
>
> (*b*) As we depend so much upon the parts of the body affected, every attention must be paid to the localization of symptoms.

Let us dilate somewhat upon these several points:

1. That officinal names are needed is self-evident. Equally apparent is that euphony requires the adoption of a fixed pronunciation of drug names; and this can be utilized by proper syllabic marks.

The origin of a remedy is often very suggestive. So soon as it is known that *Duboisia* belongs to the Solanaceæ, our familiarity with the mydriatics of this order, enables us at once to interpret the dilated pupil and dry mouth of the new plant. When *Bothrops* is found to be an Ophidian, the general nature of its effects is almost pre-determinable.

Composition is often more suggestive even than origin. Two or more substances, which contain the same active principles, must, of necessity, possess similar properties.

A knowledge of the source and of the constituents of drugs, is all important, then, as it leads to an intelligent unification of the Materia Medica.

2. Before any schema of symptoms is devised, the drug should be prefaced with a concise statement, not of its vague generalities, as has been the custom, but of peculiarities which are essentials, and which, con-

sequently, must enter the thought as qualifications of what is to follow.

3. But the chief task is that of arranging the symptoms of a drug. To render a work practical, it must be free from all verbosity, unnecessary repetitions and vague, unimportant symptoms. But condensation is so frequently effected at the sacrifice of valuable matter, that if we would avoid such loss, we must proceed cautiously and intelligently. Whenever in the provings we find two or more symptoms differing only in fullness of expression, we may select that one which is nearest complete in phraseology. But if two symptoms agree in the main, but offer in addition entirely different modalities, both must be employed.

In selecting symptoms which are local, those are preferable that are most characteristic. But since a drug, when fully proved, acts somewhat on nearly all parts of the body, completeness requires that all parts should be represented in the abridgment.

Clinical experience has taught us that local symptoms are of inestimable value. For instance guided by the splenic pains of *Ceanothus,* leucorrhoea has been cured by that remedy. Influenced by the sour stomach of *Robinia,* one physician learned to value that drug in ulcers on the legs. And so on indefinitely. But since such indications are frequently derived from practice, we must not neglect clinical symptoms.

Our estimate of these latter symptoms should depend, it seems to us, upon their agreement with the provings, with the genius of the drug to which they are assigned, and also upon the reputation of the physician who reports them. If they disagree with the provings, they can form no part of a precise Materia Medica.

Those clinical symptoms are most trustworthy, which are evident developments of imperfectly expressed provings; or, which have been so frequently confirmed as to have become indisputable facts. *Xanthoxylum* has not caused pains along the anterior crural nerve, and yet it seldom fails to relieve. But as it has caused neuralgic pains in the thighs, and also uterine and overian pains, we have a right to conclude that its clinical estimate in crural pains is just. *Hepar* as a remedy in suppuration has no foundation in provings, other than in certain subjective sensations, which led to its trial; and yet no one to-day, not even an allopath, will deny its efficacy.

Having made choice of the material to be used, the next step is the adoption of a schema of arrangement.

All plans hitherto employed are open to the serious objection that they violently sever symptoms and so impair or destroy the natural sequence of drug effects. We do not quite agree with those who assert that a remedy is of no use unless selected according to the order of its symptoms. Nor do we coincide with those who affirm that parts of one series of symptoms cannot be transferred to another series. For instance, if a drug causes headaches on the right side, worse from motion, and, in another prover, headache on the left side, with nausea it does not follow that the qualifying phrase in the first may not also qualify the second, and *vice versa.*

It seems to us that the most efficient schema is one which begins, as we have already observed, with a description of the universal qualities of a remedy, which next considers symptoms as to their respective localities and concomitants, and which finally displays such rational combining of subjective and objective, physiological and pathological symptoms as will enable the reader to make practical application of them. It is useful to say that *Hepar* may be employed in that pathological condition known as pus formation; but it is more practicable to say that *Hepar* may be employed when, in addition to the presence of forming pus, there are also present throbbing pains, rigors and the extreme sensitiveness to touch, so characteristic of the remedy.

But, further, an intelligent arrangement of drug effects requires a knowledge of anatomy, physiology, pathology and indeed, of many branches of a scientific education. Symptoms are not merely empty words, they mean something, and to determine that meaning one needs all the culture a complete education can afford. A "model" materia medica demands more than the vague statement that, for instance, "slimy yellow mucus covers the tongue," if that so-called mucus is actually pus hanging from Steno's duct!

But, though very useful, the ordinary means of investigation employed by the old school are often too gross to fulfill the requirements of our molecular drugs. A thermometer will tell us whether or not a medicine taken is affecting the temperature; chemical analysis will reveal the nature of the red deposit in the urine, and the miscroscope will tell when the sputa contain pus cells, lung tissue, etc.; but we need psychology to teach us to estimate relations between mental and bodily symptoms; we need such delicate machinery as the volumenometer and the French graphic method of determining the separate and combined effects of cerebral, pulmonary and cardiac motions; and, above all, we need a firm reliance upon a pathology which teaches not merely the ordinary course of diseases, but also such molecular changes as are set forth in the totality of the symptoms of a given case. Lastly, to complete the schema, the several symptoms employed must be compared with one another that analogies and differences may be clearly seen; and there great discrimination is required. It does not follow that because a drug acts upon the heel (*Natrum Carb* for example), that therefore it can cure the same symptoms when located upon the instep. Still, just as metastases are apt to take place in tissues of similar function, so are analogous parts prone to be affected by a drug. Reasoning from such premises, *Arum Triphyllum,* which causes rawness of the corners of the mouth, was successfully employed by Dr. B. F. Betts for a similar condition of the os uteri; and upon the same principle, drugs which disease the testicles have been used when the ovaries are affected.

In the hope of making ourselves better understood, and also in compliance with the instructions of the Chairman of Bureau, we essay an application of our several "points to the study of *Nux Vomica.* At the risk of prolixity, we shall explain our steps by numerous annotations, observing here, however, that of course no such addenda should mar the pages of a fully prepared "model."

NUX VOMICA.

Strychnos Nux Vomica.

Natural Order, Loganiaceæ. It yields Strychnia, Brucia, Igasuria.

Nux Vomica owes its chief effects to the Strychnia which it contains. It causes in small doses an increase in the heart's action and a general increase of functional activity. In large doses, its action upon sympathetic nerves and also upon the spine, by which it induces an exaltation of reflex functions, leads to a train of symptoms, varying from a very characteristic over-susceptibility to impressions, to tetanus and trismus; also dilatation of the pupils, erection of the hair follicles, tinnitus, sweat, marked rise in the arterial pressure, and finally death from tonic spasms of the respiratory muscles or from exhaustion. Paralyses are not direct effects, they arise only from exhaustion following the intense excitation. Cerebral and spinal softening have been observed *post mortem* after the patient had suffered from intense congestions.

Nux Vomica likewise causes changes in secretions and some structural alterations.

In nearly every case in which it is indicated, gastric and enteric disturbances are present. Functions are performed defectively, not so much from atony, as from derangement in the normal order of muscular contractility with over-susceptibility to even normal stimuli. This universal quality arises from the tendency of the drug to increase reflex-action (1).

Many ailments are worse in the morning and are made worse by exertion, by exposure to cold air, by leading a sedentary life (1), and for mental exertion (1, 19). Complaints originating in an excess of stimulants, condiments, or in so-called "high-living". Hence, many ailments are due to abdominal plethora, or to sudden suppression of hæmorrhoidal flow.

Mind and Sensorium (3).

Over-impressionable from internal or external sources, hence irritable, and even if sad and tearful, still morose or angry.

Feels faint, nauseated, and has flushes of heat with the mental symptoms.

Intellectual labor impossible or effected with difficulty; many ailments result (19).

Anxiety with delirious fancies at night—with orgasm of blood, worse in the morning (18)—with suicidal impulse in hypochondriasis.

Delirium tremens with over-sensitiveness and malicious vehemence; marked trembling of the hands. Can bear no contradiction or even gentle persuasion. Reproaches others; quarrelsome; angry; scornful. Dreads intellectual work, if it requires thinking; worse in the morning; slow flow of ideas; makes mistakes in speaking. Cerebral hyperæmia in vigorous, tense-fibred, irascible persons, or when caused by mental labour, abuse of alcohol, coffee, highly-seasoned foods, etc.; also from suppressed hæmorrhoidal discharges; apoplexy from similar causes (5). Softening of the brain. Feeling of intoxication, dizziness, with heaviness; worse in the morning or when stooping. Confused feeling and dullness; worse after a carousal in the morning (18), after dinner; worse when the head is erect, though bending forward causes heaviness in the forhead.

Vertigo (6), as if the brain was turning in a circle, momentary loss of consciousness; feels like falling to the side or backwards. Caused by abdominal plethora, and then worse in the morning (18) or after meals; the face is red or the cheeks flushed on a sallow ground. Also caused by mental exertion, by drinking wine, etc. Nervous vertigo from strong odors, after loss of sleep, after loss of animal fluids with obscuration of sight, ringing in the ears, and fainting.

Head (3, 7).

Headaches originate in irritation of brain tissue; or more commonly reflexly from hepatic and abdominal plethora, from gastric affection and constipation. They are most frequently situated in the forehead, or in the occiput. Characteristic sensations are: fullness; bursting; bruised soreness; tension; pressure. The pains increases from morning (18) to noon, and then decrease towards evening.

Stunning headache after eating, in the sunshine, in the morning (18). Pains seem to be in the middle of the brain. Internal soreness as from the blows of an axe.

Congestive headaches; burning in the forehead, whole head, with hot and bloated face, body chilly; feels as if the skull would burst; throbbing. Worse mornings (18) moving the head, walking in the open air, studying (19) and after eating. Better at rest and in a warm place.

Clavus, worse from coffee. Headache in the middle of the brain, worse on awaking in the morning (18). Periodical headaches.

Tension, drawing in the forehead as if pressed in; worse at night and in the morning (18) and from exposing the head to cold air.

Headache pressing in the forehead; stitches in the left temple, left eye, or in the occiput; worse in the morning (18) on awaking, or, begins early and reaches the acme at noon. All worse from late suppers, mixed diet, debauchery, mental labor (19), sedentary habits; accompanied with nausea and sour vomiting.

Head feels full, heavy, worse from stooping, worse from want of sleep.

Brain seems to shake when one walks.

Scalp sensitive to touch; liable to take cold from dry winds or drafts. Fetid sweat of one side of the head and face, with dread of uncovering the head; sweat relieves the pains; parts feel cold to the touch.

Special Senses (3).

The senses are rendered over-sensitive, are perverted and finally are destroyed. The sense of taste is not intensified proportionately to the others, though even here natural taste of food despite perverted taste from disordered stomach, shows the characteristic tendency of the drug.

Eyes.

Retinal hyperæsthesia with pains at the top of the head; sleeplessness. Vision sensitive. Sees objects more distinctly.

Bright, glittering objects in the field of vision.

Photophobia worse in the morning (18); in keratitis, scrofulous ophthalmia, etc.

Dilated pupils with irritation of the spine.

Amblyopia potatorum. Blurred vision, worse when over-heated. (See also Headaches). Atrophy of the optic nerve. (*Nux* or *Strychnia*).

Biting, as from salt (17), worse in the external canthi, with lachrymation.

Conjunctivitis, especially if the cornea is involved; also when ecchymoses are found in the conjunctival tissue, or when blood oozes from between the lids. Eyes swollen, red streaks in the whites, pressive-tensive pains.

Blepharitis, smarting and dryness (17); margins of lids feel as if rubbed sore. (See Skin). Worse from touch, and in the morning (18).

Spasms of the muscles. Eyes wild, upturned, or in constant motion. Paralysis of the rectus externus.

Ears.

Sounds reverberate.

Noises: ringing; hissing; roaring in the morning (18).

Earache; lancinating, pinching pains.

Nose.

Over-sensitive to odors, even fainting.

Illusory smells; of sulphur, bad cheese, a smoking candle-wick, etc.

Nose-bleed during sleep or in the morning; preceded by red cheeks, headache; or accompanying abdominal plethora. Catarrh (18): mucous membranes are irritated and inflamed, with a sensation of smarting (17), conjunctival, roughness and rawness (throat). Discharges are scanty, watery and acrid, thick and adherent, or bloody and clotted.

Colds are contracted by exposure to dry, cold air, or by a draft. Gastric symptoms are usually present. The air passages feel stuffed. Diphtheria has been relieved when the breath was putrid, and an undisturbed nap relieved.

Stuffed nose even with watery or thick mucous secretion. Severe pains in the frontal sinuses. Sneezing. Itching along the eustachian tubes. Pharynx feels constricted. Throat and larynx as if scraped and raw.

Small aphthous ulcers in the mouth, stomacace.

Cough dry, painful, caused by irritation about the palate, in the throat or larynx, by constriction, or by adherent mucus in the trachea, or by eating; worse when exerting the mind (19), on ascending, in the evening on lying down, or in the morning (18); with bursting headache, bruised pain in the abdonimal walls, tightness of the chest.

Gastro-enteric Symptoms (3, 9).

Irritation of stomach and bowels leads to irregular and perverted functioning, and to obnormal cravings (10). Hence arise excesses with consequent over-stimulation, with abnormal plethora, resulting in dyspepsia,

SUGGESTION FOR "A MODEL MATERIA MEDICA"

neuroses, piles and many reflex phenomena. There are many nervous symptoms; such as cardialgia, colic, bearing down, etc. The mucous membrane is affected very much as in other parts, with smarting (17), rawness and scanty secretions or clotted bloody discharges. Most of the ailments are markedly exacerbated in the morning (18).

Face pale, yellow; flushed red, the skin being still sallow; yellow about the mouth.

Toothache, stinging in decayed teeth; tearing in cold air; worse from exerting the minds (19). Gumboils.

Tongue dry in the morning (18) without thirst; still there may be much saliva in the fauces. Tongue white or yellow-coated, worse near the root. Saliva increased.

Taste bitter, putrid, sour; food has a natural taste. The mucus hawked is bitter or putrid.

Appetite wanting, though there may be hunger. Hungry 24 hours before a dyspeptic attack. Craves sauces, condiments, beer, fats, meats, lime (11). Aversion to food. Ailments from coffee, milk, beer, brandy, cold foods (11).

Thirst, but water nauseates. Aversion to drinks (11).

Eructations sour, bitter; also with spasmodic constriction of the œsophagus. Heartburn. Waterbrash.

Hiccough; also when worse from hot drinks.

Nausea, qualmishness and faint-like weakness. Vomiting with marked retching (12) and deathly nausea. Vomit is sour, bilious, fetid, slimy, bloody, or excrementious.

Distended stomach and abdomen (14), worse after eating. Cannot bear the pressure of the clothing about the hypochondria. Flatulency, abdominal plethora, etc.

Pains (13) pinching, clawing, spasmodic; *cramping;* pressing as from a stone; accompanied with nausea; with pains in the back, pressure between the scapulæ, etc. Gastralgia. Colic, flatulent, hæmorrhoidal, from cold or from indigestion.

Flatus incarcerated; presses up under the ribs or downwards or to rectum and bladder, with tormenting but ineffectual urging to defecation and micturition.

Liver swollen, sensitive, painful. Congested liver of drunkards (15).

Throbbing pain, as from an ulcer.

Jaundice, with faint spells; caused by anger, by cold, "high-living," debauchery, etc.

Dragging in the abdomen as from a load; weak feeling in one of the abdominal rings as if a hernia would protrude. Piles, bleeding or not; constricting pain in rectum and anus; worse after a meal and after exerting the mind (19): Burning, smarting (17), sticking, pressive pains. Proctitis; evacuation of dark-coloured mucus.

Stools hard, dry; with ineffectual urging, or with incomplete evacuation, and followed by a sense of constriction of the rectum.

Diarrhœa scanty and attended with irregular, unsatisfactory urging and tenesmus, with smarting and burning in the rectum. Mucous and bloody stools.

Urinary Organs (3).

From imperfect action of the liver, etc., the urine contains lithic acid; and so the remedy is useful in renal-colic when the characteristic pains obtain. The same irregular, spasmodic action observed in the rectum occurs also in the bladder.

Renal colic, worse on the right side, with ineffectual urging to urinate.

Ineffectual urging to urinate; strangury. Burning, tearing pain during micturition. Tenacious mucus in the urine. Dirty yellow sediment. Hæmaturia.

Genital Organs (3)—Male.

Irritable weakness, hence sexual desire is easily excited, but erections are too short or the emission is too speedy. Therefore, useful after excesses. (See Spine).

Chancroid. Gonorrhœa with thin discharge and strangury. Orchitis, when there is spasmodic contraction with retraction of the testicle.

Soreness on the margin of the prepuce; biting, itching of inner surface.

Genital Organs (3)—Female.

The usual bearing down, cramping pains of the remedy, with exquisite over-susceptibility; hence many reflex symptoms; but irritability, faintness and weakness predominate.

The menses are too early and long lasting, though not necessarily profuse; flow dark, clotted.

Displacements of the uterus; recent cases after lifting, over-exertion, etc. Bearing down in abdomen and back, with ineffectual urging to stool and urination. Labor pains, metrorrhagia, etc., with the same concomitant.

Internal swelling of the vagina, like a prolapsus, buring pain; touch intolerable.

Lungs-Heart (3).

Chest symptoms are usually reflex. Thus, there are asthma, tightness, dyspnœa and congestion, caused by spinal irritation, dyspepsia, suppressed hæmorrhoidal flow. The asthma is worse after midnight and is felt more in the lower part of the thorax.

Spasmodic palpitation of the heart, fluttering at the pit of the stomach. Palpitation on lying down after dinner.

Spine (3).

By increasing the reflex action, *Nux Vomica* causes many motor symptoms. These are inharmonious, in-co-ordinate, and finally followed by paresis. Hence, the symptoms are spasmodic, paretic and mixed, giving the so-called irritable weakness: tetanus, trismus, renewed by touch, a strong light or a draft of cold air. Tonic spasms. Spine symptoms from loss of fluids with dyspepsia, constipation, etc.

Spasmodic trembling.

Burning, tearing in the back. Bruised pains; worse 3 A.M. (18). Pains in lumbar and sacral regions.

Gait tottering, inco-ordinate as in ataxia. Sense of sudden loss of power. Bruised, tired pains in the legs; irresistible desire to lie down. Numbness, stiffness and tension in the limbs. Cramps in the calves.

Muscles and Joints.

Are bruised, swollen, tense; overlying skin, pale, with tearing pains; affects generally the large joints and the muscles of the trunk. The tearing pains compel a change of position, but with only momentary relief; the bruised sensation, the swellings, etc., are made worse by motion. Tension, shortening of the tendons, jerks on going to sleep, cramps and numbness, point to co-existing nervous irritation.

Skin.

As in mucous membranes, so here, there are soreness, as if ulcerated, especially on the margins (17) of skin and mucous membrane, crawling, itching and burning. There is also extreme sensitiveness of the skin to slight touch (see Senses), to drafts of cool air, etc. Painful desquamation, especially of the lips, whenever fatigued or after excesses.

Acne on the face, after excessive use of liquor; also after cheese.

Ulcers with raised, pale edges; pain as if beaten; itching worse in the evening; feeling of tension; burning and sticking of flat ulcers in the mouth and throat. Boils. Abscesses.

Sleep.

Falls asleep early in the evening; awakens at 3 or 4 A.M., and cannot sleep again; or dozes for a while, and on again arousing (18), feels tired, sore and sleepy. An uninterrupted nap relieves him very much. (See Diphtheria).

Fever.

Not synochal, but intermittent, with accompanying gastric or bilious symptoms. Heat and chill are intermixed or paroxysms are irregular, intolerance of uncovering, even when hot; and yet covering does not relieve the coldness.

Chill preceded by aching in the limbs; blue nails; vomiting.

Chill and coldness with blue nails; skin painful as if frozen; limbs numb.

General heat, burning hands, thirst for water and then beer; heat, headache, roaring in the ears and nausea; hot and chilly.

Sweat sour, offensive; one-sided or only on upper part of body; alternate with chill. Bathed in sweat. Worse after midnight and in the morning (18). Relieves the pains.

Relationship (16).   Antidotes, &c. (16).

Similar to *Bryonia, Ipecac, Sulphur, Zinc*.

Distinguished from the tetany of *Aconite, Cicuta* and *Hydrocyanic Acid* by its marked increased reflex excitability; from that of *Cocculus* by the spasmus glottidis of the latter; and from traumatic tetany, by the interruption of spasms and the late onset of trismus.

Antidoted: large doses, by *Chloral, Potass, Bromide,* and by the maintenance of artificial respiration. Small doses, by *Coffee, Cham., Pulsat.*

Incompatible with *Zinc*.

At considerable sacrifice, we have reduced *Nux Vomica* to the prescribed limits. It will occupy about six and one-half pages, *brevier, leaded.*

It will be seen that our plan of procedure enables the reader to keep ever before him the entirety of drug action. If, now, he reads consecutively the generalizations which preface the various headings, he will find a brief but important abridgment of the remedy, that will enable him to apply it intelligently. Particular characteristics may mislead him.

We have purposely avoided such synthetic study as would tend to present the remedy already for application to a given disease. However desirable such studies may be, they can form no part of a Materia Medica, which should leave its readers free to prescribe according to the rules and laws of Institutes.

NOTES.

(1) There are numerous instances of this in the symptomatology of *Nux Vom.*, *e.g.*, irritable, irascible, worse from slight disturbances—cannot bear light, noise, touch (spasms renewed) or odors (faints)—stomach rejects all food—retching predominates over vomiting—ineffectual urging to stool—strangury, etc., etc. Here, too, we may find a reason for the efficacy of *Nux* after abuse of drastics; it calms the irritability they induce. Sedentary habits and mental exertion aggravate, the first because they lead to the irritability of fibre so characteristic of *Nux*; the second for this reason, and also because it wears out the brain and spine just as does *Nux* in its prolonged effects. Hence, *Nux* is useful in fatty degeneration of the brain, *cæteris paribus*.

(2) Periodicity since it shows how a drug acts upon the nervous system, cannot but be of universal value in a nerve-affecting drug like *Nux*. So characteristic is this morning aggravation, that we shall see it guiding us even in scrofulous ophthalmia.

(3) Each heading should be as comprehensive as possible, and should include a full symptom record. *Just as the entire remedy is prefaced with a brief general account of the action of the drug upon the part under consideration.* They should follow particulars under these generals.

(4) Ailments of the mind may be comprised under those of the will on the one hand and those of the understanding on the other. Hence, we mention one group and then the other. If there are opposite phases, as when a function is at one time exalted and at another time depressed, the contrast should be shown.

(5) Nux causes irritation and congestion of the brain and spine, and also induces congestions reflex from abdominal plethora. It is therefore suited for the initial symptoms of apoplexy. But since the ultimate effect of irritation is paralytic weakness and degeneration of tissue, *Nux* bears some relation to the apoplectic seizure, especially when the history reveals such causes as abuse of alcohol, etc., and when the attack is associated with gastric symptoms.

(6) Veritgo belong to hundreds of drugs. To be of any practical value, then, it must be considered as to its form and origin.

(7) In arranging headaches, we refer to congestions, then to nerve forms, then to reflex kinds, and then to two sorts expressive of relaxation and depression. Catarrhal headache is referred to another place.

(8) Beginnig as usual with a general account, we proceed to mention such individual and local symptoms as characterize the remedy under consideration. Such symptoms as soreness of nostrils, etc., are omitted as vague or as necessarily implied in cases in which the specified symptoms are present.

(9) After generalizing we proceed to as brief a description of the symptoms as possible. These necessarily include the expression and color of the face, condition of the mouth, pharynx, etc. They belong together, even though we may need but one or more in a given case.

(10) It is not excess alone with calls for *Nux*. It is also the irritability of the patient which suggests the remedy. High living increases his over-susceptibility; and finally, the organs exhausted, he presents a picture of complete "irritable weakness." The stomach is too weak to digest the food, yet it is still irritable.

(11) Symptoms marked "11" have been many times confirmed and cannot be omitted.

(12) Symptoms marked "12" are indispensable, since they show the neurotic effects of *Nux*.

(13) These pains characterize the gastralgia and the colics.

SUGGESTION FOR "A MODEL MATERIA MEDICA" 337

(14) This distended feeling means more than flutulence. It is indicative of portal stasis, abdominal plethora, etc., and so as central in importance, cannot be omitted.

(15) Large liver, when not cirrhotic, has often yielded to *Nux*.

(16) In an abridged *Materia Medica*, "Relationships" should be confined to drugs intimately related, and not to mere symptom-resemblances.

Under this heading should be mentioned homœopathic antidotes, and also antidotes in cases of poisoning. The allopathic law of "antagonism", which is half true, because half a law, cannot apply in homœopathic prescribing; but it can in choosing antidotes to poisons.

(17) Symptoms thus marked are selected, not as an exceptional illustration; but as a good example of that harmony of action, which is to be continually kept uppermost in arranging a medicine. All marked "17" have "smarting", or its equivalent, as characteristic; hence, they are particulars of one general effect. Speaking figuratively, they show the warp and woof of the cloth and so reveal its quality.

If the reader takes the pains, he can follow any other thread of the remedy in the same manner. Take, for instance, symptoms marked "18". This number repeats itself nineteen or twenty times; and as this was not premeditated it becomes a sort of test. See also "19" repeated eleven times, and so on.

A PROVING OF NATRUM PHOSPHORICUM

Synonyms: Phosphate of Soda, Sodi Phosphas, Sal Mirabile Perlatum, Alkali Phos., Tasteless Purging Salt, etc.

The Phosphate of Soda exists in minute proportions in all solids and fluids of the body. Like all the alkaline phosphates, its quantity is greater in flesh-eating animals.

Its function in the blood is not conclusively known; but it has been recently demonstrated that it conveys carbonic acid from tissues to lungs. If this is so, it must have a nutritive value, and is well worthy of a therapeutical study. Schussler, so impulsive in therapeutics, is an excellent student of physiology. According to him, it plays an important part in the lymphatic system; hence in the blood genesis.

In 1800, Dr. Pearson introduced this salt into allopathy. He considered it a mild purgative, suitable to children, and persons of a delicate stomach. It has sometimes been given medicinally by substituting it for common salt.

Dr. William Stephenson (Edinburgh Medical Journal, 1867, Vol. xiii, p. 336) recommends it for "infants who are being artificially reared, and who are liable to frequent derangement of the bowels....where, from the character of the motions, there is a deficient or defective secretion of bile....chalky stool, or white, fluid motions, and in many cases of green stools," etc.

In our school, several partial provings were made years ago by Dr. Hering. In 1873, Schussler mentioned it as a tissue remedy. Von Grauvogl lays more stress

A PROVING OF NATRUM PHOSPHORICUM 339

on the Muriate and Sulphate of Soda, preferring the Phosphate of Potash in the saponifications of fats, change of gases, etc., as the most active. But potash salts exist more in the blood-cells, muscles, etc., soda, in the liquor sanguinis, Potash salts, when proved, show an aggravation when awakening, that is, when we begin to use oxygen, which was stored up during sleep; soda salts are worse during sleep, while oxygen is accumulating (C. Hg.). Hence, even though as alkalies they have many similarities, we shall find sharp differences, depending upon variations in function. Potash must be present to insure an amount of oxygen calculated to keep muscles in their full power of contraction; soda must be present to carry away carbonic acid, a resultant of oxidation.

The following resume is collected from nineteen provings made by twelve provers; nine males, three females. The potencies range from the sixth to the 100,000th. No prover knew the name of the medicine, nor did any two have opportunities of conversing or comparing notes. In no case was a single dose given, but at least twenty were taken. The first proving was made in 1869, the last in August 1875.

I am well aware that prejudice will lead some to refuse these provings because they were made principally with the high potencies. This, however, will in no wise alter their truth or falsity. If four or more persons, in different seasons of the year and in different latitudes, experience the same effects from any given potency, we have an indisputable right to claim these effects as resulting from the medicine taken. If only one prover develops a certain symptom, or set of symptoms, they may be fallacious or they may be true. Who shall decide from preformed opinion? The advocate of the high or of the low potencies? Neither. There is no court of appeal for the homœopathician but that which Hahnemann was the first to establish, *viz., experiment.* So with the symptoms here offered for trial. If they fail when tried, let them go. If they do not fail, let us use them, however our prejudices may question their origin.

Great care has been exercised in preparing the accompanying resume. Symptoms which had been previously experienced by the provers have generally been omitted. Something may thus have been lost, especially as illustrating the reawakening of latent disease; but much has been gained in precision and certainty. For the same reasons obscure or indefinite symptoms have been reserved until more clearly expressed.

Provers.

Each symptom has the initial of the prover and the potency used. Mrs. P.; Miss F.; A., a doctress; Dr. V.; Dr. H.; Dr. K.; Dr. D.; Dr. S.; Dr. Hn.; Mr. H.; Mr. M.; Mr. J.

NATRUM PHOSPHORICUM.*

Mind.

Melancholy, especially after emissions. J., *10m.*
Depression; too apt to dwell on annoyances. J., *50m.*
Frequent attacks of gloominess, evening. Dr. D., *cm.*
Apprehensive of some approaching evil. J., *50m.*
5. Worries about his health; about the future. Dr. D., *10m.*
Vexed at trifles; disposed to be irritable. M., *50m.*
Ill-humor, mostly forenoons; no ambition to do anything; inclines to study in the evening. Dr. D., *10m, cm.*
Imagines he hears footsteps in the next room. M., *50m.*
Study makes him so nervous he must get up and walk about. M., *50m.*
10. Study is burdensome, it is so difficult to remember what is read. Dr. D., *cm.*

---

* Every fifth symptom of this proving has been marked with numerals like 5, 10, 15 and so on.

A PROVING OF NATRUM PHOSPHORICUM

Easily startled by the least noise, especially at night, causing palpitation. See Sleep. Dr. D., *cm*.

Sensorium.

On rising in the morning, dizzy, as if he would fall; objects turn around; gone feeling in the stomach; nervous. Dr. S., *cm*.

Internal Head.

Tensive headache, with dullness and heaviness, accompanied by dim sight, as from a veil before the eyes. P., *30th*.

Frontal headache, sharp over the left eye every forenoon. Dr. S., *cm*.

15. Pain in right temple extending to right eye and ear, at noon; better by 5 P.M. (after eating grapes). In evening pain over left temple while riding in a street car. P., *6th, 30th*.

Immediately after dinner, sharp tearing in left side of head, front of ear and temporal region particularly. Dr. D., *cm*.

Pressure over the right eye, with sighing as if room were too close; later over left eye; worse before and after, better during menses. F., *30th*.

Pinching in left temple descending to left ear and tonsil. P., *6th*.

Heaviness and fulness of the head, with flushes of heat in the afternoon, followed by sweat. P., *2c*.

20. Empty feeling in the head; stomach feels empty. Dr. S., *cm*.

Frequent sensation of fulness in the head, with pulsating pain on stepping. Dr. D., *10m, cm*.

Pain in centre of left eyebrow.

Pain in left orbit, with pain in bowels, extending up into the chest; flatulence.

Headache 9 A.M., preceded by gagging and faint feeling; pain all over head, better at first from pressure; no better after dinner or siesta, but suddenly leaves at 8 P.M. Dr. V., *1m*.

25. Headache at 10 A.M. M., *10m*.

Eevery afternoon, after menses, headache. F., *30th*.

Headache better after breakfast; worse after dinner. Dr. S.,

External Head.

Rheumatic drawing up left side of occiput into the forehead. *50m*.

Very severe pains in the temples nearly all the morning. Dr. S., *cm*.

Sight, Eyes.

30. Mist before the eyes; halo around the gaslight; eyes feel sore, weak. Dr. S., *cm*.

On rising, 5 A.M. flickering of sight in left eyes. A., *10m*.

Dim sight, as from a veil over eyes, with dull, heavy headache. P., *30th*.

Quivering of right eyelid while reading, before sleep, and on awaking. Dr. Hn., *30th*.

On using the eyes, dull, aching pain in the orbit above the ball; eyelids feel sore, itch, and burn. Dr. S., *cm*.

35. Eyes feel sore when reading in evening. M., *10m*.

Eyes as if bathed in hot water; drowsy. M., *50m*.

Eyes bloodshot, M., *10m*.; feel as if sand was in them, mostly the left eyes. M., *50m*.

Burning lachrymation; drowsy, 10 A.M. M., *50m*.

Inner canthus of right eye feels sore, he wants to rub it; slightly injected. Dr. S., *cm*.

40. Aching in right eyeball. M., *1m*.

Dryness of left eyeball, with pain in same as if bruised. Dr. K., *1m., 10m*.

Scrofulous ophthalmia. Schussler.

Lids feel heavy and itch along the margins; pain over the eyes. Dr. S., *cm*.

Hearing, Ears.

Tickling from middle ear into the Eustachian tube. J., *10m*.
45. Whille lying down, sensation as of water dropping from a height into a long, narrow vessel. M., *tm*.

Lobe of right ear burns and itches so intolerably he has to scratch until it bleeds; face burns; joints itch. M., *50m*.

Smelling, Nose.

Offensive odor before the nose in the morning, two days. Dr. D., *cm*.

Slight epistaxis in the morning; irritable. Dr. D., *10m*.

Tough, clear-white phlegm from posterior nares. J., *10m*.

A PROVING OF NATRUM PHOSPHORICUM

50. Dropping of thick, yellow mucus from the posterior nares; worse at night; awakens him, he must sit up to clear his throat. J., *1m, 10m.*

Left nostril stopped up; accumulation of mucus in the throat. J., *1m.*

Left nostril stopped up; worse in open air. M., *50m.*

Left nostril sore, painful; picks it continually; scabs form. Dr. S., *70m, cm.*

Itching of the nose. A., *10m.*

Teeth, Gums.

55. Teeth in the morning and mouth all day covered with a brownish mucus. J., *10m.*

Taste, Talking, Tongue.

Coppery taste, 5 A.M. A., *10m.*

Bad taste in the mouth, morning, on awaking; gastric symptoms. Dr. D., *cm.*

Tries to say a word, but it will not come out; feels as if something closed in the throat, preventing speech. J., *10m.*

Sensation of hairs on the tip of the tongue, followed by prickling numbness of whole mouth, next day a small pimple. P., *2c.*

60. Tongue coated dirty-white with a dark-brown centre. Dr. D., *cm.*

Blisters on tip of tongue. M., *10m.*

Palate, Throat.

Sensation as of a pin pricking the right side of the throat; worse swallowing liquids; better from solids. Dr. S., *70m.*

Accumulation of mucus in the throat, causing hawking, afternoons; this causes a tickling and slight cough. Dr. D., *cm.*

Right side of throat sore. Dr. S., *cm.*

Desires, Aversions.

65. Desires strong-tasting things, even alcohol. Dr. Hn., *30.*

Desires strong-tasting things. J., *1m.*

Desire for beer; it relieves the goneness. M., *50m.*

Desire for fried eggs, J., *1m.*; for eggs, M., *50m.*

Aversion to bread and butter, yet formerly fond thereof; very persistent for weeks. Dr. D., *10m., cm.*

70. Not very hungry for meals, yet enjoys them; most appetite for supper. Dr. D., *cm*.

No desire for food; sick, gone feeling. Dr. S., *cm*.

Eating, Drinking.

Before breakfast; pressure from spine to stomach, A., *10m.;* headache better. Dr. S., *cm*.

After breakfast; nervous, went to bed again. Dr. S., *cm*.

Before dinner: 11 to 12 o'clock, sick feeling, nervous; empty, gone feeling; pulse quick, jerking. Dr. S., *cm*.

75. After eating a little, feels full. M., *50m*.

After dinner, headache. Dr. S., *cm*.

Fulness in the stomach all the time, but worse after eating. Dr. D., *cm*.

Sensation of heaviness in the epigastrium, better after eating. P., *30th*.

Feels weak and cross after dinner, would like to lie down, Dr. D., *cm.;* empty feeling in the chest and abdomen, M., *1m.;* empty, gone feeling all day, but worse after eating, Dr. S., *cm*.

Eructations, Nausea.

80. Eructations after eating. M., *1m*.

Eructations frequent, tasteless. *10m, 50m*.

Stomach.

Heavy feeling in the stomach, causing a restless feeling; third day after tea. A., *10m*.

Constant feeling of fulness. Dr. D., *cm*.

Awakens, 2 A.M., with pressure in the stomach; feels as if a stick was pressing up and forward from about the last dorsal vertebra into the stomach. A., *10m*.

Goneness in the stomach and abdomen, even in the chest. M., *1m, 10m, 50m, cm;* H., *10m*. See also symptom by Dr. S.; goneness at 4 P.M., M.

85. Goneness in stomach and abdomen, with a feeling of weight above the ensiform. See Chest and Arms. M., *50m.;* H., *10m*.

Abdomen.

Anxiety felt through the abdomen, lasting only a few moments. Dr. K., *1m*.

A PROVING OF NATRUM PHOSPHORICUM

Bloated feeling, worse evening; wind in the bowels; must loosen the clothing; urging to stool. Dr. S., *cm*.

Pain in the bowels ascends to the stomach; flatulence; at the same time return of pain in left orbit.

Goneness. See 85.

90 Colic, as from wind pressing on the bladder, causing frequent micturition; urging to stool. M., *50m, cm*.

Rectum, Stool.

Distressing, burning, contracting pain in anus and lowest part of rectum; feels it after awaking from a troubled dream. Dr. D., *cm*.

Diarrhœa, colicky pains before morning. M., *50m*.

Three or four diarrhœic stools a day, with much flatus; crampy pains in stomach and abdomen; is afraid to pass flatus lest fæces escape also. Dr. D., *cm*.

One day costive, next day diarrhœa. M., *50m*.

95 Costive. M., *1m, 10m;* Dr. D., *10m, cm*.

Urging to stool two evenings, 8 P.M. in succession. M., *10m, cm*.

While at stool, sensation as if a marble dropped in left abdomen (descending colon) two evenings, 8 P.M. M., *10m*.

Itching of the anus. Soreness. M., *50m*.

Urging to stool; feels often as if bowels would move, but they do not.

100 Itching about the anus.

Kidneys, Urine.

Fine stitching pains in left renal region. Dr. D., *cm*.

Urine dark-red; no sediment. *1m*.

Constant urging. M., *10m*.

Burning during urination; urine apparently normal. M., *50m*.

105 Obliged to urinate, but pressure not thereby relieved. A., *10m*.

Frequent micturition, *90m, cm;* Dr. S., *cm*.

Male Parts.

Sexual desire, but no erections. *1m;* later, total absence of desire. M., *10m*.

Great sexual excitement. Dr. S., *70m*.

Sexual desire diminished; drawing in the right spermatic cord. M., *50m*.

110 Seminal emissions without erotic dreams; two in one night. Dr. S., *cm*.

Emission of semen some hours after coitus; no dream or erection. M., *50m, cm*.

Emissions almost every night (married man); preceded by slight pains in the testicles, mostly left. M., *50m*.

Three emissions in one week; unconscious thereof until morning. J., *1m;* M., *10m*.

Emissions every night; no lascivious dreams; semen thin, watery, smells like stale urine. J., *10m*.

115 Emissions every other night. Dr. S., *cm*.

After coitus, burning and itching at meatus urinarius; urging to stools, and urine; bowels loose; stools small. M., *50m*.

After emissions, melancholy; pain through right groin next day. M., *50m*. For weeks dull drawing in testicle and cord. M., *cm*.

Pains in left spermatic cord. M., *cm*.

Pain in left testicle and about the chin. M., *cm*.

120 Itching of the prepuce. Dr. D., *cm*.

Female Parts.

Great and unusual excitement; not able to get to sleep until near 1 A.M.; awoke at 5 unrested. A., *10m*.

Three nights later sexual dreams; thinks she is with her husband, but the act is prevented by the unbidden entrance of some stranger. A., *10m*.

Menses five days too early. A., *10m*.

Menses five days too early (always regular before); feet icy cold by day, burn at night in bed; flow pale (dark in health), with pressure over right eye, and desire to take a long breath, as if room was too close. Three days later, headache over left eye; all worse 3 to 4 P.M. Fifth day, flow dark as usual.

125 After menses much worse. Trembling about the heart; worse walking upstairs; pressure in pit of stomach; better eating; headache returns every afternoon, now over one, now over other eye; sleep restless, tosses from side to side. F., *30th*.

A PROVING OF NATRUM PHOSPHORICUM 347

Next period three days too early. Same symptoms as before, but flow stopped two days and returned with headache, chilliness, restless sleep, and paralytic aching in right wrist; knees felt as if the cords were shortened. F., *30th*. (Was under treatment eighteen months before symptoms were all removed.)

Breathing.

Constant tendency to sigh; menses. F., *30th*.

Cough.

Cough after drinking water. J., *10m*.
Cough from tickling in the throat. See 63.

Inner Chest, Lungs.

130 Like a weight above the ensiform, with empty feeling in stomach and abdomen. M., *50m*.
Empty feeling in the chest and abdomen after a meal. M., *1m*.
Heaviness in epigastrium and lower third of sternum, worse going upstairs; during menses. F., *30th*.
Lower third of sternum pains as if torn in two. J., *10m*.
Sudden feeling of fulness in upper part of chest. P., *6th*, *200th*.
135 Burning deep in chest, worse right side; evening in bed. Dr. S., *cm*.
Pain from right clavicle diagonally to stomach, so intense that it made her start, followed by hoarseness. P., *6th*.
Pain through left chest and in left shoulder. Dr. S., *cm*.
Pain through chest after dinner, especially left side. Dr. S., *cm*.

Heart, Pulse.

Trembling about the heart going upstairs; after menses, F., *30th*.
140 Heart feels uneasy and pains especially about its base when pains in limbs and great toe are better. P., *6th*. (Twenty years ago had pains in toe and heart relieved with *Lycopod.;* no return until now.)
Every strange noise causes palpitation. Dr. D., *cm*.

Lying down at night, hears the heart beat as though it came from under the pillow. M., *cm.*

Feels the pulse all over the body. J., *1m.*

Pulse is felt in different parts of body, as if shot were rolling through the artery. M., *50m.*

145 Feels as if a lump or bubbles started from the heart and were forced through the arteries. J., *10m.*

Pulse quick, jerking. See 74; Dr. S., *cm.*

Outer Chest.

Intercostal muscles feel sore and as if drawn when sitting erect or moving chest, not in ordinary breathing. M., *50m.*

A spot in right chest feels bruised. P., *200th.*

Sore, pressing pain, as after a contusion, about cartilages of fourth to sixth ribs, right side; worse from deep breathing, deep pressure; later in the evening, cannot breathe deeply, or move the arms, or bend body backwards. Dr. D., *cm.*

150 Contracted feeling in walls of right chest, lasting only a few moments. Dr. D., *10m.*

Neck, Back.

Rheumatic pain in right shoulder; feels nervous. M., *50m.*

Crick in both sides of neck. M., *1m, 50m.*

On taking a deep breath, stitches to right of spine, morning. Dr. D., *10m.*

Lying in bed, 11P.M., weak feeling in small of back, most felt when lying in back, but not relieved by lying on the side; diminishes in a few minutes, and is followed by an annoying deep-seated twitching in left inguinal region. Dr. D., *cm.*

155 Pain in the articulation of the lumbar vertebræ and sacrum, left side; pressing the spot causes a pain down the thigh to knee, *10m.* Later this spot grew more painful, and the leg seemed to give way walking, as though knee was weak. J., *50m.*

Upper Limbs.

Slight drawing in the left deltoid, morning. Dr. D., *cm.*

Heaviness of the right arm. M., *50m.*

Numbness of right hand and arm. P., *200th.*

Arms (left) feel 'gone' tired. J., *10m.*

A PROVING OF NATRUM PHOSPHORICUM

160 Arms so weak she must let them drop. P., *6th.*

Synovial crepitation. P., *6th;* J., *10m;* M., *1m, 10m, 50.*

Drawing in right wrist-joint. Dr. D., *cm.*

Sudden drawing crampy pain in left wrist, at various times, extending over dorsum of hand to fingers; index finger intensely painful. Dr. D., *cm.*

Slight crampy pain in left hand, particularly index finger. Dr. D., *cm.*

165 Pain in right index finger in an old gouty joint. P., *6th.*

Deepseated pain in right wrist going to centre of palm. P., *6th.*

Sharp pain, like a needle, in middle finger of right hand. Dr. D., *cm.*

Rheumatic pains in joints of little finger, left hand. M., *50m.*

Pains darting in little finger of left hand, then in the right; worse riding. P., *6th.*

170 Pain in little finger of right hand. M., *5m, 10m.*

While writing cannot keep the hand from trembling; the pen moves further than he designs; thus he makes a 't' or a 'y' too long. J., *10m.* See also Skin.

Lower Limbs.

Sudden giving way of legs while walking, as though they would be paralysed; fears she will have typhoid fever. P., *6th, 200th.*

Unsteady gait. Hn., *10m.*

After getting up for several mornings, legs feel from knees down heavy as if paralyzed. M., *cm.*

175 On getting up after sitting awhile, knees tremble. Dr. S., *cm.*

Tired in the morning, weak feeling in the legs seemingly relieved by forcibly stretching. Dr. D., *cm.*

Slight drawing in left ischiatic nerve from foramen to middle of thigh. Dr. D., *cm.*

When walking, calves feel as if pulled tight. M., *10m.*

Muscles of left knee pain as if hamstrings were too short. M., *10m.*

180 Feeling as if cords were shortened; after menses.

Hamstrings feel stiff when he attempts to rise; he 'kicks out' to limber up. M., *cm.*

Drawing in the hamstrings of left leg while walking. J., *10m*.
Twitching in joint of left knee. Dr. D., *cm*.
Pain in left popliteal space going upstairs. P., *6th*.
185 Synovial crepitation. P., *6th*., J., *10m;* M. *1m, 10m, 50m.*
Bruised pain inside of thighs when walking upstairs. M., *10m*.
Pains about the patella. M., *cm*.
Dull aching in right thigh, very severe. M., *10m*.
Drawing in inner side of left thigh. M., *50m*.
190 Sensation as of a needle piercing the calf while walking. M., *10m*.
Right calf feels as if tightly bandaged. M., *1m*.
Pains between knees and ankles when walking fast. M., *cm*.
Slight pains about shin and left testicle. M., *cm*.
Aching along the shins while walking. P., *6th*.
195 Big toe pains. P., *6th, 200th*. When rubbing it, it prickles as if going to sleep. P., *200th*.
Right big toe pains; as this gets better pain in heart. P., *6th*.
Pain in ball of left foot. M., *cm*.
Pain in hollow of left foot, worse walking or exercising; alternates from foot to foot. M., *50m*.
Muscle pain when flexing left foot. M., *cm*.
200 Ball of left foot pains; pain in calf, worse on first rising. M., *cm*.
Pain in ball of left foot walking. M., *10m*.
Pain in hollow of right foot after going upstairs; also while riding. P., *6th*. See also Skin.

All the Limbs.

Right wrist and left ankle weak, and ache as if paralyzed; after menses.
Drawing in hands, feet, wrist-joints and left shoulder. Dr. D., *cm*.

Rest, Motion, etc.

205 Ascending: chest 132; heart, 139; hollow of foot, 202; inside of thigh, 186; pain in popliteal space, 184; heavy feeling in epigastrium, 132.
Descending: knees ache.

Walking; shins, 194; between knees and ankles pains, 192; legs give way, 172; like needle in calf, 190; calves, 178; hamstrings, 182; ball of foot pains, 201: crepitation of joints; pain in hollow of foot, 198.

Motion: crick in neck; intercostals sore; worse moving arms, 149; must move, 9.

209½ Stepping: pulsating pains in head, 21.

Stretching: relieves legs, 176.

210 Flexing: foot, muscles pain, 199.

Stooping: pain over right eye.

Standing: legs weary, tired, 216.

Sitting erect: intercostals sore, 147; falls asleep while sitting, 219.

Lie down: desire to, 79.

214½ Lying: in bed, feels pulsation all over; ears, 45; lying on back, back weak, 154; lying down at night hears heart beat, 142.

215 Rising: hamstrings, 181; stiff; knees tremble, 175; on first rising legs feel paralyzed, 174; pain in calf, 200; flickering of sight, 31.

Nerves.

Weariness of the legs while standing. M., *50m*.

General lassitude. C.Hg., Ha., M., P., Dr. S., Dr. D., H.

Languid in hot weather (hitherto indifferent to summer heat). M., *cm*.

Very tired in the afternoon, falls asleep while sitting. Dr. D., *10m, cm*.

Sleep.

220 Sleepless after 12 P.M. until 3 A.M. Dr. Hn., *30th*.

Cannot get to sleep; feels so hot; thoughts crowd on his mind. Dr. D., *cm*.

Restless sleep during and after menses. F., *30th*.

Restless sleep all through the proving. Dr. Hn., *30th*.

Could not get to sleep until 4 A.M.; then had a tiresome sleep until 5 A.M. A., *10m*.

225 Drowsy all day, mostly forenoon. M., *1m*.

Drowsy afternoons, must lie down; after dinner, so sleepy can hardly keep his eyes open; tired, weary, not disposed to do anything. Dr. D., *cm*.

Sleepy from 3 P.M. until bed time, then sleepless from thoughts; finally on going to sleep, dreamed of these thoughts. Dr. Hn., *30th.*

Sits up in bed, seizes the sheet, and folds it precisely along the hems. M., *50m.*

Wide awake from the least noise. Dr. D., *cm.*

230 Awakens after 12 P.M.; soon after, a sensation as from an electric shock through the body, trembling and palpitation as from fright. Dr. D., *cm.*

Awakens in the night and imagines pieces of furniture are persons. M., *50m.*

Awakens, fears his child, who has a trifling ailment, is dead; he goes to her room to relieve the otherwise ineffaceable impression (never nervous before in sickness). M., *50m.*

Dreams of sexual excitement.

Troublesome dreams. A., *10m.*

235 Vexing dreams. Dr. H., *1m;* J., *50m.*

Dreams of the dead; tired on awakening. Dr. D., *cm.*

Times of the Day.

Night; easily startled, 11; mucus from post. nares, 50; emissions, 110, 111, 112, 113, 114, 115; feet burn, 124; hears heart, 142; imagines furniture people, 231.

After 12 P.M., 2 A.M. pressure in stomach, 83; cannot sleep until 1 A.M., 121; sleepless, 220; awakens, 230.

Morning; dizzy, 12; temples, 29; on rising, 5 A.M., flickering of sight, 31; offensive odor before nose, 47; epistaxis, 48; mucus on teeth, 55; coppery taste, 56; bad taste, 57; diarrhœa, 92; awoke, 5 A.M. unrested, 121; stitches rear of spine, 153; legs feel weak, 173, 176; drawing in deltoid. 156.

9 A.M. headache, 24.

240 10 A.M. headache, 25; drowsy, lachrymation, 38; 11 to 12 A.M., sick, nervous, gone feeling, etc., 74.

Fore-noon, ill-humour, 7; drowsy, 225.

Afternoon: heavy head, flushes, 19; headache, 26; hawking, 63; tired, 219, 226; sleepy, 227; flushes of heat, 251

4 P.M. goneness, 84.

5 P.M. pain in temple; better.

A PROVING OF NATRUM PHOSPHORICUM 353

Evening: gloomy, 3; inclined to study, 7; eyes sore, 35; bloated, 87; pressing, sore pain in chest, 149; 11 P.M., weak feeling in back, 154; flushes, sweat, 252; itching of skin.
8 P.M. headache suddenly leaves, 24; urging to stool, 97.

Warmth and Cold.

Feels warm weather more than usual.
245 Nervousness, goneness at the stomach, headache, crick in the neck, worse in a thunderstorm. M., *50m.*
Desire to take a long breath, as if room was too close; menses.
Worse in open air; left nostril stopped up, 52.

Chill, Fever, Sweat.

Chilly, felt mostly in the chest. *1m.*
Chill, followed by hot flushes around the body. Dr. H., *1m.*
250 Feet icy cold, but burn at night, menses.
Flushes of heat and sweat; evening. M., *10m.*
Flushes every afternoon, headache in a lady who, though 50, never had them before. P., *30th.*

Sides.

Right: temple, 15; pressure over eye, 17; lid quivers, 32; inner canthus sore, 39; eyeball aches, 40; lobe of ear itches, 46; pricking throat, 62; throat sore, 64; drawing in cord, 109; pain through groin, 117; burning in chest, 135; clavicle to stomach, 136; bruised spot in chest, 148, 149; walls of chest feel contracted, 150; shoulder pains, 151; stitches to rear of spine, 153; heaviness in arm, 157; hand numb, 158; drawing in wrist-joint, 162; index finger, 165; wrist to centre of hand, 165; like needle in index finger, 167; pain in little finger, 170; dull aching in thigh, 188; calf feels as if bandaged, 191; big toe, 196; hollow of foot, 202; right wrist, left ankle, 203.

Left: Headache, 14; temple, 15; tearing in head, 16; pinching in temple, 18; centre eyebrow, 22; orbit, 23; drawing up the occiput, 28; flickering in eye, 31; like sand in eye, 37; eyeball dry, 41; nostril stopped up, sore, 51, 52, 53; like a marble in left side of abdomen while at stool, 98; stitches in renal region, 101; pain in testicle, 112; in cord, 118; in testicle and shin, 119; in chest and shoulder, 137, 138; deep twitches in inguinal region, 154; soreness about sacrum, etc., 155; drawing in deltoid, 156; arms, especially left, feel 'gone', 159; drawing, crampy pain in wrist, 163; crampy pain in hand, 164; pains in joints of little finger, 168; drawing in ischiatic nerve, 177; hamstrings short, 179, 182; twitching in knee, 183; pain in popliteal space, 184; drawing in inner side of thigh, 189; ball of foot,, 197; hollow of foot, 198; muscles pain, flexing left foot, 188; ball of foot, 200, 201; drawing in hands, feet, left shoulder, 204; itching pimples, 265.

255 Right—Left: temples, 15; pressure over eyes, 17.

Left—Right: Darting in little finger of left, then of right hand, 169.

Worse from touch, rubbing, etc.: Big toe prickles when rubbed, 195; must loosen clothing, 87.

Pressure relieves: Head at first, 24; want to rub eye, 39.

Riding: Headache, pains in right foot, knee, left hand.

Skin.

260 Intense itching of the face, especially of the nose, also spots on body and limbs, etc.; feel like insect-bites; she wants to tear the flesh. A., *10m.*

After going to bed, itching here and there, and lumps similar to hives raise up; scratching relieves itching, but is followed by burning; could not sleep. Dr. S., *cm.*

Itching of the skin, particularly lumbar region and hips; rubbing causes an eruption of papules about the size of lentils and of the colour of the skin. Dr. D., *cm.*

Itching about the joints, elbows, knees; at the same time, itching of right external ear; vesicles form. M., *50m.*

Small, round, reddish papules about the tendo-Achillis and, later on, lower limbs, mostly in bend of joints, itching terribly. Dr. D., *cm.*

265 Pimples on left leg itching, burning; loss of appetite. Dr. S., *cm.*

Burning, stinging lump, like hives, on the second joint of ring finger. J., *10m.*

Itching about mouth and neck all through the proving. J., *10m.*

Itching about mouth, neck; vesicles form; pimples like nettle-rash. M., *50m.*

Itching of prepuce; of arms; of coccyx. M., *50m.*

Other Drugs.

270 Apis removed hives.

Sepia aggravated, but finally relieved, eruption about joints.

SALICYLIC ACID

(Additional Proving)

(On the 15th of June I began a proving with *Salicylic Acid*. Not venturing to expose myself to any very serious action of the drug, having had a sufficiently troublesome experience of its power in the 10th potency, I only took a small part of a drop of the 30th, repeating the dose four times at intervals of about two hours. Here are the results which I observed for twenty-five days after, when I started on a vacation trip, from which I did not return until Friday, July 22.)

Proving.

First day: 2-30 P.M.—About fifteen minutes after the first dose, a burning and scratchy feeling on the tongue. Drawing pain in the calf of the left leg, extending up into the thigh, and then transferred to the left arm. Later, a similar pain for a short time back of the right temple.

4-30 P.M.—Nervous excitement after gentle exercise or walking.

6-30 P.M.—Pain in the knuckles of the right hand.

6-45 P.M.—Third dose.

8-45 P.M.—Fourth dose. During the night, pain on the top of the head, in one spot, as if struck by a hammer.

Second day.—Swelling under the skin of fingers on both hands; with a burning itching on the inside of the left hand. Itching on the back, below the jaw bones, and under the chin. The rheumatic pains feel worse when walking outdoors.

Third day.—After a good night's rest, awake dull and nervous, with a ringing in the ears, especially the left, and a fulness in the head. Dizziness. Pain in the bones below the left eye, as if bruised. Rheumatic pains in the upper and lower extremities continue. Nervous headache characterized by a bruised feeling in the head (not aggravated by exposure to a very hot sun). General lassitude and weakness, worse indoors, relieved in the open air. Stoppage of the ears, especially of the left. Much sexual excitement

Fourth day.—Dull headache on the left side of the head. Feel very uncomfortable and indisposed to any exertion, mental or physical. Difficulty in voiding urine—it flows slowly and seems less in quantity. Pain in the sinews of the left forearm, extending into the third and little fingers, followed by a tingling sensation. Pain in the left inferior maxilliary bone; the parotid gland is painful when touched by the finger, affecting the inside of the throat. Burning pain inside the joint of the thumb. Scratching sensation in the left side of the throat. After lying down in the afternoon stiffness and aching in the muscles of the back along the spinal column. The morning headache, better during the day, is aggravated in the evening. Palpitation of the heart. During the night following an unconscious, profuse and somewhat bloody discharge of semen (or prostatic fluid) staining the linen a brownish colour, and followed on awaking, by a pain in the genitals, as if overstrained.

Fifth day.—Headache, continuing during the night, better in the morning. Tedious and insufficient stool. Headache returns in the afternoon on the right side. Pressive pain in the forehead, above the right eye. Itching of the left upper eyelid. Itching of the skin after undressing; better in bed. Sexual excitement, more physical than mental. Very restless at night, longing to sleep, with inability to do so.

Sixth day.—During the night, rheumatic pains in the lower limbs and feet. A kind of burning sensation in the ball of the great toe. On awaking in the morning, pain in the right shoulder, as if from a strain, continuing some hours. Still some headache with a dull, bruised feeling in the right side of the head. During the day all symptoms disappear, returning again in the evening. Itching of the head, with feeling as if the hair stood on end.

Seventh day.—Awake during the night, with stiffness in the back, so as only to be able to turn with difficulty. Severe pressing pain in the lower abdomen and bladder, without urging to urinate, and only small discharge. In the morning, stoppage of the ears returns. In the afternoon a sharp, stinging pain in one of the toes of the right foot. In the evening, sore feeling on both sides of the lower jaw, under the tongue.

Nineth day.—The rheumatic pains and headaches have disappeared. Itching pimples here and there on the body; one on the right cheek.

Tenth day.—The eruption continues. After removing some ear wax from the left ear, pain and feeling of stoppage.

Eleventh day.—Stoppage in both ears, early in bed and after rising. Eruption continues, red pimples here and there; and small whitish ones, the latter in groups, itching and filled with water. In the evening, feeling as if I had taken a long walk.

Twelfth day.—Pain in the groin, as if from a strain, on the right side. Constriction in the anus shortly after stool. Much flatulence in the evening. Hacking cough, with scratching in the throat and hawking up small pieces of thick, yellow phlegm, with occasional sneezing and discharge from the nose. Boring pain in the left eyebrow, the place tender when pressed. Pain above the left ear.

Thirteenth day.—Much difficulty in voiding urine in the morning on rising. Itching in the anus, and ineffectual attempt at stool. Six hours after, slimy, insufficient stool. When coughing pain in the groin. Pain in the muscles of the middle of the back, with stiffness. Much itching, especially over the breast and stomach. Burning and feeling of dryness in the eyes. Aching in the left collar bone.

Fourteenth day.—No special new symptoms noted, except stoppage of the ears when walking out, relieved by drawing breath strongly through the nostrils, yet almost instantly returning. Sexual excitement. (Coition about once in two months.)

Fifteenth day.—During the night, again amorous dream, with bloody emission, followed by erections in the morning. Dull feeling in the head and oppression on the chest. Sometimes after moderate physical exertion, palpitation of the heart, with intermittent pulse. Pulse continues somewhat higher than the regular beat (62) running up to 74.

Sixteenth day.—As for several days past, much audible rumbling in the bowles, and a feeling of dryness, with itching in the nostrils.

Seventeenth day.—During the night much voluptous itching of the skin. On scratching, a pimple appears in the place; the itching is relieved by scratching, with, sometimes, a burning of the skin after it. Soreness at the right corner of the mouth. Eruption between the fingers of the right hand; little watery pustules that itch violently.

Eighteenth day.—A.M.: Bitter taste in the mouth, with tenacious saliva, hawked up with difficulty. Dull feeling in head and general oppression. After mental labor and nervous excitement, great nervous prostration. On lying down to rest, cough as if occasioned by flow of mucus from the Eustachian tube into the throat, which causes a scratchy feeling. A nervous headache seems imminent, but does not come.

Nineteenth day.—After having eaten some salad at dinner, suffer from weight and oppression of the stomach for several hours (could formerly eat salad without inconvenience). The cough seems to return every afternoon from 3 to 5 o'clock. In the evening, pain and discomfort in the bowels, aggravated by pressure. Flatulence, with inability to expel it. Itching and burning in the inner corners of the eyes.

Twentieth day.—Free from pains all day, but gloomy and depressed; don't know what to begin. General lassitude; feeling as if I had walked a long distance. Not much itching of the skin during the day; the eye symptoms return in the evening, with severe itching on the toes of the right foot.

SALICYLIC ACID (ADDITIONAL PROVING)

Twenty-first day.—Group of little itching vesicles on the little finger of the left hand. Bloated feeling in the bowels towards noon.

Twenty-second day.—Continuance of eruptions.

Twenty-third day.—Eruption worst on the left arm, from the wrist to the elbow joint and above; single small itching pustules; the skin becomes rough when scratched. Catarrhal symptoms continue. A burning sensation in the throat after a very plain supper.

Twenty-fifth day.—The eruption has disappeared. No other special symptoms except fits of frequent yawning several evenings in succession.

REMARKS:—The proving seems to have established the fact that *Salicylic Acid* is a powerful antiseptic. A lady of my acquaintance after I had given it to her for bad nervous headaches a year or two ago, and had derived considerable benefit by taking it persistently for several weeks, became affected with an eruption of the skin. I have also read that its external application to ulcers and sores has proved beneficial, and that it has been successfully used in inflammation, if not ulceration of the breasts. Near the close of my first proving with the 10th, I had several pustules on my face and head, but took no particular notice of them; it requires a higher potency, I think, to bring out the psoric symptoms. Probably provings of a lower potency than the 5th would develop little or nothing—as in the case with *Natrum Mur.* and other drugs. *Salicylic Acid* is freely used in many parts of the country as a preservative for fruits and vegetables without cooking or boiling and it is claimed that no injurious effects result.

LAC CANINUM.

(Additional Proving)

I gave *Lac Caninum* 10m (Swan), four doses daily for three or four weeks, to a lady of 25 years of age, in excellent health, except that she had never mensturated.

October 19.—Dizzy, nausea, as after rich food; worse after standing, must sit down; feels as if she would fall if she closed her eyes.

October 26.—The same nausea. In stomach feeling as if something pushing up.

November 6.—Acute pain across over eyes and bridge of nose. Cannot clear the head, nose stuffed. Soreness from nose through into throat. Feeling of a lump in throat, which goes down when swallowing, but returns; throat worse right side, worse on swallowing saliva. Tired, totters when walking.

From Nov. 8th until Jan. 5th suffered from the following. They were so evident to her that she came into my office crying, fearing she was contracting consumption. I give them in their order of appearance:

Clavicles sore to touch. Feels as if she wanted to fix shoulders so it would not feel strained. Pain and stiffness up right sternocleido-mastoideus. Throat, which had been getting well, suddenly one evening grew rapidly worse, but this time on the left side. Soreness from right clavicle down to third and fourth ribs, worse on moving, less on left side. Fears consumption. Soreness through chest to back. Cramped feeling in chest, wants to stretch up and back. Lungs feel as if fastened to chest, worse while writing. Right clavicle feels as if out of place, worse by moving shoulder. Pains down right arm and in fingers, which feel cramped. Does not seem to have the same power in right hand. Sore across mid-chest during forced expiration; feels just as if she had been struck. Veins in hands look bluer than usual; they are swollen. Every scratch gets sore. Sore spot just to right of mid-sternum, worse from lifting or from pressure. Right cheek burns like fire and is red after coming in from the cold. (She remarked: "If this was the cold alone, why wasn't my left cheek red?")

PROVINGS OF LINARIA VULGARIS.

PROVER No. 1.—Took a dose of the 1x alcoholic dilution at 8 o'clock, P.M.

At 12 P.M., had colicky pains in abdomen over region of bladder, with a desire to urinate; these pains lasted about fifteen minutes, then passed away a few minutes after urinating. The urine passed was highly coloured and normal in quantity (not accustomed to pass urine at this time of the night. Have done nothing to account for high colour of urine).

At 8 A.M., of the following day, after second dose of remedy has been taken I have sharp pains running from elbow to wrist, and from knee to ankle on left side, while at rest.

Second day.—Violent itching between toes, compelling me to take off shoe and rub them (on right foot). Better from rubbing.

Sensation as if stick was crosswise in throat. Dry sensation in pharynx.

Fourth day.—Shortly after dinner, slight chill running up back.

Sixth day.—Tickling and severe irritation in urethra, awaking me out of sleep in morning between 2 and 3 o'clock.

PROVER No. 2.—About fifteen minutes after taking medicine, have dry sensation around glottis and posterior nares, compelling me to swallow frequently. The parts looked inflamed, epiglottis felt dry and stiff, compelling me to swallow to keep it moist.

Frequent passages of urine, which is highly coloured and very profuse.

Distressed feeling in lower part of abdomen.

Third day.—Slight aching pain down in line of ureters on left side. I could not tell whether this pain went into testicle or penis, or terminated at base of bladder, as there was a general aching feeling with which the pain seemed to mingle.

Fourth day.—I took a dose of medicine last night. Had no symptoms other than frequent urination, which seems to be constant—with emissions of urine at night, until 12-45 P.M.

About twenty minutes after eating and a walk of four squares to office, I was suddenly attacked with violent palpitation of the heart. Pale face, oppressed breathing, every artery in the body seemed to pulsate. Pulse could not be counted. Could not take a deep inspiration. No pain of any kind. I never felt like this before. Pulse increased, and I grew faint. The doctor who was with me, becoming alarmed, gave me a dose of *Verat. V*

I took no more notes after this for about four weeks. When I again took a dose of *Linaria*, I obtained the following symptoms:

Frequent passages of fetid flatus. Heavy distressed feeling in lower abdomen. Slight tickling sensation in urethra, which did not last long.

Third day.—Stitches in region of fourth costal cartilage on right side, later on left side. Frequent and copious emissions of urine.

Being afraid of reproducing those heart symptoms, which I so much dreaded, I suspended my proving.

SUPPOSED POISONING BY TOAD STOOLS.

(Agaricus Muscarius)

Mr. S. —— dined on beefsteak and stewed mushrooms. Felt a heaviness in abdomen, as if dinner had not been digested. Retired at 12 p.m., sleep restless. In morning, on rising, a diarrhœa, sudden, followed by retching and vomiting; desire to lie down with *an aching along the spine, from head to coccyx, the pain extending into the thighs.* Head felt dull, no desire to read, or talk, or move; felt sleepy; *eyes burn like fire;* the whole body *gave one convulsive twitch;* mouth dry, but no thirst; feels an unconquerable anxiety; dreads a fit of sickness, body now *aches all over, as if tired;* can't find an easy position to lie in.

Puls. 30, was given in water, every half hour, as an antidote.

Tired feeling disappeared within one hour; pains moved from back into legs; patient very nervous; burning in eyes continued.

The next morning all well, except a feeling of goneness, which did not disappear even after eating. Next day, felt as usual.

Agaricus Musc. 2c, given to a patient, caused the *same aching along spine and in limbs* as described above.

The patient was not a new one, and never exhibited such symptoms before.

IS LAUGHING GAS INJURIOUS ?

(NITROUS OXIDE)

About a year ago, a coloured woman, long under treatment for a scrofulous disease of the glands and skin, had several teeth extracted while under the influence of *Nitrous Oxide Gas.* Although she had never before shown any hysterical or spinal symptoms, yet new symptoms followed alarming in their nature, and refusing to yield to treatment for two months. Recently she again had teeth extracted under the gas, and the same symptoms returned, thus conclusively showing that they were caused by the *Nitrous Oxide,* for they commenced to appear *before* the teeth were extracted; hence they were not the result of the shock. *Nitrous Oxide* bears the same relation to Nitrogen, that the *Ethers* do to their respective radicals, and may be complementary to the aromatics among which I searched for an antidote. The symptoms in both attacks were precisely the same:

Became so violent in dentist's chair could hardly hold her. Headache and aching along spine as if they were asleep. Spells of semi-unconsciousness, preceded by a numb feeling in head, spreading thence over the body. She falls *backwards* to the ground. If she can get to the open air, the spells are postponed, but are all the harder when they do come .When busy at her work they will not appear, but as soon as she goes to bed, or sits down unoccupied, she is at once attacked. Between the paroxysms she has coldness of feet and legs to the knees; pressure in the epigastrium; begged me to give her something to kill her or else to make her better; mouth and head feel numb as though asleep; fever every afternoon from 3 to 6. Drawing in neck as though skin were contracted or cords shortened. All during the spells she is partially conscious, knows she is sick, but cannot help herself like one in nightmare; afterwards her whole body throbs. *Tinct. of Camphor* 3 drops, in a half tumbler of water, two doses to be taken one hour apart. Slept well; next day symptoms almost gone. *Camph. 200* was left to be taken in case of a return.

RHUS POISONING.

J. J., poisoned in the woods, by *Rhus Tox.* Left eyelid swollen, dark red, œdematous; exuded pus of a yellowish-white colour, from the tarsal margins. Right forearm covered on its anterior surface with minute vesicles, burning and stinging. They were preceded in their spreading up the arm by a plain line of inflammation. Gave *Croton Tiglium 30.* The next day the right eye became involved. On the third day the right eye was again well, the left improving. The eruption ceased to spread, and blisters half an inch long, appeared on the fingers, which, bursting, discharged a yellowish-white serum, and then rapidly healed. On the fifth day the eyes were both open, and a yellowish-brown scab had formed on the arm. On the seventh day the eyes were perfectly well, with no photophobia, and the cuticle on the right arm and fingers were peeling off.

I reported in the Journal, the above case of *Rhus poisoning* for which *Croton Tiglium 30,* was given, and the question was asked did the *Croton* antidote, or did it run its course?

Since then the same medicine antidoted an almost identical case of *Rhus* poisoning in shorter time than the case before reported, the potency here used being the *200th.* Hence I answer my own query, *Croton* did cure both cases, and hence is an antidote to *Rhus* poisoning.

MERC. IOD AND MERC. BINIOD.

WHEN DOCTORS DISAGREE, WHO SHALL DECIDE?

WHEN Dr. A. says that the *Iodides of Mercury* are not useful in diphtheria and Dr. B. declares that they are, who shall decide? Our impartial tribunal is the Organon.

Looking at the provings we find: "Pricking in the throat; mucous patches on tonsils easily detached; superficial ulcers; sense of a lump in throat, with hawking; much mucus collects, he is continually hawking; tonsils swollen; mucus through posterior nares into throat; nose and throat dry and feel closed up: septum naris sore and swollen; tired, weary feeling in limbs."

Clinical study has determined the following characteristics:—

MERC. IOD.

Tongue yellow with tip and edges clear and red; coppery smell from the mouth; must swallow from a constant sensation as of a lump in the throat; worse from empty deglutition; glands engorged, salivary and cervical; much painful hawking of stringy mucus; fetid discharge from fauces and nares.

MERC. BINIOD.

Must swallow from a collection of saliva or mucus or from feeling of a lump in the throat; sometimes livid, purplish patches; discharge thin, offensive; hawking up mucus, white and tough.

Thus exhibited we need never fear to give either remedy notwithstanding the fact that it does not cause such debility as we usually find in true diphtheria. The

Iodides correspond more to the early stages. When, with patches on the left tonsil and engorged glands the *Biniodide* will often check the whole disease. If the tongue presents the well known buff-yellow back, the *Proto Iod.* will be preferable. But these preparations of *Mercury* have often been used simply because the disease is diphtheria and not because of any individual similarity. Why have such cases so frequently ended favourably in open contradiction to the precepts of the Organon?

Possibly Œrtel may help us to an answer. According to his investigations, the method of treatment, which will favour suppuration, will be successful, because it will form a layer beneath the diphtheritic membrane which is practically impenetrable. Through it the cryptogamic fungi cannot pass. Now whoever has given *Merc. Iod.* must have noticed how readily a muco-purulent expectoration is formed, as annoying to the patient, as it is fortunate for the empiricist.

But to return to homœopathy. When after the administration of *Merc. Iod.* the expectoration becomes thicker, more stringy and yellow, we must at once change to *Kali Bich.;* for the mucous membrane is becoming more involved and a croupous formation is imminent. In some instances, it is difficult to distinguish from *Lachesis,* because both *Mercur. Iod.* and *Lachesis* have aggravation from empty swallowing, and after sleep; and extreme tenderness of the neck. The *Mercury.,* however, lacks the superficial sensitiveness to light, touch, or pressure of clothing, and also the sudden constriction of the throat, which seems to threaten suffocation. And too extreme prostration and cardiac debility are the peculiar property of the snake poison.

A SYNOPSIS OF QUILLAYA SAPONARIA.

THE California physicians have, for some time past, used a new drug, called *Quillaya Saponaria.* It has gained quite a reputation through the West as a certain remedy in common colds and in influenza.

As a seperate plant it has never, so far as I know, been proved. But its alkaloid, *Saponin,* has received a thorough examination by Dr. Hills, of New York.

The QUILLAYA is a genus of plant belonging to the order Rosaceæ. The bark of some of the species, notably of the *Quillaya Saponaria,* is used in South America, and quite generally, too, among the Spaniards, Mexicans, etc., in California, as a substitute for soap. Its saponaceous qualities are due to the Saponin, contained in the bark.

Dr. William Bœricke, who for eight years had charge of the San Francisco Pharmacy, informs me that he has had frequent calls for the tincture of the *Quillaya,* and that several physicians have pronounced it an invaluable drug in the beginning of coryza and sorethroat. He adds his personal experience also in its favour. It is claimed to cure when there are sneezing, stuffed feeling in the nose, soreness and rawness in the throat, aching all over the body, chilliness, etc.

Now, in the absence of proving of the individual plant itself, our next best thing is to examine into the produced symptoms of the *Saponin.*

Allen, vol. viii, tells us that *Saponin* is a 'glucoside, the active principle of many plants belonging to the Caryophyllaceæ, Polygalaceæ, etc.; principally obtained from *Saponaria Officinalis, Gypsophila, Struthium, Polygala, Senega,* and *Quillaya.*'

From the symptoms collated in his Encyclopædia, I glean the following:

Frontal catarrhal headache; sneezing; cannot breathe through the right nostril; dull pain at the root of the nose, and at the temples; tongue yellow-white on the back, edges red and papillæ elevated; hard palate rough when touched with the tongue, the papillæ are raised. Tenacious mucus from the posterior nares; throat raw, scraped, sore, with feeling of constriction on swallowing. Tonsils swollen, bright red. Cough at every forced inspiration through the nose. Muscles ache, feel weak, as after great exertion; numbness; tingling especially of fingers and soles of feet; chilly, feel faint; feel as if covered with cold stockings; head hot, skin dry. Diarrhœa, painless but urgent, 4 P.M.

In the New York State Transactions, 1875, Dr. Hills records that *Saponin,* when locally applied to the heart, retards its action, like *Digitalis.* When applied to muscles, it paralyzes them. Given in appreciable doses to act, it caused dysphagia, rattling of mucus in the larynx, flow of saliva, loose cough, clay-colored but formed stools or green and offensive; stupidity and inclination to keep quiet. Death is said to result from paralysis of respiratory centres, of cardiac nerves, and of the muscles.

It has been used accordingly for local anæsthesia, consistently with its recorded symptoms of formication, numbness, etc.

The depressing effects of the drug account for the general feeling of muscular soreness and want of energy, and remind us of *Gelsemium,* which, too, is indispensable in catarrhs, occurring in spring and summer,, when the heat so depresses both the muscular and nervous systems. It would seem, then, that the *Quillaya* ought to relieve colds, which are produced by a damp, relaxing atmosphere, such as is common enough in our latitude, from May to mid June, and from mid August to far into October, or even November. It exhibits quite a contrast to *Aconite, Nux Vomica, Belladonna, Cepa,* etc., but seems to concord with *Ferrum, Gelsemium, Mercurius, Ipecac., Bryonia, Carbo Veg.,* etc.

Like *Nux Vom.,* it is said to be adapted mainly to the initiament of a cold; but the *Nux* is curative when the cause of the cold is exposure to dry cold air, sitting or lying on cold stones, etc. Like *Mercurius,* there are rawness and soreness in nose and throat, and general muscular soreness; but *Mercury* suits late in catarrh, when the discharge is thick, yellow or green; or, in the beginning after exposure to wet, to damp evening air, to foggy weather, and when the discharge is watery, burning, and excoriating. There is, also, generally present fever and sweat, the latter exhausting rather than relieving the patient.

Like *Gelsemium,* the *Saponin* (*Quillaya*), cures colds contracted in warm, relaxing weather. Both have muscular languor, desire for rest and quiet, general bruised feeling, even of the eye-balls, etc. The one, however, has more a stuffed sensation in the nose.

Gelsemium, cures a fluent, excoriating coryza; and there is generally neuralgia of the face, and even of the head, with pains rising from the occiput to the forehead.

NOTES ON TARANTULA.

THE translation of *Tarantula* from the Spanish of Nunez, received so severe a criticism from Dr. S. A. Jones, that professional opinion may vary as to its efficacy. Dr. Lilienthal's kind reply must do much in its favour, and a thorough study of the provings can not but exhibit how beautifully each part harmonizes with every other; a sure test of the truth of the whole.

As a mite on the side of confirmation, I venture to subjoin the following case:

Mrs. C., aged 40, long under treatment for "Irritable Spine" and its consecutive troubles. After a fruitless trial of *Conium, Cimicifuga, Nat. Mur., Sepia,* etc. *Tarantula 30* was employed, indicated by excessive hyperæsthesia; the least excitement irritates, to be followed by ennui and sadness; slight touch along the spine provoked spasmodic pains in the chest, and indescribable distress in the cardiac region; at times the heart feels as if twisted over (spiral fibres). On the third day, there appeared an intense headache, as though thousands of needles were pricking into the brain; the body burned all over. Headache was better by rubbing the head against the pillow; she trembled so, she could hardly talk. On the following day her menses appeared without her usual suffering and a leucorrhœa of years' duration, disappeared (I can scarcely think permanently since so suddenly). The spinal and heart symptoms, however, gradually ceased, leaving no apparent structural changes. How permanent these effects will be, time only can decide.

It is worthy of remark, that *Tarantula,* besides causing cramps of the circular fibres of the heart, like *Cactus, Iodine, Kali C., Lachesis* and *Digitalis,* differs from them in producing contractions of the spiral fibres. Herein it stands almost alone. These spiral fibres end in the columnæ carneæ and hence influence the capillary muscles thus causing the murmurs spoken of in the chronic symptoms.

The symptoms of the aorta, distension, sensation as if torn or squeezed or stretched or bursting, remind one of aortitis. Dr. Bright found extreme sensitiveness of the surface, as prominent in aortal inflamation, and we find this especially over the left chest and down the left arm, in the proving of *Tarantula*.

If rheumatism is checked by putting the extremities in cold water and there follow, panting respiration, anxiety, cramps in the heart or twisting pains; pulse full, hard, frequent; and especially if the aorta feels full, tense, stretched, with stitching pains; morning and night, cold extremities, *Tarantula* may do more than *Verat. V., Lachesis* or *Belladonna*.

In regard to the relief the patient experienced from rubbing her head against the pillow, we see here expressed one of the most characteristic indications for the medicine. The termini of the nerves become so irritated, that some kind of friction is resorted to, in order to obtain relief. All through the proving, we find this irritation, varying with the part affected; "must move hands or legs; must rub head against something; must roll something between the fingers; must put fingers in mouth, etc."

The mode of "working off" over-excited nervous states, will often give us accurate indications for medicines. For example,

Belladonna drinks hastily; tears his breasts.

Verat. tears his clothes.

Bufo runs or jumps in preference to walking.

Kali-Brom., gives us, "constantly busy, tying his shoes, fumbling in his pockets, or picking threads from his clothes."

Nat. Mur., Puls., Stann., etc., seek relief in weeping.

Zinc corresponds to many serious diseases, when "fidgety-feet" is a marked symptom.

So we may hope to rise from the "simile" or "similius" to the "similimum" which, being the outgrowth of individualization, becomes forever the faithful index to successful cure.

CLINICAL CASES, ETC.

A CASE OF PUERPERAL CONVULSIONS.

MRS. —— engaged me to attend her in confinement. She anticipated some trouble as she had not conceived before for fourteen years.

At the seventh month I was hurriedly summoned to her, the messenger informing me that she had a stroke of apoplexy. I found her with suffused face, thick speech, heavy eyelids, and considerable drowsiness. She evidently had had a convulsion and not apoplexy. I gave her *Gelsemium,* and as she lived several miles from my office, left word to call in Dr. Chas. H. Smith, if she should be taken worse. I had it in mind to leave a note for the doctor, suggesting *Belladonna* if spasms should set in, as she was a stout lady, full blooded and had previously complained of a throbbing headache over the right eye. But on second thought, I concluded to leave his mind unbiased. My object in prescribing the *Gelsemium* was to endeavour to prevent spasms, rather than relieve them if they should occur. The immediate symptoms seemed to demand it. About midnight I was again called, and found my patient in convulsions. Dr. Smith, who lives but two squares from the patient, had arrived before me and very properly gave *Belladonna 40m.* The spasms began with flushing of the face, rolling up of the eyeballs, with biting of the tongue and violent jerkings of the whole body. As the convulsive symptoms subsided, the face became purple and swollen and she went off into a deep, snoring sleep. The medicine was given every half hour all night and until our visit the next forenoon. We then found her in a continued deep sleep, from which aroused she would answer mechanically, but seemed not to recognize any one. The convulsions had ceased. Three questions presented themselves to us. Shall we change the remedy, discontinue it, or repeat it? A change was absurd, for every symptom was still for *Belladonna.* Since her stupor was more profound, though the spasms had stopped, it was evident that either she was feeling the effects of her attacks or was going into a worse condition of coma. In either contingency, it would be best to suspend the remedy, so that the system might have opportunity to react in the one case, or that we might await developments, which would lead us to a new remedy if the case grew worse. She accordingly received *Sac. Lac.* At my afternoon visit I was met by the husband with the cheering words: "Doctor, she's much better, that last medicine acted like a charm!" And better she certainly was. Her face was still swollen, but had lost much of its turgid appearance, she was conscious and had passed urine freely. Improvement continued for three days. Our immediate concern, now, was what was the condition of the fœtus. No motions had been felt since the spasms. Camman's stethoscope, however, enabled us to distinctly hear the fœtal heart, which beat at the rate of about 140 per minute. Our next step was to examine into the condition of the mother's kidneys. At my request Dr. Smith analyzed the urine and found it loaded with albumen. There was œdema of the face and slight swelling of both feet and ankles.

On the evening of the third day of relief, our patient became more restless, complained of feeling sore and tired and of headache in the occipital region. *Belladonna 40m* was again resorted to. At about midnight she was seized with convulsions, which were not so intense as formerly, but lasted longer and caused a paralysis of the right arm. Subsequent convulsive efforts were confined to the left side. No other remedy was indicated; even this paralysis pointed to the *Belladonna,* so we pertinaciously continued, lengthening the intervals as the spasms diminished. Towards morning she became restless and though unconscious, complained and grunted as if in labor. The os externum was soft and dilatable, but the os internum was as firm as gristle. No attempt at artificial dilatation was made, because the pains did not seem to threaten convulsions, and above all our trusty *Belladonna* was a better and safer dilator than clumsy instruments. A meddlesome doctor is an abomination. Daylight came and with it—not the baby, but an unwelcome cessation of all pains, while the patient sank into a stupid sort of sleep, from which she could not be aroused to consciousness. What was to be done? I examined the symptoms carefully. Pulse regular, full; breathing snoring, but not stertorous; face red; pupils failed to react to light; right arm paralyzed; urine retained. Still *Belladonna;* but it was not needed so frequently as for the acute symptoms, so it was given for every two hours, and directions left to stop it entirely so soon as consciousness should return. The afternoon brought the desired relief; she recognized familiar faces, the pupils responded to light, the urine flowed freely and the patient became annoyingly aware of the condition of her right arm. In the evening she grew talkative, it was difficult to control her. Pains made her screw her face up; she said they were in her stomach and as they were followed by belching, I thought she was correct in her statement. But towards morning she began labor in earnest. Two or three vigorous pains were followed by the expulsion of a living, seven-month's child.

The little fellow was as blue as indigo and cried with a faint voice, showing that its life had well-nigh been sacrificed by the terrible disturbances in the maternal circulation. It was wrapped in cotton batting, laid on its side, fed with milk in teaspoons, hourly doses and treated with *Laurocerasus 1m,* as a corrective of its cyanotic condition.

The mother seemed to be in excellent spirits, talking so vociferously that threats were necessary to calm her. Her lame arm was still a mystery to her; for she had not been made acquainted with the character of the disease, she had passed through. She fancied she had had a chill with congestion to the head—an illusion I was very willing to leave undisputed.

The usual post-partum prescription of *Arnica* was omitted, because the labor had been too rapid and easy to need it, and also because I desired the *Belladonna* impression to continue undisturbed.

The child died of cyanosis eight hours after birth.

The mother rallied steadily, regaining the use of her right arm in two days. Milk appeared in the usual time, but was unattended with any untoward symptoms. For several days the mother had occasional diarrhœic stools composed of fæces and offensively smelling bile; but as they seemed to relieve rather than aggravate the patient, it was deemed unnecessary if not meddlesome, to interfere.

The patient is now convalescing rapidly. She has regained the use of her arm and the symptoms of albuminuria are subsiding also.

A CASE WITH COMMENTS.

An intelligent patient came to me complaining of a singular heart trouble; several experts had pronounced him free from organic disease. There were various subjective symptoms, but the most marked was "a sensation after exercise, as if the heart were loose." Physical examination showed no signs of hypertrophy or valvular lesion; but the heart muscle evidently lacked tonicity. When lying on the left side, the apex could be felt one inch to the right of a line drawn vertically from the axilla; and yet, the actual area was not over one inch and hence so far normal. Most authorities state that the heart falls to the left when lying on that side, only sufficiently to bring the apex an inch or less to the left of a line through the nipple. But here was a variation of several inches, and yet no alteration in the size of the heart. Neither did there exist any disease of any neighbouring viscus to displace the heart.

By turning on to the right side, the apex could be felt within or to the right of a line through the nipple. I inferred a relaxed condition of the pericardium and of the connective tissues, producing great mobility, such as has been described in "movable kidney" (Flint's Practice), and in other viscera. As confimatory evidence, the patient related that often the muscles of the lumbar region and also the pectoral muscles would shake so on walking, that they would greatly inconvenience him.

If we trace the morbid tract still deeper, we shall find a weakened action of the motor nerve of the spine from central nervous exhaustion; and this in turn may arise from many sources. To determine the primal cause and so trace intelligently the disease from beginning to the present state, was the next step. I have often found that such a course of examination, unrolling as it were the panorama of the past, not only gives anamnesis of pathological importance, but, also exposes many long forgotten characteristic symptoms of vital interest, in the selection of the curative remedy. Prescribing for the latest characteristics, is undoubtedly a positive key which unrolls the problem, until the cure is completed by eventually disclosing the whole picture.

This is the usual safest course, but if we can find a shorter way, we must follow it. And just here lies the advantage of pathology, physiology and the differential study of diseases. We know albumen in the urine points often to congestive kidney. We know excess of phosphates points to the nervous system. We know how ague is indexed by a swollen spleen. Thus far, we have no guide whatever as to the remedy, but we do know where to look for characteristic symptoms even though the present picture shows none of importance or of distinctive value. If we discover phosphatic urine may we not hope to find what we desire in the subjective phenomena of nervous exhaustion with its many causes, excesses, mental fatigue, emotions, etc.? If we discover a caked spleen may we not examine into suppressed ague, abuse of quinine, large doses of elixirs, not one tangible key-note? If there are well-known indications of psora, or syphilis, or sycosis, or with Grauvogl, if we suspect hydrogenoid constitution, etc., may we not review the medical and pathological histories of the case, and perhaps find therein key-notes, which unite with the latest (totality), confirm them or even supersede them in importance? Thus we find, that medical research into the nature and course of diseases, unties the gordian knot, but here it stops. The error of the day is in searching here for the remedy and not in the symptoms which this process reveals. Pathology recalls the past and points with approximate certainty to the future, but no more. Therapeutics picks out the characteristics from the revealed panorama and says, "these characterize the whole disease; find the remedy covering these and all inferior symptoms vanish." Thus we find the basis remedy, so to speak, of the case; the remedy which is to be given long and carefully, under the strict

L.24

rules of our practice. If troublesome symptoms appear, one of its analogues may act as an intercurrent remedy, as Hahnemann often employed *Arnica, Chamomilla, Aconite,* etc.

So in the case before us, my mind carried me analytically to some affection of the spine, so I inquired if his back troubled him now or ever had. His reply was that it was rather weak, for some years ago, he wrenched it trying to lift a heavy weight in a gymnasium. The present key-note was "weak, loose feeling about the heart from exertion" the first was, "a strain from mechanical cause"; the latter symptom belong to *Arnica, Bryonia, Rhus., Lyc., Calc.,* etc., etc., the former only to *Rhus,* which is thus seen to cover the whole. It was given first in the 200th, raising the potency with each prolonged aggravation after a relief, until finally the 60,000th seems to have restored the patient.

Now, even though my explanation of the case proves erroneous, the result was correct, and we may say with Darwin, who though absurd in argument is excellent in observation: "False facts are highly injurious to the progress of science * * * * but false views do little harm, as every one takes a salutary pleasure in proving their falseness"—(The Descent of Man, p. 368, Vol. II).

A POINT IN THE ETIOLOGY OF OPHTHALMIA NEONATORUM.

Three years ago, we attended a lady in confinement whose new-born baby suffered terribly from purulent inflammation of the eyes. The cause was, we presumed, a purulent leucorrhœa with which the mother was affected, and the existence of which we were not informed of until after her labor.

A few weeks ago it again fell to our lot to attend the same patient in confinement. Labor followed so closely upon our engagement, that she had time to take only two of the daily injections we had ordered.

Always quick in parturition—and this was her fourth pregnancy—we instantly obeyed the summons to visit her, and found labor well advanced. The "waters" had not broken, and it occurred to us that if the child could be born with an entire amnion, it would necessarily escape direct contact with the maternal tissues, and so leucorrhœal infection would be prevented. Our wish was gratified, and we lifted the caul from off the struggling child after its safe removal from the mother.

Upon the fourth day after delivery, the very same time that ushered in our trouble with the previous child, the little one's eyes presented unmistakable signs of inflammation. We administered medicine, and cleaned the eyes frequently with *Calendula* and warm water, until the case was cured.

Now, the interesting point for consideration is, what caused this disease? That leucorrhœa is a common cause is undeniable. But in the case referred to, the child was protected and, moreover, was cared for by the most competent nurse we ever employed. Every effort was taken to shield the child from strong light, and to protect it during bathing. It has been suggested that some purulent matter may have been inadvertently transferred from the child's legs to its eyes, and this is a possible elucidation of the case; but still the face was the first part bathed and dried.

Defective nutrition cannot be urged as a cause, for the child, from birth, was plump and well-nourished.

Probably, then there is a tendency in some to such inflammations, that light cool air, or some other slight cause, may arouse into active disease. That the eyes of the new-born are sensitive is well known, and, according to Noyes, "a red and sticky condition of the eyes is common to many infants when they begin their extra-uterine adventures."

It behoves us to watch with scrupulous care the eyes of our little charges, and endeavour to protect them from needless and perhaps fatal disease. Nurses should be taught to cleanse the eyes, not with a wash-rag or sponge, nor with a weak solution of *Nitrate of Silver*, now advised as universal preventive; but with an ordinary medicine-dropper and warm milk, milk and water, or, if matter already exists, with warm calendulated water.

AN INTERESTING POST-MORTEM.

Mr. E., aged 50, came under treatment for jaundice. The liver was found enlarged, the movements from the bowels were clay-coloured and the skin deeply dyed with the colouring matter of the bile. The most distressing symptom was the intense itching of the skin.

There were no evidences of malignant disease, yet the persistency of the jaundice, in spite of medical treatment, proved that it arose from more than mere duodenal catarrh.

By and by ascites developed, though it was at no time extensive. Appetite was good, and hearty meal of non-fatty food never caused any distress.

Merc., Nux Vom., Sulph., Podophyl., etc. gave little or no relief. *Nux Juglans*, selected by the nightly itching and burning of the skin, palliated more than any other remedy.

Suddenly one evening in December, he was seized with an agonozing pain in the left groin, followed by rapid swelling of the affected region. The temperature began at once to sink, and this together with a rapid but weak pulse and the suddenness of of the onset, led to the conclusion that perforation had taken place. He sank rapidly and died in fourteen hours.

The post-mortem was performed for me by Dr. Jhon E. James.

The liver was somewhat enlarged. The ductus choledochus was indurated and considerably narrowed by a scirrhus deposit. This, evidently, was the cause of jaundice. As stated above, there was no external evidences of such an affection, as no cachectic symptoms had as yet developed.

The peritoneal sac was intact, so there had been no perforation into its cavity, as was inferred. But in the left groin was seen a mass of dark coagulated blood, forming a tumour as large as a child's head. Dr. James, proceeding with great caution, traced the swelling to the deep vessels. But none of them showed any rupture or any pathological changes, which could have resulted. The femoral vessels were also healthy.

Some small vessel, probably one of the hæmorrhhoidal, was undoubtedly the source of the fatal hæmorrhage. On careful enquiry we found that shortly before he felt the pain, he sat up in bed and indulged in "a good long scratch", swaying to and fro and exclaiming: "I feel as if I could scratch my legs off." It is quite probable that this effort ruptured some small blood-vessels, which were overdistended by the abdominal congestion and which were unable to withstand pressure.

Judging from the condition of the various viscera, the muscular strength of the patient, and his digestive powers, it would have taken months for the jaundice to destroy a life which so quickly ebbed away from the rupture of the vessel, too deep for a ligature.

ALBUMINURIA.

Miss L. F., aged 15. Retention of urine; right kidney sensitive, no urging to urinate; no tenesmus; cutting, burning, crampy, pains in the bladder; *Canth. 30,* every two hours. Then followed twitchings, cough, hoarseness, asthma; *Dros. 2c,* no relief. Restless, anxious, worse at night; *Ars. 2c,* relieved all except kidney symptoms. Urine contained albumen, but miscroscope discovered an abundance of triple phosphates without any lithates, casts, etc. She now reluctantly informed me that her menses, although over-due, had not appeared. A new symptom appeared; cramp in the bladder causing her to bend double; *Coloc. 30,* three doses gave speedy relief. The soreness in back lessened, urination increased from one to three times daily. The next month the menses returned, but the flow was scanty, with heaviness, languor, drowsiness and the urine still albuminous; *Helonias 6,* three doses daily. The urine became normal.

This case illustrates a congested state of the kidneys from amenorrhœa, the congestion being sufficient to cause albuminuria.

The twitchings I regard as reflex symptoms from an irritated bladder and kidneys and not uræmia. The cough and hoarseness were very likely from the cause which suppressed the menses. But the chief feature is the complete relief following the use of *Helonias*. Whether it would be of use in genuine Bright's Disease remains to be seen. It must be carefully distinguished from its analogue, *Senecio*. The latter is of service in nervous, restless, sleepless females, who always complain of nausea with usual symptoms. *Helonias,* on the other hand, gives us dullness, drowsiness, languor; kidneys heavy, sensitive; pains less intense than under *Senecio*.

ATONY OF THE UTERUS.

Mrs. —— had long been troubled with retroflexion of the uterus. At about the third month of pregnancy, she was taken with symptoms that indicated an impending abortion. Digital examination detected the uterus so retroflexed as to be almost inverted. Its replacement was followed by instantaneous relief of the threatening symptoms. By frequent replacements, danger was averted until the uterus had grown out of the pelvis. The labor, which ensued in full time, was tedious, the pains exciting but very imperfect contractions. *Caulophyllum* did no good; *Pulsatilla* also failed. The labor, however, terminated without other artificial interference than some manipulation of the fundus uteri to excite its contractions. Hæmorrage followed, which *China* controlled. The after-pains (this was her third pregnancy) was intense and seemed to call for *Caulophyllum*. This relieved for two days; but on the third, they again became worse, and this time were accompanied by ineffectual urging to stool and entire suppression of the lochia. There were no head symptoms, no fever, nothing to explain the cessation of the flow, except this persistent atony. *Nux Vom.*, repeated with each new paroxysm of pain, relieved and developed the lochia; but it would again cease and finally at the end of three days, stubbornly refused to reappear. The case had now reached its eighth day. The intermission of the lochia suggested *Sulphur,* but its use was followed by no relief; on the contrary, the symptoms grew more serious. There had been no lochial discharge for forty hours. The patient was weak and feverish. She complained of an agonizing headache. It felt as though the face was being drawn towards the root of the nose, and then backwards towards the occiput as if by a string. *The eyeballs were sore and pained on the slightest attempt at motion.* The italicized symptom is found under *Paris Quadrifolia* (see Allen, vol. vii, and also Allen & Norton, p. 100). After the first dose of the 30th, the discharge returned. Two hours later, following the second dose, the headache perceptibly diminished, ceasing entirely after the third dose. The remedy was then suspended. The lochial discharge, though somewhat fitful in its flow, continued the usual two weeks.

BAD COLD.

One cold, blustering day, a poor woman brought her child to my office to be treated for a "bad cold". She had given it magnesia and rhubarb to "work the cold off". The child, a well-nourished girl of, perhaps, three years, was lying in a semi-conscious state, skin pale; eyes half-open; an excoriating nasal discharge reddened the upper lip; the cervical glands were swollen, and cellular tissue about the throat markedly infiltrated. The lips were covered with black scabs, and the mouth and throat internally so swollen, that an examination seemed impossible. I diagnosed the case as scarlatina and gave *Nux Vom.* 2c, 3 doses, to prepare the way for *Lycopod, 2m.*

Next morning no better. Child started from sleep as if choking. *Lachesis 2c,* every 2 hours. On the following day an eruption appeared over both face and body; child conscious. At the next visit the rash had turned purplish; the child was lying with its head thrown back, the neck terribly swollen. The breathing was accelerated and labored. Mucous rales could be heard all over the chest. Urine suppressed. Unconsciousness was complete. *Ailanthus 6th,* every 2 hours. The first sign of improvement was a diminution in the engorgement of the throat; the breathing became consequently more easy and the child returned slowly to consciousness.

It is quite possible that the above case was not scarlet fever, as diagnosed. The rash, which very much resembled measles and which appeared quite plentifully on the face, reminded one of the Roseola, now quite prevalent in Philadelphia.

And, besides, in three days two other children in the same family developed an unmistakable Roseola.

Nevertheless to the prompt action of the *Ailanthus* the child owes its life, the blood having become poisoned by an undeveloped disease. Poverty together with the impression that her child had merely a cold, prevented the mother from seeking medical advice until eight days after the initial fever. *Lachesis*, while it seemed to bring out the eruption, did not relieve the blood of its contamination.

CASES FROM PRACTICE.

Mr. ——, subject to attacks of rheumatism every spring, suffered a year ago from complication of diseases. While in the West he contracted chills and fever, and travelling over the prairies added the itch. Thus he combined rheumatism, itch, chills and fever, and asthma. The characteristic picture called for *Sulphur*.

Evening spells of asthma, with rush of blood to the chest and constriction; stinging between the shoulders; chill in the forenoon, followed by long-lasting heat, flushes of heat in the afternoon. Rheumatic pains erratic; vesicles on the hands between the fingers itching intolerably.

All the symptoms were soon relieved, and finally removed. The prairie itch lasted the longest.

About a month ago, just a year after his previous attack, I was summoned to visit him, the messenger stating that he was suffering from asthma. Being engaged in the office at the time, I sent *Sulphur*, as it had relieved before. An hour later, on seeing the patient, I found not asthma, but rheumatism of the

CLINICAL CASES

diaphragm. The agony was intense. Respiration jerking, numbness of the limbs, coldness. As well as he could, he described his sensations. There was a *feeling as of a cord around the hypochondria; rush of blood toward the chest; shooting pains through to the back and up each side of the chest;* cannot lie down; dry tickling cough, as from dust in the throat. *Sulphur* had done no good. *Cactus 30* relieved. Another attack in the night again yielded to *Cactus 2c.* On the following evening, the symptoms reappeared, though not so severely. *Cactus 2c* quickly relieved.

Miss ——, aged 48, nervous temperament. Troubled for 6 years with diarrhœa, which occurred only in the morning and *hurried her out of bed.* She had a severe attack when I saw her, aggravated by a *suppressed perspiration.* Gave *Sulphur 900.* No apparent relief in several weeks. From the fact that, if she composed *three lines even, in the afternoon, she would wake up the next morning with diarrhœa,* showing the preponderating influence of *mental labour,* I gave *Nux Vom. 1000.* The diarrhœa disappeared and *congestive headaches, to which she was formerly subject,* reappeared. They in their turn went away without any other medicine. The patient remained unusually well for three months, when an undue amount of mental work brought it on again, but it readily yielded to the remedy.

Miss ——, aged 21, complained of headache, which was *improved by looking cross-eyed.* There were no other symptoms that would guide me. Knowing that *Oleander* was improved by *looking sideways,* I gave two doses of the 200th. The result was a cure. She had had no return to date.

Mrs. C. ——, dark complexion, dark brown eyes, has had for years uterine troubles; cancer of the left mamma, and was taking medicine for these general ailments. In the course of treatment she caught cold and exhibited the following condition:

Headache in occiput and *right temple; intermittent.* Eyeball aches and feels as if there were a *"shot in it."* Darting in right eye *at intervals* during the day; but in *both eyes, and much more severe at night.* She says, *"I shall go crazy."* Involuntary twitching of eye-lid. Worse from light, especially gas-light.

Worse from least noise, as others walking, etc. Gave *Spigelia* 30. No relief. I then studied *Cimicifuga*, which I gave two doses of the 30th. The neuralgia was well the next day, and with it the following improvement: A heavy pain in right ovary disappeared. She could lie on right side, which she hadn't done for two months, and a troublesome leucorrhœa of several months' standing, ceased entirely.

Mr. —— had Syphilis nine years ago, for which he received large doses of *Mercury*. On December 24, 1869, he came to me complaining of shooting pains from above the *left ear to the root of the nose;* the nose was swollen at its base, and so also were the eyelids, especially in the inner angles. The similarity of the headache to that described by Dr. Neidhard (A. J. H. M. M., Vol. No. I, page 106), together with the swelling of nose and inner corner of eyelids, induced me to give *Sarsaparilla 2c,* one dose.

Two weeks later. Headache well; rheumatism in every joint. On enquiry I found this was an old symptom, felt *before* the headache supervened. I, of course, gave *Sac. Lac.*

February 21st. Rheumatism and headache gone, but swelling not much diminished. He had suffered from headache almost constantly for 6 years.

CHOLERA INFANTUM.

Some years since, Dr. Neidhard noticed as a symptom of *Calc. Phos.,* "longing for bacon, ham, fat, etc.". At the time I concluded it would hence be a good remedy in cholera infantum, when there existed an abnormal craving for fat, etc. All through the last summer I had been struggling to keep a little one year old boy from succumbing to this disease. *Hydrocephaloid* set in, the body was cold, respiration scarcely perceptible, and even a loose stool was followed by fainting. *Phos.* 2c worked like a charm. But in three weeks a second attack was but partially relieved by *Phos. Arsenic* seemed to revive the little fellow. But on one occasion, I found him propped up in his crib, his skeleton fingers clutching a piece of raw ham, which he was endeavouring to masticate with all the power of his four tiny teeth. I gave him (remembering Dr. N's remark) *Calc. Phos. 2c*, and from that time his uninterrupted improvement dates.

CRAMPS.

Whatever may be said against the class of remedies, or remedies of which this is a sample, I, for the one, will ever feel grateful towards Dr. Jeanes for introducing this bile of the Terrapin, *Cholos. Terrapin.* He recommends it for "cramps in the calves," a symptom it has often removed. Quite recently I gave it in a case of secondary syphilis with these cramps as a prominent symptom. In three weeks the sorethroat, pains in bones and cramps disappeared, and four or five vesicles formed at the site of the old chancre. These have disappeared, leaving the patient apparently well. In olden times, *Terrapin* was used in venereal diseases.

CURE OF A HYPOPYON.

Dr. A. Korndœrfer and myself succeeded in permanently curing a case of *Hypopyon.* The patient was a stone-cutter; who a year before, had been allopathically treated for gonorrhœa. He had taken among other drugs, much mercury. While working in his trade, he was struck in the eye by a piece of stone. A violent inflammation followed, which he attempted to subdue with tea leaves, laudanum and acetate of lead, the latter of which *always causes opacity of the cornea*, when directly applied. The *sclerotica* looked like raw beef and light was intolerable. The patient meditated suicide, *especially in the evening.* There was a feeling of sand in the eye, and examination revealed in the anterior chamber a collection of pus, *apparently* about two lines in diameter. *Hepar 30* was given as suited to the symptoms and as the proper antidote for mercury and acetate of lead. The result was a perfect absorption of the pus and removal of the opacity of the cornea with the return of normal vision.

DIZZINESS.

Mrs. —— complained of nausea, vertigo and headache, all decidedly worse from the slightest motion. *Bry.* 6 every two hours. No relief. Further enquiry elicited the additional symptom that *any noise made the dizziness and nausea intolerably worse.* This last, with the former mentioned symptom, can call only for *Theridion.* Three doses of the 1000 cured in 24 hours. The patient in previous attacks, taking *Nux, Ipecac, Bry.,* etc., according to a supposed similarity, was always sick in several days.

DROPSY.

Early in the autumn of 1881, Mr. —— returned from the sea-shore, expecting soon to fall a victim to dropsy.

Coming under my care, I found his heart dilated with mitral insufficiency. The whole body was anasarcous, the legs being enormously swollen. The scrotum was very much distended, though its size had been somewhat modified by an incision, from which continually dropped serum into a bucket, placed conveniently in front of the patient's chair.

Unable to lie down, owing to water in pleuræ and pericardium, as well as peritoneum, the poor sufferer was compelled to remain seated, catching snatches of sleep in brief intervals of rest from severe dyspnœa.

The surface of the body, especially the nose, lips, finger tips and legs, was bluish-red. The pulse was rapid and intermittent. From the legs oozed a small quantity of water, not enough to give much relief.

The cardiac weakness, blueness of the skin and dyspnœa when falling off to sleep, led to the selection of *Lachesis,* which was given in water, a dose every three hours.

The first potency used was the 5th, taken from the original stock procured by Dr. Hering, more than 50 years ago.

In a few days the colour of the skin changed decidedly. The pulse strengthened, though it still remained intermittent, and the legs and scrotum discharged copiously of their redundant water. Soon the patient could lie down, though sleep was broken by cardiac, instead of what we may term "dropsical" dyspnœa.

Relapses occurred during the winter, but no other remedy was needed, the only change being in the potencies used, from the 5th to the 30th.

Here is an instance in which an incurable disease was for months almost entirely relieved of distressing dropsy with medicine alone. The man is still living.

DROWSINESS.

A coloured woman complained of an *unconquerable drowsiness, whenever ceasing from her work she sat down to rest.* I could not obtain any other symptom, and physical examination revealed no abnormality of the heart. *Nux Moschata 2c,* one dose, entirely cured the symptom.

DYSPEPSIA.

Mr. F.——, aged 46, had for 15 years suffered from dyspepsia. His general health seemed good, but his pulse was soft, and every attempt to eat meat would be followed by headache, eructations and itching all over like an undeveloped nettle-rash. Fat could be eaten with impunity, and even a small amount of meat could be tolerated, if he also ate apples; that is, so far tolerated, that only a slight headache would follow. Hence the case was one of insufficiency of gastric juice, partly obviated by the mallic and other acids of apples. Liver and pancreas were normal, as shown by the easy digestion of fatty and starchy food. The next point was, what could have caused this gastric inertia?

The patient had always been remarkably temperate. It appeared, that some 15 years since, while helping to carry a heavy iron beam upstairs he tripped, straining his stomach. For months he was forced to walk bent. Thus, this accident had so impaired the stomach, that it failed to secrete sufficient gastric juice. Only one medicine covers the *cause,* and the aggravation from meat, with eructations and itching—*Ruta Graveolens,* which was given in the 2c potency, before each meal. Cure complete in 3 months. The only obvious symptoms produced from such persistent use of the medicine, were an itching of the eyelids and forehead, and watering of the eyes when attempting to read—symptoms, which clearly belong to the drug.

EPILEPSY.

Miss B. ——, a coloured woman, aged 24, suffered for more than a year with epilepsy in spite of treatment. During the last examination I discovered a phlyctenoid eruption on the skin, discharging a thin yellow fluid, and a similar fluid appeared in the vomit and in the leucorrhœa. The laryngoscope displayed a like eruption in the pharynx, and it may be presumed it was present in the stomach. The speculum showed enormous bilsters on the tumefied uterus, discharging the same serous matter. Further, during the spasm, the face was bathed in sweat, the eyes sunken and the subsequent coma very profound. The attacks were ushered in by numbness of the brain, a jerk in the nape of the neck, and then the spasm, differing in nowise from ordinary epilepsy.

In reading the pathogenesis of *Bufo,* I was struck with the apparent connection between suppuration of internal parts and the spasms it produced, and I was determined to test its virtues in puerperal spasms following peritonitis, suppuration or suppurative ovaritis, or even in suppuration of the kidneys. Here was an opportunity in epilepsy with uterine tumor and destructive inflammation of both skin and mucous tissue, to confirm my opinion and so give more confidence to trust its use in the more dangerous puerperal convulsions. After three doses of *Bufo 30,* the spasms which had been of daily occurrence, ceased, and with them the troublesome eruption. The uterine tumor, however, remained apparently unchanged.

Bufo may become invaluable in the treatment of those forms of epilepsy which follow onanism; for we see in the provings such symptoms as: "Longs for solitude to give himself up to onanism"; (a symptom of *Sulphur* also, according to Jahr); "Quick ejaculation, without pleasure, sometimes with spasms, and painful weariness of the limbs."

Compare with *Plumbum* in epilepsy with destructive suppuration; with *Sulphur* in that on onanists: and with *Calcarea* and *Silicea* when the attack commences in the abdomen, or concurs with the changes in the moon.

FEVER.

Miss A. ———'s case illustrates how easily we may spoil a cure. She was attacked with chill and fever of the following description: Anteponing type; chill followed by burning fever as if the veins were on fire; great restlessness, even delirium; thirst unquenchable; sweat comes later, lasting all night, leaving her prostrated in the morning. Face during apyrexia waxy-yellow; great weakness, yet restless. *Arsenic 40m* relieved in four days, leaving only heat at night and sweat. Thinking that possibly *Sulphur* interpolated might complete the cure, three doses of the *Sulphur 2c* were given. The next day the chill returned precisely as above described. *Arsenic.* was again resorted to.

The abdomen seemed to be the centre of attack. She complained of burning heat there which was almost constant. One week after returning to *Arsenic.*, the patient described the burning as concentrated across the lower abdomen, hence it had descended. The medicine was discontinued. On the following day a diarrhœa substituted itself for the chill; the abdominal heat ceased and the patient convalesced from that hour.

It is comparatively easy to select the first remedy in an acute case, but only the *master* knows when to change for another.

GELSEMINUM IN ALBUMINURIA.

Mrs. ——, during her first pregnancy, complained of great lassitude, with pains in the limbs, and scanty urination. About the seventh month, the urine examined, showed an abundance of albumen. As yet there was no dropsy. She had cough, worse lying down, before 12 P.M. weakness from the shortest walk; flushed face, especially cheeks, afternoons; anxiety before a thunder-storm or during sultry weather. *Phos. 2c* was given, three doses per week.

At the ninth month, the condition of the urine was unaltered; but still there had been no dropsy. At the beginning of labour, the patient sank into a semi-stupid state, out of which she could be aroused by shaking, but she would soon relapse. If any answer could be forced from her, it was spoken with a thick tongue, like one intoxicated. She had had no labour pains, yet on examining her per vaginum, the os was noticed fully dilated with the unbroken membranes protruding. The face was pinkish, as if uniformly blushed, and the pulse was slow, full, about 60 per minute. The semi-comatose condition, the colour of the face, and the atonic condition of the uterine walls being characteristic of *Gelsem.* this was given in water every fifteen minutes in the *200* potency.

Hoping that an erect position might excite labor pains, she was seated in an arm chair. In about half an hour, the nurse thought that the child was partly protruding from the vulva.

The patient was returned to bed and a soft fluctuating tumour, about four to five inches long, was left exteriorly. The exploring finger was easily pushed between this and the labia, and the head found buried in the perineum. The child by its own gravity, had fallen, until the resisting perineum checked it. The bulging tumour was, of course, the unruptured amnion. Slight twitchings of single muscle were noticed. In fifteen or twenty minutes, she complained of sharp pains, running from before backwards and upwards (very marked in *Gels.*). Hence the medicine was discontinued.

The pulse increased to 80, and genuine pains began to announce the distension of the perineum. The labor was successfully terminated. One month later, no traces of albuminuria were to be found. In a subsequent conversation, the patient related that, at times, when in her dreamy state, she had felt, as though her head was "growing big". Such ominous symptoms may well lead one to fear puerperal convulsions.

MENTAL DERANGEMENT.

Mr. C. ——, after severe brain work, developed a long train of symptoms, requiring patient and lengthy treatment. The most satisfactory effects were obtained from potentized *Alcohol,* the indications being very similar to those recorded on pages 138, 139 and 140 of the Encyclopædia of Materia Medica, Vol. I.

Quarrelsomeness, even from imagined insult. Impatient of contradiction. Headache, with stupidity. Memory weak, forgets what he was about to say. Congestive headaches. Sensation benumbed here and there, especially about the scalp; even his brain feels hard and numb. Mental inquietude, compelling change of work frequently during the day. Apprehensiveness; thinks some one will injure him, that he is in danger, etc.

So decided was the improvement after *Alcohol,* that it was, no doubt, the remedy for the case. The symptoms were almost in the very words of Dr. Allen's collection. It will be seen that they closely resemble *Hyoscyamus* and *Kali Bromatum*.

OVARIAN TUMOUR.

Mrs. —— after her last confinement in December, 1874, complained of intense soreness in the left inguinal region. *Hamamelis* externally, and the 30th internally. Relief only temporary. When she began to menstruate, which happened when her child was four months old, her suffering was extreme. The ovarian region was swollen; pains burning as from fire; agony; restlessness; numbness of the left limb; cold sweat; fainting. *Arsenic 2c* in water, every half hour, seemed to relieve. During the succeeding month, an examination was permitted. Left ovary was found enlarged, rising above the bones and laterally pushing the vaginal wall in towards the median line, and pressing the os firmly against the right side of the vagina. The tumour was extremely sensitive. It seemed to be about the size of a baby's head. *Sepia 2c* was given twice weekly for the following symptoms: Irritable temper; at times indifferent to her household; headache every few days over the left eye, with intolerance of light or noise; sallow complexion; gone feeling at the stomach; dragging pains, heaviness in the abdomen; better sitting. Feeling in the rectum as if for stool, yet none passed; smarting, cutting during urination. The next period was ushered in with even worse distress. The bladder became involved, and with the burning ovarian pains there was frequent urging to urinate, with tenesmus and burning; urine passed in drops. *Canth. 30* relieved, and the menstrual flow became established. Some emotional excitement, however, stopped it on the second day, and the following symptoms resulted:—

Bearing down in the uterine region, worse walking, better holding up the abdomen with the hands; tenderness over the swollen left ovary; stinging, burning pains from ovary up into the abdomen and down the thigh; shooting pains from left ovary across to the pubes; urine causes a smarting sensation. Digital examination determined a prolapsed and sensitive uterus.*Lilium*

Tig. 30 twice daily. In three weeks ovarian swelling entirely disappeared. Has since menstruated with very little pain. On two or three occasions, when the pains returned severely, the *Lilium* effectually removed them.

PARALYSIS FROM SPASMS.

The following case, lasting through a year, presents several points of interest and profit. It is given as succinctly as possible.

Miss H, aged 17, was found in a comatose state. Her brother had died of uræmia, her mother and father each of heart disease. *Bellad., Opium* and *Gelsem.* were given respectively. Still there was but partial relief until the ninth day. The return to consciousness was, however, only temporary; for, the afternoon found her in spasms. Previously she had *complained of hunger,* and on eating, went into a convulsion. This led to the choice of *Hyosc. 2c.* Changed to acute mania, declared she *was being poisoned,* was crazy, was in an asylum. *Hyosc. 10m* relieved, but on the 18th day she commenced *singing, praying, reciting poetry;* eyes injected; wild look, *Stram. 2c.* The mind became quiet, but the inevitable stupor returned, interrupted by occasional whispering: "ice, ice." Thinking that perhaps such a succession of narcotics had injured, she was allowed to suck a lemon by way of antidote. Within an hour she became conscious, and so remained for over a week. Inquiry now revealed something of her history. Menstruation either did not come on at all or remained but a day, followed by *blood-spitting, cough, tightness across the chest.* The day she was taken sick was the proper time for her menstruation, but hard study had prevented its onset and determined the cerebral congestion, which had ended in coma. *Phos. 2c* was given and the next menstruation was nearly normal. At its close however, the patient was seized with spasms, varying in number from three to six a day. They were not followed by prolonged stupor, but by left-sided hemiplegia, seemingly intensifying at each new attack of spasm. After a week, only the right half of the body would be convulsed. There were total blindness, loss of speech, and dysphagia. For twelve days nothing could be swallowed but ice cream. The breathing was rapid, and so increased the painful dryness of the throat and mouth. As water could not be swallowed, a plan was tried which proved very grateful to the sufferer. Over the mouth was laid a thin piece of muslin, from which extended a wick into a tumbler of water. By capillary attraction, the cloth was kept damp and the in-going air bore enough moisture to diminish the all but intolerable thirst. At the approach of a spasm, she would make signs that she desired water. Of course, she could not swallow, even powdered ice choked her, but she would angrily bite at the proffered tumbler, a symptom, which, with the paralysis following, led to *Cupr. 2c,* and higher. Swallowing soon became normal, but the spasms persisted, menstruation remained irregular and finally both legs lost sensation and motion. *Sulph. cm* helped. Later, by the advice of Dr. M. Macfarlan, who had seen paraplegia result from the persistent use of *Sulphur cm,* this preparation was given *every three or four hours for several weeks.* Soon the sight returned, menstruation became regular, the attacks of spasms grew less and less frequent, until now they appear to have ceased entirely. Locomotion is still imperfect, but each day adds new strength and renders crutches less needful.

Pathologically, this case owes its phenomena to congestions of nervous centres.

After beating about the bush with medicines, selected according to *their* characteristics, but not according to the *characteristics of the case,* or at least medicines but partially similar, *Sulph. 100,000,* cured. It relieved the congestion in the *corpora quadrigemina,* and restored the sight; it constricted the spinal vessels, relieving the paraplegia; it caused absorption of such effusion as generally follows venous stasis and so removed undue pressure on important nervous centres. It may be that the *pons varolii* (so called convulsive centre) was influenced. Most certainly were the vaso-motor nerves affected. We know this because *Sulphur 100,000 has repeatedly produced such a state when given to the healthy.* More than this, repeated experiments have demonstrated to the writer that *Sulph. 1,000, 000* will, frequently given, cause congestions of nervous centres. And if this occurs in different seasons, on different constitutions, and in both sexes, where is the unpardonable sin in accrediting these "moonshine" potencies?

We have no doubt but that the hemiplegia was not cerebral but spinal; that the pressure was on the left half of the anterior column (motor) and the right of the posterior (sensory). This decision finds some confirmation in the subsequent change to paraplegia (congestion *across* the spine). The objective probability is enhanced by the fact that the deltoid, upper half of the trapezius, all the cervical and facial parts preserved their sensibility and motility. Hence, after the removal of the dysphagia, that is, after the medulla and parts above were relieved, the hemiplegia was sustained by spinal, not cerebral, pressure. It was a mistake to treat the first stage with such a succession of nearly allied narcotics. No more forcible example than this could be found to prove Hering's law of Conjunctive and Disjunctive Relationship. The lemon seemed to mitigate the symptoms, but on the disease went; slipping from sensorium to medulla and spine, leaving blindness, dysphagia and hemiplegia; yet the oft recurring spasms showed that the causes were still at work.

PERICARDITIS.

In the spring of 1881, Mr. ——, aged seventy-two, was attacked with pericarditis. Under the skilful care of Dr. O. S. Griggs, the disease rapidly subsided. But the patient, who had always been rheumatic, and who had probably suffered in former times from similar inflammation of the pericardium, began now to manifest serious symptoms, indicative of disturbed heart action. The pulse ranged from 130 to 150 per minute; there was short breathing, and the feet and ankles became œdematous.

Dr. Griggs, in June, called me in consultation, the case by this time having developed into general anasarca, with hydrothorax.

Physical examination showed that the pleural cavities contained water, which, on the left side, was as high as the third rib, and on the right side, as high as the fifth rib. There was no evidence of hydropericardium. And although the abdomen was very large, the increase in size was considered to be due to anasarca, and not ascites, for the physical signs of the latter were obscure or absent.

The legs were enormously swollen, presenting the scaling and oozing, with other alterations of the skin, incidental to such cases.

The points of interest in this case are the ready response to medicines, offering thus excellent opportunities to study drug-action; and the remarkable fact that the pulse, for more than ten months, never sank below 130 beats per minute, while it often arose as high as 160 to 170.

The medicines employed were principally *Antim. Tart., Digitalis, Laurocerasus, Sulphur* and *Bryonia*.

The first was selected for the following group; cough, drowsiness, nausea and white-coated tongue; cough always followed by gaping and yawning; urine scanty. These well-known *Ant. Tart.*, symptoms would rapidly disappear after a few doses of the 30th potency. And not only this, the general improvement would be striking. The heart, which being bound down by adhesions, was visibly pulsating in the epigastrium, would beat less perceptibly, the pulse would fall 20 to 30 beats and the water entirely disappear from the serous cavities. Even the legs would lessen in size, leaving great folds of stretched tissue, which, but a few days before were tense with serous effusion. Frequently such a respite as this would last from a week to two or three, when the embarassed heart, unable to work as it should, again permitted blood stasis, with a renewal of dropsy.

It should have been mentioned before, that painstaking and oft-repeated examinations of the heart, failed to acquaint us with the *exact* changes which the interior of the heart had undergone. That some valvular defect existed was evident from the murmurs which we heard. They were apparent over the mitral valve and also over the aortic. There was no regurgitation detectable.

As the symptoms returned after a more or less lengthy period of remission, they rarely yielded to the medicine which last relieved. Thus, after *Ant. Tart.*, the returning symptoms were as follows: dyspnœa, on falling off to sleep he would be aroused with gasping or a sense of falling. Terrible, distressed, nauseated feeling at the epigastrium, lips livid, face anxious. *Lachesis* would not help, but *Digitalis*, which plainly suits the entire group, would again institute a period of relief and comfort, effecting an almost complete removal of the dropsy and decided increase of the urine. Then, perhaps, the following phase would call for *Sulphur* 200: cat-naps, flushes of heat, must have air; feet burn, so he must have them cooled. Relief was certain, and certain, too, was a diminution of the attendant dropsy.

On one occasion it seemed as though the poor sufferer would suffocate. None of the remedies hitherto successfully employed were now indicated. His face was livid, the eyes protruding, as with one being throttled; the breathing was gasping, and he was continually clutching at the heart. The picture pointed unmistakably to *Laurocerasus;* which, given in the 30th relieved promptly. This particular set of symptoms never returned.

Towards the close of the year, however, evidences of decreasing power of reaction were more and more manifest. We still had opportunity of witnessing over and over again the favourable effects of drugs. They would eliminate their respective symptoms with almost mathematical precision, so that we had numerous confirmations of the relation of drugs to the groups of symptoms already detailed. But the patient was weaker; the legs ulcerated, discharging more or less, and were always offensive, despite Platt's chlorides and other disinfectants.

As with many old men, an enlarged prostate interfered with free micturition. From some cause or other the urine now failed to pass. The attempt to introduce a catheter provoked urethral bleeding, though Dr. Griggs used no undue force. Even after the catheter had been introduced and retained, the patient's sufferings were not over. An urethral inflammation was set up, with thick purulent discharge. The disease travelled stubbornly along the cords until both testicles were inflamed and swollen, and the scrotum was purple and œdematous. Medicines began to fail; or, we were unskilful in their selection.

One night, however, Dr. Griggs was hastily summoned to prescribe for sharp stitching pains about the heart which prevented a deep breath, and were aggravated by respiration or motion. Of course, he very properly gave *Bryonia*. At our consultation we found the pains better. There was purple spots on the skin; the pulse was rapid and thready; skin blue. We thought of *Lachesis;* but before giving it, we bethought ourselves of the wholesome advice, "Let well enough alone." So we awaited the reaction from *Bryonia;* and we were not disappointed. Within a few hours the scrotum and the testicles began to grow smaller, the purulent discharge stopped, the urine doubled in quantity, and no more medicine was needed for three weeks! Not even the catheter was required!

But relapse followed; the urine failed to pass; there was much straining, but it was ineffectual. Dr. Griggs gave *Causticum* 30 with prompt and permanent relief. Still the trend of the disease was slowly and surely deathward. Finally the patient became restless, anxious; the skin, if pinched, remained in a fold; the legs were more offensive than ever; his strength failed rapidly, death coming at last quite suddenly.

The autopsy was performed by Prof. A. R. Thomas. The heart was found intimately adherent to the pericardium. The valves were intact, excepting some roughening of the mitral, and a calcareous mass embedded in one of the cusps of the aortic. The other viscera were nearly normal, although the prostratic gland was considerably enlarged, and a mulberry calculus was embedded in the posterior wall of the bladder. Aside from the difficult urination, there were no ante-mortem evidences of the existence of stone.

SANGUINEOUS TUMOR.

Mrs. H. —— had an easy labor of four hours. Boy, weighed ten pounds, and seemed "all right". But on the third day a tumor as large as a black walnut appeared on the right of the occipital bone. Examination showed it to be a sanguineous tumor. The anterior fontanelle was nearly closed, but the posterior was open and the tumor connected with it, showing a venous connection with the sinuses within. This condition of the fontanelles led me to prescribe *Calc. Phos. 2c.* The tumor lessened and then came to a stand still. The *anterior fontanelle opened more,* and the connection between the posterior and the tumor disappeared. No further advance was noticed until *Sulph. 2c,* one dose, completed the cure. But now the occipital bone showed a depression of the size of a silver quarter, previously concealed by the tumor. It looked as though a knuckle had indented the bone. *Calc. Phos. 2c,* three doses, brought the bone to its proper rotundity.

SCARLATINA.

A child, aged 13, threw a shawl belonging to a child who had died of scarlet fever, over her shoulders; next day she had high fever, pulse one hundred and forty; sorethroat; vomiting; headache; the next day the rash appeared on neck and chest, extending gradually over body and becoming red after pressure from periphery to centre. *Rhus Tox.* cured with no sequelæ and the stages were short.

ST. VITUS' DANCE.

Miss —— came to us from allopathy. She was suffering from St. Vitus' Dance. The leading symptoms were: Spasmodic movements of the muscles of the face and right arm and leg. Spasmodic twitchings and restlessness *during sleep.*

These two symptoms, according to the Index, are very nearly identical with symptoms under *Zizia Aurea.* The cure with this drug was prompt and permanent.

The aggravation during sleep is an exceedingly important modality, distinguishing the *Zizia* from *Mygale* and the oft used *Agaricus;* the latter of which has jerking, etc., on *going* to sleep.

SUPPOSED PHTHISIS.

Mr.——, aged 40, has been long under treatment for supposed phthisis pulmonalis. When I saw him, he was thin, sallow, emaciated; was aroused 5 to 6 A.M. every day, with a hard cough, terminating in gagging and vomitting of stringy mucus and an offensive mass, which was frothy and green, looking like soap-suds. He has had in four years, five or six hæmorrhages. The periodicity of the cough and soap-sud sputum led to *Kali Hyd.*, under which he improved in flesh and general strength, was able to resume his business; the cough became less annoying, losing its spasmodic character; and the sputum white and less frequent. It is now a year since he has had no return of hæmoptysis.

SYPHILIS.

I can testify that *high potencies will cure syphilis,* and potentized Mercurial preparations will produce symptoms similar to those of syphilis; the *Iodide of Mercury* in the one-thousandth potency has produced a pimple or papule which resembles a hard chancre; and this same *Iodide of Mercury,* given in repeated doses for days continually, has cured this kind of chancre in a number of instances. It has also cured a secondary sorethroat which was developed six or seven weeks afterwards, but which on the continuance of the medicine disappeared and for nine years has not been seen.

I have also produced similar results with the five hundredth potency, getting an ulcer that looked as though it were punched out at the top; of this I am positive from my own personal observation, and I know this to be the case in the experience of Dr. Macfarlan of this city, who has proved this thing by experiments, and whose cures I have seen.

ULCER ON CHIN.

Mrs. L. ——, aged 76. Ulcer on chin, right side, perforating to the gums, so that fluids taken in the mouth run out through the opening. Has not grown in circumference much for 2 years. All our usual means failing, I resorted to *Cundurango*, three doses, since which the following change has taken place. I give her own words: "I feel a great deal better; the medicine took away the pain in the throat; also the lumps on the chin have almost disappeared. It does not bleed any more, but there is still a continuous flow of slimy water. The sore does not heal on the outside, but it does not look so bad as it was." (Letter to me, dated July, 12th.)

This is the first time in two years *she* ever acknowledged any benefit from treatment. More anon.

VARICELLA.

During January, while vaccinating for the year just closed, a child was brought for re-vaccination, all previous attempts having proved unsuccessful. The vaccine-disease developed perfectly, and by the fifteenth day all traces of irritation had passed away. Two days later he became restless, sleepless, with a dry teasing cough, and considerable evening fever. On the following day papules appeared, which soon exhibited the characteristic vesicles of chicken-pox. The attack was mild, leaving no scars which will be permanent. A younger member of the same family, in whom vaccination had failed to take, contracted chicken-pox at the same time, and developed a remarkably severe case. Many of the vesicles became pustules.

The non-identity of variola and varicella is now generally admitted. It is regarded as a mere coincidence that epidemics of the two diseases sometimes concur. One does not protect against the other; nor are they comparable in point of virulence. Variola displays a well marked periodicity, running through three distinct stages of eruption; the varicella papules recur in crops, and either end as vesicles or quickly pustulate, selodom, pitting so deeply as small-pox.

The cases above recorded is interesting as tending to confirm the separate origin of the disease germs of small-pox and chicken-pox. Vaccination though in all respect perfect, did not prevent the development of the varicella.

It may be asked, however, what influence had the vaccination in modifying the attack, which was much milder than in the case of the younger brother in whom vaccination failed? This question is difficult to answer because individual susceptibility to the disease is exceedingly varied.

In the epidemic in Philadelphia this fall and winter all cases under our charge have run a mild course under the use of *Hyoscyamus 2c*. It was Dr. Lilienthal, we believe, who draw attention to the similarity of this remedy and the symptoms of varicella. *Hyoscyamus* develops vesicles *coming in crops;* restless sleep, slight febrile excitement, and above all it corresponds to the *dry, teasing cough, relieved by sitting up.*

Now, because of the size of the vesicles in the younger of the cases referred to in this article, vesicles which more resembled water blisters, we selected *Rhus Tox. 2c*. In two days the symptoms became provokingly violent. The fever was intense, the child could not sleep, vesicles appeared thickly over the scalp, face and back. Some of them broke, forming thin scabs; others pustulated and pitted deeply. *Hyos. 2c.* quickly relieved. In the milder case *Hyos. 2c.* was given from the beginning.

This circumstances, this error of prescription, might account for the disparity in intensity, leaving us to conclude that vaccination had no modifying influence.

VERMICULAR TROUBLE.

A boy, 10 years, came under treatment for a supposed vermicular trouble. The symptoms seemed to point to *Cina* (Artemisia Vahliana), which relieved for a time. Other medicines followed, when, on one occasion, while in my office, he suddenly grew pale, commenced a chewing motion with his mouth, *walked around the room, picked up a book and threw it forcibly on the table,* returned to his seat and became conscious again. He was then as well as usual with the exception of a slight languor. On questioning him, he stated that it commenced with a creeping (*aura*), beginning in the pit of the stomach and spreading thence to the head, causing unconsciousness, during which his automatic motions took place. In school, he has been known to walk in the same unconscious state, slam his slate on the desk, look up the clock, cry out the hour in a loud voice, and then return to consciousness without the slightest recollection of what he had done. *Artemisia Vulgaris* relieved these symptoms. Unfortunately the family has left the city, and I am unable to say how permanent is the relief. But I am certain that each attack following the medicine was lighter.

It is a singular fact that all of the tribe of Senecionideæ, ord. Compositæ, which we have proved (*Cina, Artemisia Vulg., Cham., Tanacet., Arnica, Senecio Grac.*), have relief from some form of motion.

The *Artemisia Vulgaris* resembles the *Cina* in nervous troubles, but as it is in conjunctive relationship it cannot be used immediately before or after *Cina*. As a distinctive relative, and hence one who has followed well, *Silicea* corresponds to the somnambulistic state and *Silicea, Nux Vom.* and *Caust.*, to the irritation of the solar plexus giving rise to spasm. The *Absinthium* (wormwood), another member of the Armisiæ, when drunk in brandy (a famous drink used by actors, etc., to stimulate the brain), I have seen produce the Delirium Embriosorum, which was only relieved by pacing the floor, showing again the general relief from motion.

WHOOPING-COUGH.

During last year many cases of whooping-cough appeared in Philadelphia. Some yielded readily to the usual medicines, but the following cases presented one or two interesting features, which may be worth recording:

A. Mrs. —— caught the disease from her child. At the time, she was under treatment for prolapsus uteri accompanying general debility and emaciation. Her condition greatly added to the distressing effects of the cough, the paroxysms of which exhausted her very much. Several remedies were used, but with indifferent success. One evening the husband, alarmed at her symptoms, sent for me to call at once. I found the patient too prostrate to raise the head from the pillow. She complained of a sensation of waves, which started from the pit of the stomach, and spread all over the body with trembling. Cough constant from tickling in the larynx; worse when attempting to speak. *Actea Rac.* 6 a dose every three hours cured the whooping-cough, and, naturally enough, helped the uterine disease.

B. A little boy, aged four years, was seized with whooping-cough, which developed as a croupy cough. The mother, guided by the barking cough and sawing respiration, prescribed *Spongia*. This I allowed to act for twenty-four hours; but no relief followed. The cough, though still croupy, was accompanied with frequent and well marked whooping, leaving no doubt as to its nature. With each paroxysm the child held his hands on the stomach. *Drosera* 200 was prescribed. I have often helped a croupy, evening cough with this remedy, and the other symptoms seemed to justify its selection. Relief was prompt; but the case was not cured. A week later the little fellow suffered from repeated night paroxysms, each of which culminated in profuse nose-bleed. The blood was dark and stringy. *Crocus Sativus* 500 was given, a dose every two hours. This remedy also suited other symptoms of the child. Violent exhausting dry cough, relieved by laying the hand on the pit of the of the stomach. Large quantities of mucus expectorated (see Allen, Vol. 3). The cure was speedy. This drug is not included in Bœnninghausen's list, but is doubtless deserving of a place there.

C. A little girl, aged two years, came under my care to be treated for croup. Despite *Aconite* and *Spongia*, administered three or four days before I assumed charge, the fever increased and the cough became more and more harsh and metallic. The fauces were intensely red; and during cough the child tore at the throat as if striving to remove something offending and painful.

The pulse was 160 and respiration 40 to 50. The child's face wore an anxious look, but instead of the restlessness of

Aconite, there was drowsiness. The fever, the cough and drowsiness, pointed emphatically to *Iodine*, which was given in hourly dose in the third potency.

Three days passed without apparent change, except that the breathing became deeper, and the finger, placed on the box of the larynx, could detect a decided strumming sensation. This, I presumed, was caused by partly loosened membrane, though I was unable to employ the laryngoscope to confirm the diagnosis. On the fifth day, I was informed that the vibratory sound had been much more marked during the night. The cough was more moist, and after a violent chocking spell, the child swallowed something, and since then the breathing was more natural.

Still fever and cough continued; the tongue became dry and red; the lips parched, and the drowsiness constant. The persistency of the fever led to the use of *Sulphur* 500 a dose every three hours. This was followed by remittency of fever and a more moist cough. But now the whole scene changed. Aroused from sleep with paroxysms of cough, the child would give forth long-drawn whoops. I learned that before the croup, she had been exposed to whooping-cough.

What was to be done? *Sulphur* was helping the fever, and so it ought not to be changed. Within a weak the cough almost disappeared. Ten days later no trace of disease remained, during which period the child received the conventional *Sac. Lac.*